9th Edition

# Understanding Human Behavior

## A Guide for Health Care Professionals

Alyson Honeycutt, M.A., N.C.C.

and

Mary Elizabeth Milliken, B.S.N., M.S., Ed.D.
Certified Healing Touch Practitioner

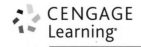
CENGAGE
Learning·

Australia • Brazil • Mexico • Singapore • United Kingdom • United States

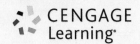

**Understanding Human Behavior: A Guide for Health Care Professionals, Ninth Edition**
Alyson Honeycutt, Mary Elizabeth Milliken

SVP, Product & Market Strategy, GPM:
Jonathan Lau

Product Director: Matthew Seeley

Senior Product Manager: Laura Stewart

Senior Director, Development:
Marah Bellegarde

Product Development Manager:
Juliet Steiner

Senior Content Developer:
Debra Myette-Flis

Product Assistant: Deborah Handy

Vice President, Marketing Services:
Jennifer Ann Baker

Marketing Coordinator: Andrew Ouimet

Senior Production Director: Wendy Troeger

Production Director:  Andrew Crouth

Senior Content Project Manager:
Kara A. DiCaterino

Managing Art Director: Jack Pendleton

Cover and Interior Design Images:
szefei/Shutterstock.com
Barabasa/Shutterstock.com
Sergey Nivens/Shutterstock.com
iStockPhoto.com/michaeljung
iStockPhoto.com/kupicoo
iStockPhoto.com/AnthiaCumming

For product information and technology assistance, contact us at
**Cengage Learning Customer & Sales Support, 1-800-354-9706**

For permission to use material from this text or product,
submit all requests online at **www.cengage.com/permissions**.
Further permissions questions can be e-mailed to
**permissionrequest@cengage.com**

Library of Congress Control Number: 2016953427

ISBN: 978-1-3059-5988-0

**Cengage Learning**
20 Channel Center Street
Boston, MA 02210
USA

Cengage Learning is a leading provider of customized learning solutions with employees residing in nearly 40 different countries and sales in more than 125 countries around the world. Find your local representative at **www.cengage.com.**

Cengage Learning products are represented in Canada by Nelson Education, Ltd.

To learn more about Cengage Learning, visit **www.cengage.com**

Purchase any of our products at your local college store or at our preferred online store **www.cengagebrain.com**

**Notice to the Reader**

Printed in China
Print Number: 02     Print Year: 2017

# CONTENTS

# PREFACE

## INTRODUCTION

*Understanding Human Behavior: A Guide for Health Care Professionals* is designed to assist students in health occupations education programs to learn basic principles of human behavior. These principles provide a basis for increased self-understanding and improved interpersonal relationships. With technological advances in diagnostic and therapeutic procedures, it is easy for a health care professional to focus on procedures and routines. Patients, however, want personalized care that conveys respect for the patient as a person.

Patients' expectations are more likely to be met when health care professionals aim for effective interaction with each patient. By consciously attending to each interaction with patients, the health care professional will experience greater job satisfaction.

## ORGANIZATION

*Understanding Human Behavior: A Guide for Health Care Professionals,* Ninth Edition, is organized to proceed from relatively simple information to more complex concepts, from the known to the unknown, and from application to self to application in a variety of interpersonal situations. For that reason, Sections I through V (Chapters 1 through 18) are designed for *sequential study.* Each section builds on the previous section, and each unit within a section builds on preceding units.

Section VI does not follow the sequential pattern. Although the first three chapters of Section VI proceed from historical content to current developments in health care, each unit is self-contained and can be studied independently. Ideally, instructors will assign Unit 22 early in the program, so students can start practicing stress management. Undertaking the role of a student, introduction to the clinical setting, and care of the sick all include stressful experiences. Preparing to become a health care professional includes learning the importance of self-care, and stress management is an essential component of self-care.

Section I provides an orientation to the role of health care professional, the importance of accepting each patient as a worthwhile human being, the challenge of striving for self-understanding, and guidelines for personal and professional growth. Section II presents information about various influences on human behavior: the role of heredity, basic physical and psychological needs, developmental factors, role of the social environment, emotions and their power to influence behavior, and adjustment as a composite of all these factors. Section III presents more complex concepts related to human behavior: stressful events that occur in the lives of most people, domestic violence and bullying, and the mental and emotional effects of traumatic experiences. Many victims of a traumatic event subsequently require health care. For both personal and professional reasons, health care professionals need to be aware of the mental/emotional and physical effects of these traumatic experiences, as well as the potential for long-term adverse effects on the victim. The remainder of Section III covers other factors related to one's adjustment: common defense mechanisms, inner conflict, and frustration.

Section IV contains expanded content on the components of effective communication. Practice exercises are designed to help students become better communicators by improving their skills in sending, receiving, and observing verbal and nonverbal exchanges. These exercises can involve all students and be accommodated readily within a class period. Section V provides an overview of changing practices in relation to death and dying, the effect of these changes, and legislation related to the rights of patients to participate in health care decisions, especially those related to end-of-life care. The grief process is discussed in detail, with guidelines for assisting the bereaved.

Section VI is designed to encourage students to accept the changes that inevitably will occur in the dynamic health care system. Chapter 19 provides a historical overview that reflects the roots of current practices, including holistic health care. Chapter 21 describes the emergence of the holistic emphasis and spotlights several complementary healing modalities that have gained widespread acceptance with the public. The reader is encouraged to maintain an open mind in conjunction with a healthy skepticism in evaluating various treatment modalities. Unit 22 addresses stress management.

## CHANGES TO THE NINTH EDITION

*Understanding Human Behavior*, Ninth Edition, includes the following updates and additions:

- Chapters have been streamlined and condensed for conciseness.
- Learning Objectives were rewritten to be application-based.
- New color design, colorized cartoons, and full-color art
- New "For Discussion and Reflection" boxes are included throughout the text to encourage students to make personal connections to and real-world applications of the chapter concepts.
- **Chapter 1** describes effective study skills that have been validated by research.
- **Chapter 2** introduces the concepts of cultural bias and cultural competence.
- **Chapter 3** introduces the concept of fixed mindset versus growth mindset.
- **Chapter 6** combines former Chapters 6 and 7 to provide a more cohesive discussion of social and emotional needs.
- **Chapter 9** includes updated information about developmental disorders, including autism spectrum disorder.
- **Chapter 10** introduces the concept of trauma-informed care.
- **Chapter 11** includes updated information about the prevalence of drug use in the United States.
- **Chapter 12** combines former chapters 13 and 14, addressing the closely-related concepts of frustration and inner conflict.
- **Chapter 14** combines former chapters 16 and 17, discussing how good human relations skills can help in coping with challenging patient behaviors. Chapter 14 discusses strategies for setting limits with patients who display inappropriate behavior.
- **Chapter 15** combines former chapters 18 and 19, emphasizing the interrelated role of nonverbal and verbal communication and introducing the concept of paraverbal communication.

- **Chapter 18** examines the benefits and the limitations of Kübler-Ross's stages of dying.

- **Chapter 20** introduces the concept that all treatment takes place in a psychosocial content. The nocebo effect is also discussed.

- **Chapter 21** includes an updated discussion of alternative, complementary, and integrative medicine.

- **Chapter 22** provides an updated discussion of the causes of stress and a variety of stress-management techniques, including relaxation, exercise, mindfulness, and meditation.

## INSTRUCTOR RESOURCES

Resources for instructors include:

- Cognero®Testbank makes generating tests and quizzes a snap. You can create customized assessments for your students with the click of a button. Add your own unique questions and print tests for easy class preparation.

- Customizable **instructor slide presentations created in PowerPoint** focus on key concepts from each chapter.

- Electronic **Instructor's Manual** continues to offer suggested activities, topics for discussion, and teaching methods.

## MINDTAP

**MindTap** is a fully online, interactive learning experience built upon authoritative Cengage Learning content. By combining readings, multimedia, activities, and assessments into a singular learning path, MindTap elevates learning by providing real-world application to better engage students. Instructors customize the learning path by selecting Cengage Learning resources and adding their own content via apps that integrate into the MindTap framework seamlessly with many learning management systems.

To learn more, visit www.cengage.com/mindtap

## USING *UNDERSTANDING HUMAN BEHAVIOR*

The effectiveness of *Understanding Human Behavior* depends on the instructor's choice of activities: class time to clarify various concepts and specific activities to encourage student participation, especially the sharing of experiences, discussion of problem situations, and selection of effective behavior for real and hypothetical situations. The instructor's own creative use of the text material is the key to students' achievement.

No one ever completely masters human relations skills. Those who sincerely want to relate effectively to others must become lifelong students of human behavior. They must consciously practice human relations skills in order to improve their sensitivity to the possible meaning of observed behavior and select appropriate responses. The immediate challenge is to gain as much as possible from this course, as a foundation for the lifelong challenge of developing a high level of skill in human relations.

## ABOUT THE AUTHORS

**Alyson Honeycutt, M.A., N.C.C.**, is a National Certified Counselor, holds a License in School Counseling from the North Carolina Department of Public Instruction, and has advanced degrees from North Carolina State University at Raleigh and Appalachian State University. She has taught parenting and literacy classes, has been an instructor in English at the college level, has taught students with emotional and behavioral disabilities, and has served as a district-level behavior support coordinator in the public schools.

**Mary Elizabeth Milliken, B.S.N., M.S., Ed.D.**, was a graduate of Duke University School of Nursing. Her graduate study at North Carolina State University at Raleigh concentrated on both education and psychology. She practiced nursing in a variety of settings, served as instructor, then coordinator, of a practical nursing education program, was curriculum specialist for health occupations in the North Carolina Department of Community Colleges, and was a consultant on curriculum and effective teaching. From 1971 to 1987, she served as Coordinator of Health Occupations Teacher Education at the University of Georgia in Athens. Dr. Milliken followed the emerging holistic health movement since 1974, attending numerous workshops and conferences in which holistic concepts and complementary healing modalities were presented. She completed the curriculum sequence and certification requirements of Healing Touch International, Inc.

## REVIEWERS OF THE NINTH EDITION

Mohammad Bajwa, PhD
*Professor and Program Director*

Stacey Davis, B.Ed, RHIT, CHTS-TR, CPC-P, CPC, CCA
*National Director of Allied Health*

Margaret Garber, BA, RMA, CPC, CPPM
*Department Chair*

Hope Hinson, AA, BA
*Medical Program Director*

Erin O'Hara-Leslie, CMA (AAMA), BS, MS
*SUNY Broome Community College*
*Chairperson/Assistant Professor, Medical*
*Assisting and Health Studies*

Pamela McNutt, MA, RMA (AMT)
*Allied Health Instructor*

Amy Samuel, CMA (AAMA), AHI (AMT)
*Assistant Professor*

Bobbi Steelman, BSEd, MAEd, CPhT
*Pharmacy Technician Program Director*

Barb Westrick, CPC, CMA
*Program Chair*

# SECTION I

# On Becoming a Health Care Professional

This section introduces some of the challenges, responsibilities, problems, and satisfactions of being a health care professional. People from all walks of life require health care. As a health care professional, you will be challenged to learn how to serve each person effectively. Section I is designed to help you become aware of the realities of a health career and also to help you learn strategies to succeed as both a student and a health care professional.

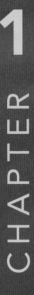

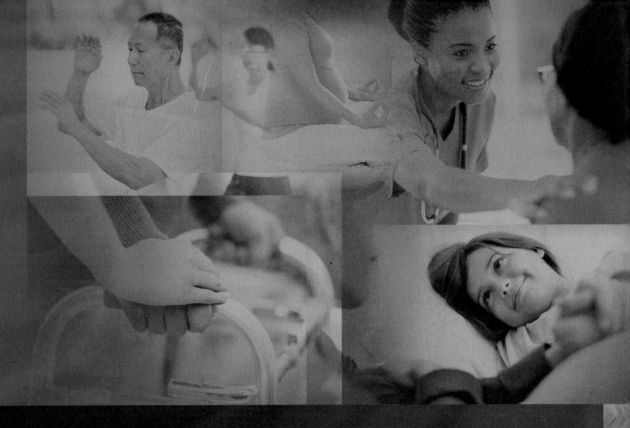

# Challenges and Responsibilities of Health Care Professionals

## OBJECTIVES

After completing this unit, you should be able to:

* Describe challenges health care professionals often face.
* Explain the importance of high standards for a health care professional.
* Explain how your achievement standards as a student relate to your future performance standards as a health care professional.
* Use effective study habits to improve learning.
* Set your own standards for achievement as a student and for performance as a health care professional.
* Explain the meaning of **empowerment** and apply the concept of empowerment to real-life situations.

## KEY TERMS

| | | |
|---|---|---|
| Empowerment | Self-confidence | Standards of |
| Excellence | Self-reliance | performance |
| Mediocre | | |

Congratulations! You have decided to become a health care professional. As you proceed through your educational program, you will have the satisfaction of learning new information and developing new skills. As a health care professional, you will be able to make a significant contribution to your community.

This chapter introduces some of the challenges, responsibilities, problems, and satisfactions of being a health care professional. People from all walks of life require health care. As a health care professional, you will be challenged to learn how to serve each person effectively.

A career in the health field differs in many ways from careers in other fields. The purpose of this unit is to help you be aware of the satisfactions, challenges, and responsibilities you face as a student and as a future health care professional.

## SATISFACTIONS

Your choice of career path indicates that you like people and have a strong desire to help others. Although you could possibly make more money in some other occupational field, a career that provides opportunities to help others may be very rewarding.

### Approval versus Inner Satisfaction

We all admire those who can do something extremely well; each of us would like to be the kind of person who is admired by others. We enjoy receiving approval from others, yet this good feeling is only temporary. Athletes may enjoy hearing the cheers of the crowd, but the deepest satisfaction comes from knowing that they performed with great skill. True satisfaction is an inner feeling of pride in doing something well, regardless of whether or not the performance is applauded by others.

As a health care professional, you will find your greatest satisfaction in trying to give each patient appropriate care. By meeting each patient's needs to the best of your ability, you will complete the day with an inner feeling of pride. The opposite approach—to view your work as a series of assignments to be completed so that you can get off work or go on break—results in finishing the day by saying "Whew, I'm glad that's over!" Stop now and consider this very important question: How will you approach your work? As a challenge that may provide satisfaction and a sense of accomplishment? Or as work you have to do to get a paycheck?

### Setting Goals for Inner Satisfaction

Performing your work well can provide **self-confidence** and a deep sense of satisfaction that is not dependent on praise from others. By working improve your performance, to do each task well, and to do better today than yesterday, you will increase your level of skill. Many of us settle for **mediocre** performance because it requires less effort to "just get by" than to do well. You have probably heard the saying, "If a job is worth doing at all, it is worth doing well." **Excellence** lies in that little bit of extra effort to achieve a superior performance. *In the health field, that little bit of extra effort may make the difference between safe and unsafe practice.*

The habits you form as a student carry over into your performance as a health care professional. Now is the time to set **standards**—the level of quality for your performance—that will lead to skillful performance, self-confidence, and pride in your work.

# CHALLENGES

## Setting Standards of Performance

Only you can set the standards that will guide your performance over the coming years. At times, you may be tempted to take a shortcut. Sometimes a piece of equipment will be contaminated; obtaining sterile materials to complete the procedure will require extra effort and time. Only you will know whether or not sterile technique was violated and the contaminated equipment was used—unless, of course, the patient develops an infection as a result. Your standards of performance serve as your conscience and determine whether you experience the inner satisfaction that comes from knowing the job was well done.

Your own standards should include accuracy in measurements, observations, and reporting. Time pressure may tempt you to take shortcuts, but erroneous reporting is not acceptable. Many health care facilities now utilize instrumentation for measurement of vital signs, but at times you will have to obtain vital signs without such aids. Suppose you are taking a patient's pulse and count for 15 seconds, then multiply by 4. If your count is off by one beat during that 15 seconds, your pulse count has an error of 4; if the patient's pulse skips two beats, the error in your count may be even greater than 4. By counting for a full minute, you obtain an accurate pulse rate. Which is more important—saving 45 seconds, or reporting the correct pulse rate?

The habits you form as a student will affect your performance throughout your career. When making that little bit of extra effort to "do it right" has become a habit, doing it correctly no longer seems an effort; it becomes an essential part of your performance. Thus, excellence as a health care professional will depend upon setting high standards of performance for yourself now.

## Excellence and Patient Safety

In the health field, all professionals should strive for excellence. *Anything less than excellence can endanger the patient.* The nurse should give the correct medicine to each patient 100 percent of the time. The medical assistant should use correct technique in 100 percent of the situations that require asepsis. The laboratory assistant should report test results correctly 100 percent of the time; the dental assistant should sterilize instruments correctly 100 percent of the time; the ambulance attendant should move the accident victim correctly 100 percent of the time. *Performance that is less than 100 percent correct can have disastrous effects for the patient.*

## Meeting Patient Needs

As a health care professional, you will work with many different people, each of whom is different as a person and as a patient. Each of your patients is a unique individual—a physical, emotional, mental, and spiritual being. Each has a history of experiences, a life within the context of a specific family and community, beliefs and values, and a unique genetic makeup. To provide the best possible care, you will need to show concern about the patient as a person (e.g., "John Smith"), rather than as someone for whom a specified procedure must be carried out (e.g., "the knee replacement").

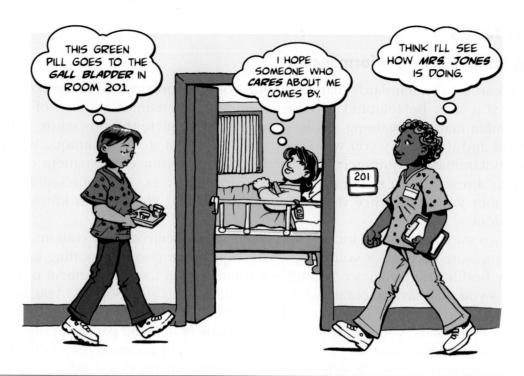

**FIGURE 1-1** Think of each patient as a person with specific needs rather than a diagnosis.

## RESPONSIBILITIES

### As a Student

Your first responsibility as a student is to take full advantage of every opportunity to learn. Try to see the purpose in each assignment; look at it as an *opportunity to learn,* rather than as a chore to complete. With this attitude toward learning, you will not be tempted to skip class occasionally without good reason.

Your second responsibility is to decide what standards will guide your performance as a student. Imagine that your school has set a certain grade, such as 70, as passing in your program. Now imagine yourself saying, "I'll study this material until I know it well enough to make 75." In many courses of study, a grade of 75 is acceptable; a deficiency in the student's knowledge of subject matter is unlikely to cause harm to someone else.

In a health occupations course, however, the implications of "just passing" are much more serious. Any gaps in your knowledge and performance skills can affect every patient served. Do you want your future services to patients to be of "just passing" quality? Or do you wish to give the very best service you are capable of giving? If your educational program is preparing you to provide health services, can you be content to learn only 70 percent

**For Discussion and Reflection**

1. Explain the importance of setting high standards for yourself as a student and as a health care professional.
2. Tell about a time you felt proud of something you worked hard to accomplish. What made your accomplishment so satisfying?

of what your teachers expect you to learn? Can you be content to develop your skills just enough to get a passing grade in a laboratory course? If you set high standards for achievement now, then these high standards will carry over into your future performance as a health care professional.

## PLANNING FOR SUCCESS

In setting standards for achievement, plan to *do your best,* rather than trying to be the best student in the class. How can you do your best? Develop a study routine and establish the habits that work best for you. In order to get started, consider the following guidelines:

- Tell family and friends that you have set aside a certain time of day as your study period. Do not allow them to violate your schedule by interrupting you unless there is an emergency.

- At the beginning of each study period, write out a list of specific things you need to complete; then, rank the items in order of importance. Complete task #1 (most important) first, and then move on to task #2. If one of the tasks is something you dislike but must get done, let it be task #1 so that you get it out of the way.

- If your list of study assignments is too long to complete today, set up tomorrow's list so today's remaining assignments come first; then put the items on that list out of your mind until tomorrow and give your full attention to today's list.

- Set up a calendar or special notebook for assignments, due dates for projects or reports, and test dates. Note on your calendar the dates/times you will work on specific assignments or study for a test. By planning ahead, you can avoid last-minute rushes to meet a deadline.

These guidelines will help you develop an organized, systematic approach to studying. In addition, you can make the most of each study session by using effective learning techniques. In a 2013 study, researchers found that the following techniques were *not effective* in increasing student learning:

- Highlighting the text
- Focusing on key words
- Summarizing
- Rereading
- Imagery (mentally picturing what is being read)

While these techniques can be used if you prefer, they are likely not the best use of your study time (Dunlosky 2013).

Study techniques which were *moderately effective to very effective* included the following:

- Explaining to yourself or a study partner, in your own words, why the information you are studying is true or important.

- Explaining to yourself or a study partner how new information relates to information you already know.

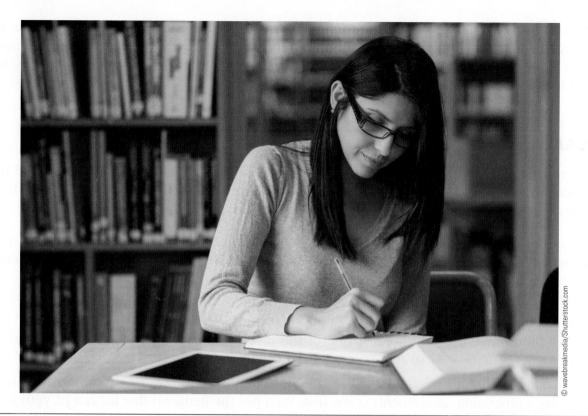

**FIGURE 1-2** Using effective study techniques will help you make the most of each study session.

**For Discussion and Reflection**

What study techniques have been most effective for you in the past? Explain how you can incorporate one or more of the techniques described into your study routine.

- Varying your study sessions so that you work on several types of information, assignments, or problems in a single session.

- Testing yourself or taking a practice test on the material to be learned.

- Spreading out your study into several shorter sessions rather than one long session.

Try incorporating one or two of these strategies into your study sessions. As you become comfortable with those techniques, try adding an additional strategy. Planning time to study is important, but making effective use of the time you have planned is equally essential to success.

## EMPOWERMENT

All adults should control most aspects of their lives. During adolescence, learning to make decisions is an important developmental task; if this is not learned, the individual enters adulthood poorly equipped to cope with life problems. If you entered adulthood with a tendency to let your parents, spouse, friends, or anyone else make decisions for you, it is time to recognize that you are giving away your power—the power to be a **self-reliant**, responsible adult.

When you are planning to eat out with a friend, who decides which restaurant? Do you usually say, "Oh, I don't care; you choose." Does your spouse or significant other give you a choice? If you do not participate in small decisions that affect you, how can you expect others to include you in big decisions? For example:

> Kate is a dental hygienist whose earnings are about equal to her husband's. Each payday, she gives her check to her husband because "he handles our finances." They have only one car, so Kate usually waits as much as an hour for her husband to pick her up. She insists on keeping the car this week so she can do some errands after work. Yesterday her husband waited 45 minutes for her to pick him up. Today, he announces proudly, "Well, I bought you your own car." Buying a car is a major decision, yet Kate's husband did not see any need to involve her in that decision. Kate has given away her power; it will take much effort to renegotiate this relationship so that she is empowered to participate in decision making.

How does empowerment affect you? Suppose you have informed the family that your study hour will begin at 9:00 each evening. During the second day of this plan, your teenager calls you to the phone at 9:15; the caller is your sister-in-law, who talks about her problems for a full half hour. Two days later, your 10-year-old opens the door at 9:30 and says, "I need a note for my teacher about the field trip next Monday." Each time you permit these violations of your study hour, you are giving away your power. You gave your two children the power to interrupt your study hour. You gave your sister-in-law the power to use 30 minutes of your study time for her own purposes. You probably responded to these requests because you are accustomed to meeting the needs of others, even if doing so interferes with your own needs.

If you repeatedly allow others to make decisions for you, then you are *avoiding the adult task of taking responsibility for your life.* If this pattern applies to you, you can start reclaiming your power by requiring others to respect your needs. For example, after informing all members of your family that a certain time period is your study time, do not permit any violations to occur. Remind those who interrupt you that you are not available during study hour. If you are consistent, the interruptions will eventually stop. Then you can use the same approach to another of your needs. You may choose to make the next decision about where to eat or which movie to see, instead of allowing someone else to make that decision. You may wish to inform your spouse or a friend that you are to be involved in any decisions that affect you. This type of change will not occur rapidly; be content with small changes initially. By persisting, you will eventually gain more control over your life. But do not be surprised if others reject your decision, especially if you are just beginning to participate in making decisions. Give your family and friends time to accept your change in behavior. Ideally, decision making is a give-and-take situation. Sometimes your decision is accepted, whereas at other times another person's decision prevails.

## For Discussion and Reflection

1. Explain what empowerment means and why it is important for adults to control most of the decisions about their own lives.
2. Sometimes even a self-reliant person has an experience that gives rise to feelings of helplessness or at least requires asking for help. For each situation below, describe one or more actions that would indicate self-reliance rather than dependence on others.
   a. You have a flat tire on the way to class.
   b. You have locked your keys in the car.
   c. You are going to lunch with two classmates and realize that you left your wallet at home.

As a health care professional, you should also recognize the importance of empowerment to patients' self-esteem and sense of well-being. Patients who are dependent on others for their personal needs may express anger about their helplessness. Many patients need help in regaining some control over their life situations. By respecting their wishes and involving patients in decisions, *when appropriate,* you contribute to feelings of empowerment.

## MAKING A DECISION

A certain grade is necessary for passing a course, but it is your decision about the desired level of achievement that influences your performance. Even more important, the *standards that guide your performance as a student will carry over into your future performance as a health care professional.*

Choosing to enter this educational program for the health field was an important decision in your life. Now, it is time to make another decision—what kind of health care professional will you be? Excellent? Mediocre? Or "just passing"? Remember, the standards of performance that will characterize you as a health care professional will be influenced by the standards you set for yourself now.

## ACTIVITIES

1. Complete each of the following using Worksheet A (see page 11) at the end of this chapter.

   a. List the things you *have to do* each day.

   b. List the things you *have to do* each week, but not every day.

   c. List the things you *have to do* occasionally.

   d. Beside each item in a, b, and c, write the name of someone who could help you complete that task, at least some of the time. For example, could you and a friend car pool so that you alternate days picking your children up from day care or school?

2. Use Worksheet B (see page 12) at the end of this chapter to develop a tentative study plan. Note times you have class, work, or other commitments. Decide when you will study each day, and when you will devote time to other tasks or hobbies. Try this plan for two weeks. If your plan seems to be effective, continue to use it. If it is not effective:

   a. List problems that interfered with the effectiveness of the plan.

   b. Modify the plan by changing the schedule, the place where you study, or other details. If other people are part of the problem, try to involve them in developing the "improved plan" to increase the probability of getting their cooperation.

## REFERENCE

Dunlosky, J., Rawson, K.A., Marsh, E.J., Nathan, M.J., & Willingham, D.T. (2013). Improving students' learning with effective learning techniques; promising directions from cognitive and educational psychology. *Psychological Science in the Public Interest, 14,* 4–58. doi:10.1177/1529100612453266.

## WORKSHEET A

### Tasks I Have to Do

Every day:

- Reading on a regular basis
- Completing all homework assignments
- Organizing time well
- Doing your best everyday

Once a week:

- Plan Study time
- Give yourself enough time
- Do Research

Occasionally:

- Spend time with fun activities to relax your mind.

## WORKSHEET B

### Study Plan

| Time | Monday | Tuesday | Wednesday | Thursday | Friday | Saturday | Sunday |
|------|--------|---------|-----------|----------|--------|----------|--------|
| 6 A.M. | | | | | | | |
| 7 | | | Wake up | | | | |
| 8 | | | Breakfast | | | | |
| 9 | | | study | | | | |
| 10 | | | study | | | | |
| 11 | | | work | | | | |
| 12 Noon | | | work | | | | |
| 1 P.M. | | | Work | | | | |
| 2 | | | Work | | | | |
| 3 | | | Work | | | | |
| 4 | | | Work | | | | |
| 5 | | | Work | | | | |
| 6 | | | Work | | | | |
| 7 | | | work | | | | |
| 8 | | | Yoga | | | | |
| 9 | | | study | | | | |
| 10 | | | study | | | | |
| 11 | | | sleep | | | | |
| 12 Mn | | | | | | | |

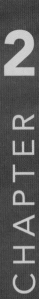

# CHAPTER 2

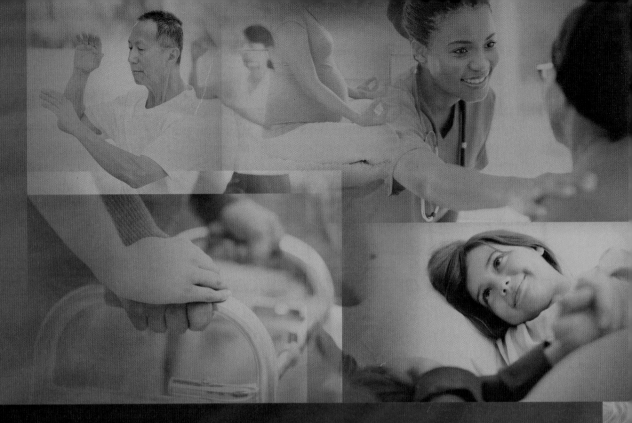

# The Philosophy of Individual Worth

## OBJECTIVES

After completing this chapter, you should be able to:

- Explain the philosophy of individual worth.
- Discuss how cultural bias can affect the quality of patient care.
- Describe examples of cultural differences that could contribute to misunderstandings between a patient and a health care professional.
- Apply the philosophy of individual worth to relationships with patients and their families.

## KEY TERMS

Affluent
Cultural bias
Cultural competence

Individual worth
Philosophy
Prejudice

Socioeconomic
Superstition
Value system

A health care professional comes in contact with people from many different backgrounds. Some patients have never known anything but poverty. Some have come from other countries or from homes in which the customs of other nationalities are followed. Some have been reared in a religious faith with beliefs very different from those of you and your friends.

If you have had little contact with people from other cultures or from other **socioeconomic** levels of society, your first reaction may be to view these people not only as "different" but also as less acceptable than people who are like you and your friends. Regardless of your personal views, as a health care professional, you are responsible for showing respect and providing quality care to all patients.

## THE MEANING OF INDIVIDUAL WORTH

The philosophy of **individual worth** is the belief that *everyone, regardless of personal circumstances or personal qualities, has worth and is entitled to respect as a human being.* For health care professionals, this means that the quality of service does not vary because of the patient's race, nationality, religion, gender, sexual orientation, age, economic level, occupation, education, diagnosis, or any other characteristic.

Each patient is an individual. Each should receive health care that takes into consideration both the person's individuality and the specific health problem. The **philosophy** of individual worth has many implications for patient care. Health care professionals who do not accept the philosophy of individual worth may interact differently with patients from a culture that is different from their own while remaining unaware of any differences in the care they are providing.

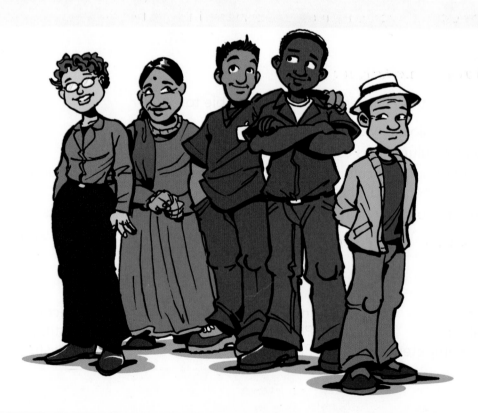

**FIGURE 2-1** Everyone has worth and is entitled to respect as a human being.

## THE HEALTH CARE PROFESSIONAL AND CULTURAL BIAS

Each of us represents a specific subclass within the larger society. The major subclasses are race, religion, national heritage, and socioeconomic level, each of which has its own beliefs, values, traditions, customs, and food preferences or prohibitions. In addition, one's occupational group is also a subclass that influences the thinking and behavior of its members. Your preparation for serving as a health care professional includes learning about cultural differences and respecting each patient's cultural heritage as you provide health care.

### Beliefs and Misinformation

In spite of the widespread availability of information about the human body, health practices, and modern methods of diagnosis and treatment through health education programs in schools, television programs, and the Internet, many people remain uninformed. People who do not have factual information are likely to believe the **superstitions** of their culture just as firmly as you believe the information in a textbook. In fact, their beliefs may be closely tied in with love and respect for their parents, since such beliefs are passed down from one generation to the next. The teachings of your parents are important to you; it is important to respect the tradition of passing knowledge from generation to generation in other cultures, even though those teachings may be different from what you think is "right."

### Socioeconomic Class

Each socioeconomic class within a society has its own customs, standards of living, **value system**, interests, expectations, and other characteristics that distinguish it from other socioeconomic classes. Members of one class generally do not understand the differences between their own class and other classes. The health care professional's expectations regarding patient behavior may be unrealistic for patients from a different cultural background or socioeconomic level. The tendency to make negative judgments about a person because of the culture or class from which that person comes is called **cultural bias**.

Most health care professionals did not grow up as a member of an extremely wealthy family, nor did they live in poverty. Although there is great diversity within the middle class, members also have much in common. One thing many of them have in common is a lack of understanding about poverty and about **affluence**. But the health care professional encounters patients from all socioeconomic groups. It is especially important that health care professionals not allow their own beliefs and value systems to influence the care they give patients from other socioeconomic levels and other cultures.

### The Patient from the Poverty Class

People who have never lived in poverty find it difficult to understand those whose lives center around survival. People who live in poverty have a daily routine that is different

### For Discussion and Reflection

Have you ever felt that another person's behavior toward you reflected cultural bias on the basis of your ethnicity, gender, religion, socioeconomic status, lifestyle, or other factors? What seemed biased about the person's behavior, and how did you respond?

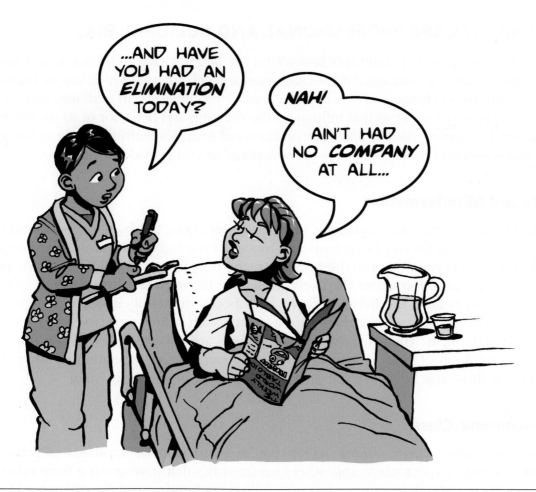

**FIGURE 2-2** The vocabulary used by health care providers may be difficult for some patients to understand.

from that followed by most middle-class people. They may lack running water or electricity in the home. As a result, they may be unable to wash their clothes or bathe regularly. Badly decayed teeth may mean poor diet and lack of knowledge about oral hygiene. Deodorants are a luxury for those who do not know today where tomorrow's dinner will come from. The language used by members of the poverty group may include words you regard as "bad," yet these words may be the patient's only means for expressing personal needs. Terminology used by health care professionals may be unfamiliar to some patients from poverty, so you may need to provide additional explanation.

## The Patient from the Affluent Class

Now consider a patient who is from the upper socioeconomic level. Perhaps this person is accustomed to the best of service and, through habit, expects to receive good service. Perhaps this person's wealth represents much hard work and successful competition in the business world. Perhaps it is inherited wealth, and this person has known a life of ease without having to struggle for material comforts.

Good health, freedom from pain, and escape from disabling accidents are not assured by wealth. Does a wealthy patient seem unwilling to put up with an inconvenient illness? Does the patient appear impatient when there is a delay in receiving an expected service or rebel against being a patient? Illness interrupts and alters patterns of living and does not respect the important matters that may await one's attention.

**For Discussion and Reflection**

How would you describe the socio-economic class in which you grew up? What attitudes did your family and you have toward others from different socio-economic classes?

Even the wealthy have problems. Though different from those in poverty, their life problems may be very demanding. Therefore, the health care professional should not conclude that the wealthy patient should lie back and be a "good patient" because he does not have to worry about how to pay the medical bills.

## Expectations of Health Care Professionals

Each patient, regardless of socioeconomic status, age, race, religion, or national origin, is entitled to the best care you can give. Each is a human being with feelings, hopes, problems, habits, and needs. All of these factors contribute to the uniqueness of each personality.

Can you, as a health care professional, expect people from other cultural groups to have the same beliefs, attitudes, hygienic habits, health practices, and understandings that you have? Are they either less worthy or more worthy as human beings because their lifestyles are different from yours?

# IMPLICATIONS FOR HEALTH CARE PROFESSIONALS

## Cultural Competence

The degree to which you accept the philosophy of individual worth will influence your practice as a health care professional. You may need to overcome **prejudice** in order to apply this philosophy to your daily work. You may even have difficulty in understanding some patients, especially those whose cultural background is different from yours. Your responsibility as a health care professional is to *know your role and, within that role, to serve each patient effectively.* Avoid making value judgments about a patient or allowing your feelings to interfere with the quality of care you provide that person. **Cultural competence** includes two parts:

- Becoming aware of your own beliefs about and attitudes toward other cultures or groups.
- Accepting others' cultures, beliefs, and lifestyles, even if different from yours.

Developing this awareness and acceptance takes practice, but it will become easier when you make it a habit to keep an open mind when you encounter a patient or co-worker from a different background.

## The Challenge

It can be a challenge to provide health services to those who are from a different culture or socioeconomic level. Try to understand these patients in terms of their background; try to see situations as they see them. You can fulfill your role as a health care professional and at the same time adapt to the special needs of each patient. The example you set is important in teaching health habits. Your choice of words is important in helping the patient understand your meaning. Your sincerity and interest can influence a patient's attitude toward the entire health care system.

## Studying a Situation

It is not easy to serve all patients equally well. Sometimes there is a strong desire to escape—to carry out an assigned task and leave the patient as quickly as possible. If you find yourself trying to avoid a patient, consider the situation carefully: Why do you find this patient difficult to serve? Does this patient remind you of someone you dislike? Have you tried to understand this patient's personal and health needs? Have you tried to see the situation as the patient sees it? If you make a habit of studying such situations, applying your knowledge about human behavior, you will grow in your ability to form effective relationships with your patients.

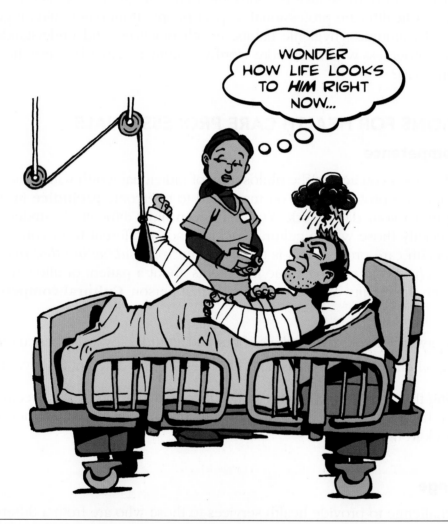

**FIGURE 2-3 Try to understand the patient's point of view.**

## PRACTICING A PHILOSOPHY OF INDIVIDUAL WORTH

It is easy to give lip service to the philosophy of individual worth; It is quite difficult, however, to practice it day after day when there is a busy schedule and a wide variety of patients to take care of, unless you form certain ways of thinking about your patients. The following suggestions provide a starting point for developing and applying a philosophy of individual worth to your relationships with patients:

- Accept each patient as an individual with a unique personality.

- Recognize that each person tries to meet his needs with patterns of behavior that have developed over a lifetime; these patterns cannot be changed easily.

- Make a conscious effort to understand each patient's behavior.

- Accept that many of your patients will not behave as you want them to behave.

- Do not expect a sick person to adapt to you. As a health care professional and as a well person, you should adapt to the patient.

- Consider each patient with a cultural background different from yours as an opportunity for you to learn about the influence of customs, beliefs, values, religious practices, and socioeconomic level on human behavior.

- Make it a habit to treat all patients with respect, regardless of their backgrounds.

## ACTIVITIES

1. Think about someone you know whose background is different from your own; describe how this person's life (past and present) differs from your life.

2. Describe an experience in which you have worked or interacted with someone from a different culture. Were there times when cultural differences led to misunderstandings or miscommunication? What did you learn from the situation?

3. Consider each of the following situations in terms of your possible feelings about each patient:

   a. You are admitting a male patient from the emergency room; he has an unkempt beard, bad breath, and his clothes smell of stale perspiration.

   b. Your morning assignment includes an unconscious patient who was admitted during the night; the report states that this person is a known drug addict.

   c. Your patient is a 6-year-old boy who looks at you with obvious distrust; he responds to your "Good morning" by looking away from you and saying "Leave me alone." As he continues speaking, he uses profanity freely.

   d. Your patient is 35 years old and weighs 300 pounds.

   e. You are admitting a patient who reeks of garlic.

4. Notice how social media, television, movies, and politicians speak about different groups of people. Can you find examples which reflect a philosophy of individual worth? Are there examples which illustrate prejudice?

## REFERENCES AND SUGGESTED READINGS

Chettih, Mindy. (2012). Turning the lens inward: Cultural competence and providers' values in health care decision making. *The Gerontologist, 52*(6), 739–747. doi:10.1093/geront/gns008.
Rosen, Dennis. (2014). How bias and stigma undermine health care. *Holistic Primary Care, 15*(4), 14.

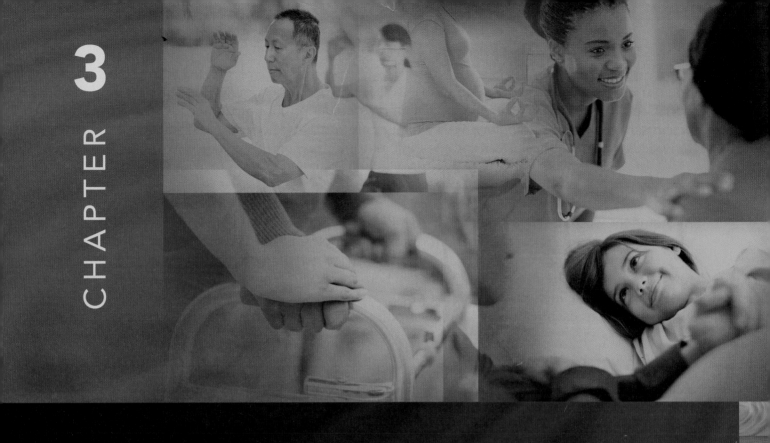

# Self-Understanding

## OBJECTIVES

After completing this chapter, you should be able to:

- Explain why learning is defined as "a change in behavior."
- Describe techniques for effective learning.
- Identify your life roles and appropriate behaviors for each role.
- Explain why role confusion is dangerous for a health care professional.
- Discuss time management strategies.
- List five guidelines for personal growth.

## KEY TERMS

| | | |
|---|---|---|
| Ethics | Learning | Role |
| Fixed Mindset | Potential | Traits |
| Growth Mindset | Procrastinate | |

You are enrolled in a course of study that will lead to your becoming a health care professional. In the near future you will graduate and assume a position in an agency that provides health services to the community. What changes are needed before you, the student of today, can become you, the health care professional of tomorrow?

## YOUR ROLE AS A STUDENT

As a student, you must acquire knowledge, learn to apply it appropriately to a wide variety of situations, and develop skill in performing certain procedures. Your teachers have organized for you a sequence of learning experiences. They will guide your step-by-step progress toward a future **role** in the field. Your teachers, however, cannot do the whole job. The desire to learn, willingness to make the necessary effort, and determination to gain as much as possible from each learning experience must come from within you.

### Learning versus Memorizing

**Learning** has been defined as a *change in behavior*. If you can answer the questions on a test, but do not apply that information in appropriate clinical situations, have you *really* learned? Do you approach assignments as though you are storing information that can be played back on demand? Simply memorizing information is not true learning.

### Developing Mental Skills

Do you constantly ask yourself how a new idea can be used? Does new information guide you in selecting appropriate behavior for situations where that information is relevant? If you can answer "Yes" to these questions, then you are truly learning. You are using mental processes such as thinking, reasoning, selecting, decision making, and evaluating for conscious control of your behavior.

### Developing Learning Skills

Chapter 1 discussed guidelines for developing effective study habits. Learning new skills begins with studying but does not end when a test or an assignment is complete. Each time you begin a new topic of study in class, ask yourself the following questions:

- What do I already know about this topic?
- What do I want to find out about this topic?
- How will I apply this information now? In my future career?

When you connect new information to ideas you have previously learned, the new information becomes more meaningful and easier to remember.

### Developing Your Potential

Think of yourself for a moment as a person who loves music, but does not have a musical instrument or teacher. Suddenly, your family obtains a piano, and a gifted piano teacher moves next door. After an appropriate period of study under the guidance of your teacher, you become an excellent pianist. Thus, through a combination of the right circumstances and effort, your **potential** for becoming a pianist has been fulfilled and you *are* a pianist.

This period as a student is your opportunity to develop your potential as a health care professional. The circumstances for learning are being provided in the form of many learning experiences, each designed to help you acquire new knowledge and develop skills. The effort necessary to develop your potential can come only from you.

Let's explore some of the ways you can strive to develop your potential for learning. These same approaches, applied to your future career, will help you develop your potential for becoming a health care professional.

## TAKING A NEW LOOK AT YOURSELF

A first step to developing your potential is to take an honest look at yourself. "But," you may say, "I already know myself." Do you really? As Richard Barbieri states, "Very few of us have an accurate view of our own strengths and weaknesses. Most of us overestimate our ability to multitask, our driving skills, our intelligence, and, most of all, our sense of humor" (Barbieri, p. 108). True self-understanding is difficult to achieve. Even a beginning effort—just taking an honest look at yourself—may make you decide on some changes.

### Will to Change

The first question to ask yourself is, "Am I willing to make changes in myself?" When someone criticizes you, do you nurse your hurt feelings or express anger toward your critic? Do you reject the criticism or make excuses for your behavior? Or do you see criticism as a possible indication that you need to change some aspect of your behavior? Willingness to change is necessary so that you can learn and grow as a person. Remember, learning was defined earlier as a change in behavior.

### Strengths and Weaknesses

Your next question might be, "What are my strengths and my weaknesses?" To develop your potential, you must know your weak points, for these will need your attention and greatest effort. For example, do you have a habit of putting off a task until the last minute? This habit can lead to many undesirable results: being late to class, not being prepared for a test, not practicing a skill until you have achieved a high level of proficiency. By correcting a tendency to **procrastinate**, you can spare yourself the emotional strain of doing things at the last minute. You may even escape the irritation others express when your last-minute efforts inconvenience them.

An honest appraisal of your personal **traits**, including your work habits, is the key to planning ways of developing your potential. If you eliminate those behaviors that interfere with good performance, you will improve your ability to perform well in a variety of situations.

> **For Discussion and Reflection**
>
> Regarding your habits and personal traits, which of the following statements best reflects your attitude? What are the pros and cons of each of these attitudes?
>
> a. "This is just the way I am; other people need to accept that."
> b. "I try to learn from each experience and become a better person over time."

## Adapting to New Conditions

A third question to ask yourself is, "How well do I adapt to change?" Are you still clinging to ineffective habits formed early in your school years? If so, these habits are probably not working very well in your current educational program. No longer can you depend on the teacher. No longer can you expect the teacher to go over the same material until you have passively absorbed it. Time is short, and there is much to be learned before you qualify as a health care professional. *You* must assume primary responsibility for learning.

In the future, you may be in a new situation and find yourself saying or thinking, "But I learned to do it a certain way, not the way they do it here." For most tasks, there is more than one acceptable procedure; adapting to the new setting requires that you perform according to the procedures of the new setting. *Basic principles, however, do not vary.* For example, aseptic technique requires certain steps and certain precautions, regardless of the setting or the precise sequence of steps for the total procedure.

## Using Experience to Learn

A fourth question is, "Do I learn from my experiences?" Let's take a look at how two people reacted to an embarrassing experience. When Maria and Kim gave oral reports, they both showed signs of nervousness and performed poorly. For each of them, this was a very embarrassing experience.

Maria reviewed the situation, admitted to herself that she had put little effort into this assignment, and made plans to be well prepared for the next oral report. She decided to have her information better organized, to study the material until she understood it, to prepare good notes, and to rehearse her presentation until she could present the report with minimal use of notes. She also spoke with her instructor after class about ways to improve her performance.

Kim, on the other hand, used the same approach to prepare her next oral report, which proved to be another poor performance. She was no better prepared for the second report

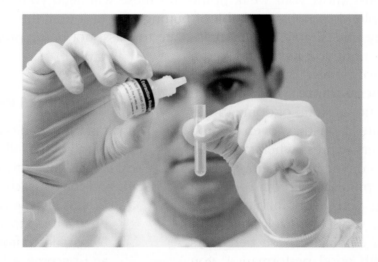

**FIGURE 3-1 Adapting to a new work setting requires that you carefully follow the procedures of the new environment.**

than she was for the first. In addition, she was developing a fear of oral reports that would have a negative effect on her future efforts to speak in front of others.

Maria used her experience constructively, making careful plans to prevent a recurrence of this particular embarrassment. With additional practice, Maria will give oral reports with confidence. Kim, on the other hand, allowed the experience to create self-doubt and fear of oral reports. Do you think she will develop either skill or confidence? Which of these students will grow as a person?

## Developing a Growth Mindset

Stanford researcher Carol Dweck (2006) popularized the term **growth mindset**. Dweck found that students who believed that their abilities and intelligence were fixed, or unchanging, traits were less successful than students who believed that they could develop and increase their abilities through effort and practice. Statements such as "I'm just not good at math" indicate a **fixed mindset** and can make it more difficult to learn new skills.

Students with a growth mindset, on the other hand, tend to have the following attitudes and beliefs about learning:

- While not everyone will become a "genius," anyone can learn and improve their skills.

- By reviewing what has or has not worked previously, we can determine whether a new strategy or approach is needed.

- An unsuccessful attempt should not be viewed as a failure, but as feedback about how to improve future efforts.

Dweck (2015) cautions that while effort is an important part of the growth mindset, effort alone may not lead to improvement. Rather, Dweck says, "Students need to try new strategies and seek input from others when they're stuck" (Dweck, pp. 20, 24).

## Role Perception

An additional question to ask yourself is, "What is my role?" The present program of study will help you understand your future role as a health care professional. For every role there are appropriate and inappropriate ways of behaving. Whether a particular manner of behavior is appropriate depends not only on the specific *type* of health care professional you are preparing to become, but also on the *level* of that role in relation to other health team members.

Certain behaviors that are appropriate for a specific health care role may not be appropriate for personnel in a different role. For example, the behaviors appropriate for laboratory personnel are distinct from those appropriate for nursing personnel. Also, within individual departments there are differences in roles based on level: Within nursing there are nursing assistants, licensed practical nurses, registered nurses, head

### For Discussion and Reflection

Do you have a particular subject area or skill that you tell yourself "I'm just not good at?" On the other hand, do you have skills that you have worked hard to develop through effort and practice? How do the concepts of a fixed mindset and a growth mindset apply to either of these skills?

nurses, and supervisors, all of whom have specific roles; similarly, within the hospital laboratory, there are numerous roles such as pathologist, medical technologist, clinical laboratory assistant, laboratory aide, and others. The same is true of other hospital departments such as physical therapy, radiology, food service, and so on, as well as for medical offices. In the dental field, dentists, dental hygienists, dental assistants, and dental laboratory technologists are all concerned with oral health. Their roles have similarities, but vary according to the specific functions and educational preparation of each.

Knowing one's role is essential to effective functioning; it is also essential to self-understanding. Most roles within the health field require accepting instructions from someone at the next higher level. If you do not like "taking orders," then you may not be happy as a health care professional. If you feel anger or distrust toward persons in authority, you are likely to resent the **ethics** of the health field; the policies of your health agency; and relationships with those on the health team who have responsibility for giving instructions, making assignments, and evaluating performance. On the other hand, if you can accept a defined role, function within that role to the fullest extent of your educational preparation, and accept the limitations of the role without feeling "put down," then you are likely to find much satisfaction as a health care professional.

## YOUR LIFE ROLES

How many roles do you play? Probably several. You are a student now and hope to have a role as a health care professional in the future; you may be an employee, a husband, father, brother, wife, sister, or mother. Within each role, you have a set of behaviors and responsibilities to fulfill.

### Role as an Influence on Relationships

There are similarities in the child-parent relationship and the teacher-student relationship during the school years. In a health occupations education program, the teacher-student relationship is between two adults, even though one adult is a student. What difficulties in role perception might occur if the student is a mature, 50-year-old person, and the teacher is a 25-year-old health professional? Or if a doctor is 35 and the medical office assistant is 55, with 20 years of experience?

### Making a Distinction between Roles

The roles you play at home, in your church activities, as a health occupations student, and as a neighbor are all different. To some extent, each role requires different behavior patterns. Do not confuse the health care professional role with other roles in your personal life. Some friends may try to get "free medical advice," but the role of friend and the role of health care professional are different. Medical practice acts, which are state laws, make it illegal for non-physicians to diagnose and prescribe. Therefore, this type of role confusion is dangerous.

### Guidelines for Growth

Becoming an effective health care professional is a process that extends over a period of time. It requires continuous effort throughout one's career.

## The Value of Self-Study

In undertaking a self-study, you will be making an investment in your own future. Hopefully, this study will start you on a lifetime process of striving for personal growth. You should continuously evaluate your habits and modify those that do not get the desired response from others. There will always be some people with whom you do not "hit it off," but you can learn to relate to most people in ways that promote understanding and minimize unfavorable feelings. As you become skillful in using a large repertoire of human relations skills, you will grow in self-understanding, in tolerance, and in your ability to accept others as they are.

## The Value of Studying Human Behavior

Note that the sequence of growth is from understanding self to understanding others. Therefore, *the ability to understand others is limited until you have begun to understand yourself.*

Human behavior is very complex. In any situation, the behavior of a person is influenced by many different factors. The remainder of this course will introduce some of these influences. Understanding of oneself and others must be based on knowledge about human behavior in general.

## Managing Your Time

An important aspect of understanding yourself is to recognize how you use your time. Have you ever asked yourself at the end of the day, "Where did the time go?" Have you ever wondered why some people seem to get everything done, whereas others are perpetually late or behind on their assignments? Learning to manage your time can make you more effective as a student and a professional.

To help you identify how you spend your time, try for a day or two to write down hourly what you are doing. You will gain a realistic estimate of how long household tasks or childcare actually take as well as how much time you spend on nonessential activities, such as watching television, talking on the phone, or surfing the Internet. Once you know how you are spending your time, you can decide what changes you would like to make in your daily routine.

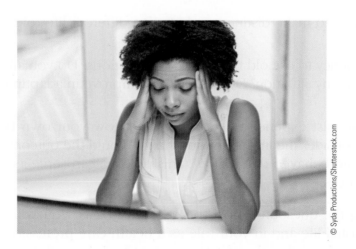

© Syda Productions/Shutterstock.com

**FIGURE 3-2  Learning to manage your time will reduce stress and help you meet deadlines.**

The following strategies may be useful in using your time more effectively:

- Write down tasks or goals you hope to accomplish each day.
- Prioritize your goals so that you tackle the most important or most urgent first.
- As much as possible, focus on completing one task at a time.
- Throughout the day, stop periodically and ask yourself, "Am I working to meet my goals? Am I doing what I am supposed to be doing?"
- Review your list of goals each evening, mark off those that were completed, and plan the list for the next day.
- Start tasks well ahead of time to avoid the stress of having to rush.
- Break large tasks into small chunks and tackle one chunk at a time.

## Personal Growth

Consider the following strategies you can use to understand yourself and set goals for personal growth and achievement as a student and health care professional:

- Recognize that learning occurs only if you make the effort to learn, if you are willing to change, and if you recognize opportunities for learning.
- Study yourself in relation to specific traits, such as willingness to change, ability to be honest with yourself, and readiness to correct weaknesses and change habits.
- Identify your strengths and make full use of them to achieve your goals.
- Identify your weaknesses—the traits or habits you need to change in order to be more effective in each of your roles.
- Study your various roles in terms of desirable behavior. Identify differences, such as habits used at home that are not appropriate at school, interpersonal relations between a parent and child that are not appropriate between the health care professional and a pediatric patient, or relations between friends that are not appropriate between a hospital employee and a patient.
- Study your ability to make distinctions between different life roles and change behaviors accordingly.
- Study your tendency to use old habits in new situations. Do you allow habits to determine your behavior in any situation? Do you need to improve in adapting your behavior to each situation?
- Mentally review past experiences to understand how your own behavior contributed to the outcome. Consider the important question, "Would the outcome of that experience be improved if I had behaved differently?" This practice can serve as a "rehearsal" for future similar experiences.

By considering the questions above on a regular basis, you will identify ways you can grow in your personal life and in your role as a health care professional.

## ACTIVITIES

1. List some changes you have made in daily habits since you entered the health occupations program. Think of one additional change that may improve one of your life roles. Write out a description of the change and the steps necessary for making it part of your habitual behavior.

2. Which of the following roles do you play in your current life situation? Add other roles to the list if needed:

   Student in a health-related educational program

   Spouse or significant other

   Parent

   Daughter or son

   Homemaker

   Employee

   a. Beside each role that applies to you, estimate the percentage of time per day that you devote to that role. The total of all roles should equal 100 percent.

   b. Mark the role that you value most with an asterisk (*).

   c. If other demands (job, school) limit the amount of time you devote to the role you value the most, describe how you can improve your approach to that role so that *quality* can compensate for lack of *quantity*. For example, "When in the role of _____, I will give it my full attention and not allow concerns about my other roles to distract me."

3. Identify one habitual behavior in each of your roles that is not a desirable (or effective) behavior for your student role.

4. Identify one behavior in your personal life that is not an acceptable behavior with patients or co-workers.

5. List actions or behaviors that are appropriate in a friend/friend relationship, but are not appropriate in a health care professional/patient relationship.

6. Consider a situation in which you ran out of time to complete a task. Discuss how time management strategies might help you handle a similar situation more effectively in the future.

## REFERENCES AND SUGGESTED READINGS

Barbieri, Richard. (2015). Know thyself (if you can*). Independent School, 74*(4), 108–111.

Dweck, Carol. (2015, September 23). Carol Dweck revisits the 'growth mindset.' *Education Week 35*(5), pp. 20, 24.

Dweck, Carol (2006). *Mindset: The new psychology of success.* New York: Random House.

# Understanding Human Behavior

The interpersonal skills of health care professionals are very important to the patient. The health care professional who can build rapport with patients increases confidence in the health team, promotes faith in the treatment plan, and is more likely to gain the patient's full cooperation. If a health care professional is unable to develop rapport, then the opposite may occur. The patient may have negative feelings toward members of the health team, may distrust them, and may not comply with the health care plan. The skillful health care professional can recognize behavior indicative of negative feelings and attitudes and make an effort to correct them. Section II explains some of the many factors that are basic influences on human behavior.

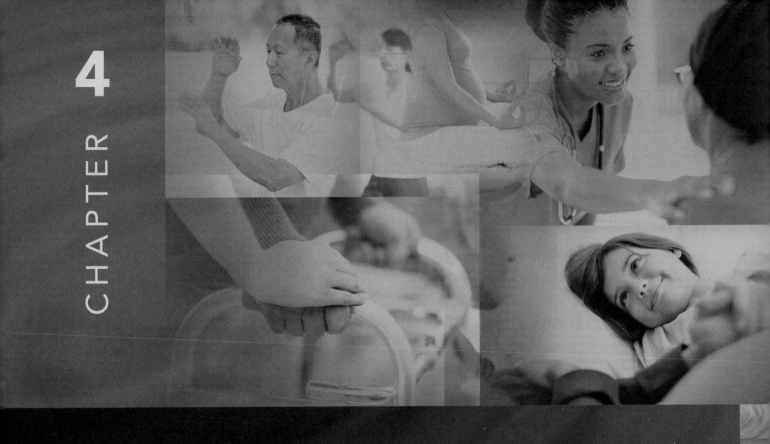

# Influences on Behavior

## OBJECTIVES

After completing this chapter, you should be able to:

- Describe how people are alike.
- Define the terms heredity, chromosome, and gene.
- Define dominant, recessive, and sex-linked traits.
- Summarize the developmental process.
- Describe how environment influences a child's development.

## KEY TERMS

| | | |
|---|---|---|
| Behavioral genetics | Genes | Heredity |
| Chromosomes | Genetics | Human Genome Project |
| Congenital | Genotype | Phenotype |
| DNA | Hereditary | Rapport |

# THE BASIS OF HUMAN BEHAVIOR

At the most basic level, any behavior can be seen as a person's attempt to either *obtain* or *avoid* something. From birth, we instinctively seek food, warmth, and comfort. We attempt to avoid cold, pain, and loud noises. As we grow, we develop an increasingly complex repertoire of behaviors to obtain what we need or want. We also develop behaviors that help us avoid experiences we find unpleasant. But what causes different people to behave in different ways, even though they are attempting to meet similar needs?

Human behavior is influenced by many factors. Heredity, environment, and culture all play a role in shaping our behavior. Researchers continue to explore the ways in which each of these factors contributes to behavior and to our metal processes.

# HOW PEOPLE ARE ALIKE AND DIFFERENT

Behavior is influenced by factors that all people have in common, as well as by individual differences.

All of us are alike in many ways:

- We have basic physical needs for food, water, shelter, sleep, oxygen, and physical safety.
- We also share basic psychological needs, such as the needs for acceptance, belonging, love, self-esteem, and opportunities to develop our talents and abilities.

Most behavior can be understood as an individual's effort to meet one or more of these needs. However, individual and cultural differences cause us to meet these needs in diverse ways. Three major forces interact to create a specific individual:

- Heredity
- The Developmental Process
- Physical and Social Environment

# HEREDITY

Each person is a unique individual. At the time of conception, **hereditary** traits are inherited from the mother and father to form a unique combination of traits. Since thousands of traits are involved, the possible combinations are limitless. That is why we say that no two people have exactly the same **heredity**, except in the case of identical twins. You are likely learning about heredity in other courses. Therefore, our concern here is to emphasize that *each person, from the time of conception, is endowed with a one-and-only combination of traits that will affect that individual throughout life.*

## The Physiology of Heredity

At the time of conception, 46 **chromosomes** are organized into 23 matched pairs (23 from each parent). There are two sex-linked chromosomes: X for females and Y for males. The combination of chromosomes from the two parents provides the individual's **genotype**, a unique set of inherited traits. The **phenotype** is the result of all genes that, in combination, provide traits that determine the individual's physical appearance.

**Genes** are segments of DNA that occupy specific locations on each chromosome. Each gene is composed of molecules of a protein called deoxyribonucleic (de-oxy-ri-bo-nu-cle-ic) acid, or **DNA**. DNA is made up of four basic chemicals: adenine, thymine, guanine, and cytosine, arranged as strands that wrap around each other to form a spiral known as the double helix. DNA is present in every cell of the body in the form of genes. These chemicals are arranged on the gene in a particular sequence, and it is the sequence that establishes the trait or traits carried by that gene, just as the arrangement of letters makes up a specific word. The "words" are actually larger protein molecules, and each has a specific function—control of a specific cellular activity. The discovery of DNA and subsequent discovery of molecular sequences on strands of DNA were exciting scientific breakthroughs. This led to the rapid development of human **genetics** as a scientific field of inquiry and the discovery of much new information on heredity.

## The Genetic Basis for Individuality

A particular characteristic of an individual may be due to:

- One specific gene
- The sequential arrangement of molecules on each gene
- A particular pair of genes
- A group of genes interacting with each other
- The influence of environmental factors on a gene or genes

Some traits are expressed, meaning that the individual will definitely manifest that trait. Other traits are unexpressed, but predispose that individual to manifest the trait under certain conditions. A person may have the gene for a specific hereditary disease but will develop the disease only under certain conditions. A person who has the gene for a disease but does not develop symptoms is known as a *carrier*; that gene can be passed on to the children, who may manifest the disease.

Like chromosomes, genes are paired so that a given trait is determined by the contribution of either or both parents. A dominant trait will be expressed, even if inherited from only one parent; a recessive trait will manifest only if matched with a recessive gene from each parent. Some traits are sex-linked, meaning they are inherited through the X chromosome of the mother or are linked to the Y chromosome of the father. For example, red/green color blindness is expressed only in males but is inherited from the mother because the gene for color blindness is carried on the mother's X chromosome.

## Health Implications

Genetics, the study of heredity, has expanded rapidly and is making significant contributions to medicine. Research to locate the genetic basis of diseases is ongoing, with new findings announced frequently.

A genetic disorder is one that results from an individual's genetic makeup. It may be apparent at birth, may appear as a developmental disorder, or may appear later in life as a disease or health problem. A single-gene disorder is due to the absence or alteration of one gene specific to that trait. Tests are available for many single-gene disorders, such as cystic fibrosis, hemophilia, and red/green color blindness. A multifactorial disorder is one involving variations in several genes. Obviously, identifying several defective genes is more complex than identifying a single gene. There are also chromosomal disorders; for example, persons with Down syndrome have three, rather than two, copies of chromosome 21.

Gene therapy has emerged as a specialty in medicine; therapy consists of modifying a defective gene in order to treat or prevent a specific disease. Genetic testing is used to identify certain single-gene disorders, confirm a diagnosis, identify carriers, and identify persons who are at risk for developing a disease but are currently free of symptoms.

From the moment of conception, then, an individual has a unique combination of hereditary traits—a blueprint that will guide growth, development, and numerous processes throughout that individual's life. Some genes are so specific that their traits cannot be modified by environmental influences or therapy. Other genes require pairing (one from each parent) in order for a trait or disorder to develop. Some genes are sex-linked—specific to the X or Y chromosome. Some genes provide a trait that will manifest only if environmental conditions foster its development.

## Genetic Testing

In 1990, the U.S. Congress funded the **Human Genome Project**, a 13-year project to map the sequencing of all of the genes on all of the chromosomes. The project was completed in 2003. This map, or pattern, of the chromosomal and gene arrangement is called the human genome, the basis for genetics in human beings. Identification of the genetic basis for certain disorders has resulted in the development of genetic testing that surpasses the development of improved therapies. Scientific advances in genetics have raised questions about privacy rights and the right of each patient to participate in health-related decisions.

DNA tests are proving valuable in areas other than health-related genetics. An individual's DNA can be used to determine paternity, to identify a body, to prove or disprove family relationships, and to investigate crimes; DNA samples have been used as proof to establish the guilt or innocence of an accused person.

Genetic testing is expensive. It also involves certain risks that should be made known to anyone who is considering genetic testing. Insurance companies and employers (or potential employers) can demand the results of genetic testing. There are examples of people who were denied insurance or lost their jobs when genetic tests indicated the presence of a gene for some specific disease (e.g., breast cancer, Huntington's disease). Although a negative test can relieve one's anxieties, a positive test has profound psychological effects on the individual and his or her loved ones.

### For Discussion and Reflection

What have you heard about genetic testing in the media? For example, has DNA testing played a key role in solving a crime? Determining the paternity of a child? What do you see as the pros and cons of genetic testing in these situations?

If your parent died at age 49 of Huntington's disease, you may or may not develop this incurable disease. Genetic testing could remove this terrible cloud over your life if you do not have the specific gene. On the other hand, if you do have the gene, you will be faced with the certainty of developing the disease, probably during your 40s. Would you choose to live with uncertainty? Or would you want to know, even if a positive test might cost you your job, insurance coverage, and relationships with those who cannot face the prospect of caring for you through a long illness? A positive approach to knowing that you have the gene would be to acknowledge your own mortality, accept that you will not have a long life, use your remaining years of health to live life to the fullest, and make end-of-life decisions while you are still in good physical and mental health.

## Behavioral Genetics

Genetics research has also given rise to the field of **behavioral genetics**, which seeks to understand human behavior in terms of hereditary or biological influences. Researchers note that some behaviors tend to run in families. Studies of twins and adoptees have been used for some time to explore the effects of heredity on behavior. Interestingly, research suggests that some behaviors are more closely linked to heredity, while other behaviors are more closely linked to environmental influences. For example, when researchers reviewed studies of antisocial behavior in twins, they found that aggression was more strongly linked to heredity, while non-aggressive rule-breaking was more strongly linked to the child's environment (Burt & Klump, 2012). Recently, researchers have also worked to identify pieces of DNA that appear to be associated with particular behaviors.

## THE DEVELOPMENTAL PROCESS

Heredity establishes the basic physical/mental/emotional makeup and all the personality traits of each individual. But many other influences determine how these ingredients will be molded as the individual grows and develops from a baby into an adult. One important difference is the built-in developmental rate, a hereditary factor. You have likely known children who appeared "big for their age" or "mature for their age" as well as children who are smaller or less mature than their same-age peers. Thus, physical development proceeds at one rate for one child and at another rate for his sibling. The study of a child must always consider the apparent rate of development.

## Prenatal Influences

The developmental process is subject to tremendous environmental influence, especially during the prenatal period. Ideally, the mother's body provides the embryo with a physical environment that is favorable to healthful development. This prenatal environment is affected by the mother's general health, her nutritional status, pathogenic organisms such as those causing syphilis or measles, and the presence in her blood of any substance that is toxic to the embryo.

Research indicates that the mother's daily habits have tremendous influence on the embryo:

- Smoking during pregnancy increases the risk of complications of pregnancy, premature birth, low birth weight, still-birth, and infant mortality.

**For Discussion and Reflection**

Consider yourself as a child, as compared to your siblings or friends. Were you small or large for your age, or were you average size? In school did you learn quickly, or was it a struggle to keep up? Were you ever told that you were mature (or immature) for your age?

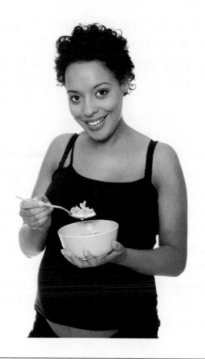

© Piotr Marcinski/Shutterstock.com.

**FIGURE 4-1 Nutrition is critical to healthy prenatal development.**

- Consumption of alcoholic beverages by a pregnant woman places the infant at risk of various **congenital** defects, including fetal alcohol syndrome (FAS).

- The role of nutrition during the prenatal p0eriod is critical to healthy prenatal development. For example, spina bifida is caused by a deficiency of folic acid. If a woman supplements her diet with folic acid *after* learning that she is pregnant, it is already too late to prevent this neural tube defect.

Every woman who may become pregnant should be concerned about nutrition, especially adequate intake of vitamins and minerals. If a couple has decided to start a family, both should practice good nutrition and a healthy lifestyle.

The experiences and emotions of a pregnant woman have profound prenatal effects. Fear, anger, and grief—normal reactions to stressful and traumatic experiences—can affect the developing fetus. If the woman has an abusive spouse, the abuse may accelerate during her pregnancy; the woman's emotional reactions to such abuse affect the fetus, even in the absence of physical trauma. On the other hand, positive experiences have a positive effect. Many expectant mothers listen to classical music daily; some read and talk to their unborn child. Studies of young children reveal that a child's personality and developmental rate are related to such prenatal influences.

## ENVIRONMENT

The environment is another major influence on the development and the expression of certain hereditary potential. Much has been written about the relative importance of heredity and environment. With increasing knowledge about heredity and with growing awareness of the power of the physical and social environment to affect the developmental process, it is now apparent that many forces interact to determine the traits of an individual. Heredity provides the basic ingredients and the blueprint, but environmental factors and events that affect the developmental process determine what aspects of the blueprint will be expressed.

## Physical Environment

Environment, in its broadest sense, means many things. The physical environment includes home conditions, climate, community conditions, means for meeting physical needs, and resources for developing one's potential. Children who live in a large city have a physical environment that differs greatly from that of children who live in a rural community. Many factors vary based on children's physical environments:

**For Discussion and Reflection**

How would you describe the physical environment in which you grew up? What activities or resources did you have access to as a result of your environment? What resources were not available to you?

- Exposure to pollution
- Access to cultural resources such as museums and concerts
- Ability to spend time outside
- Participation in team sports, clubs, or community organizations
- Opportunities to learn skills such as gardening, tending livestock, or building repair
- Ability to spend time with other children outside one's own family

All aspects of the physical environment affect personality. Some personality traits tend to develop in one kind of environment, whereas a different environment fosters the development of other traits.

Those who care for a child create the child's immediate physical environment. It may be as safe as thoughtful adults can make it, or it may contain many hazards. Unless adults make a conscious effort to control risks in the home and child care facility, the child may experience serious injuries from falls, burns, or poisoning. Although some such injuries are correctible, some are fatal and others leave lifelong scars. In addition to environmental hazards, some personal habits of adults also affect the child. Exposure to secondhand smoke increases the risk of sudden infant death syndrome (SIDS) in infants, and the chance of developing asthma is higher in babies and young children who are frequently exposed to secondhand smoke.

## Social Environment

The social environment involves people. A baby's experiences provide important first learnings about the world and people. The baby may learn that the world is a friendly place—that one can depend on others to correct such discomforts as hunger, cold, and a wet diaper. Or the baby may learn the world is a hostile place—that one cannot rely on others to relieve hunger and cold. These infant experiences lay the foundation for future relations with other people: distrust or trust, expectations of comfort and nurturing from others, or resignation to discomfort without help from others.

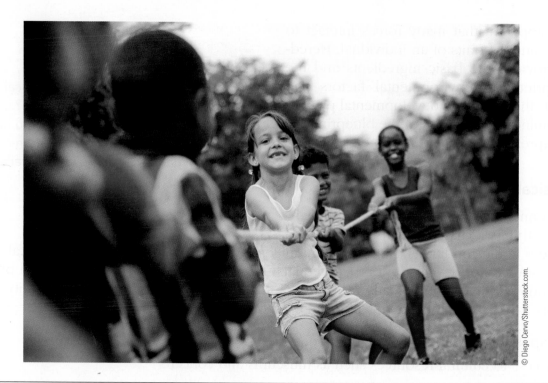

FIGURE 4-2 **The physical and social environment has a significant effect on a child's development.**

Role models are powerful influences on children. Every adult in a child's world has the potential to serve as a role model, whether they be within the home (immediate or extended family), the neighborhood, the church, or at school. Role models influence children in many ways—value system, parenting style, career choice. The role model's influence may be positive or negative. It may last a lifetime or it may be temporary. A child may have only one role model or may adopt different role models at various life stages. An adult may even be unaware that he is serving as a role model for a specific child.

## Culture and Socioeconomic Level

Children are strongly influenced by the culture in which they grow up. Culture refers to the ideas, beliefs, values, and customs shared by a group of people. These shared ideas may be based on religion, ethnicity or nationality, geographic region, or a number of other factors. Put simply, children learn from the adults around them what is important and how they are expected to act in certain situations.

Socioeconomic level also influences children's early learning. According to the National Center for Children in Poverty (NCCP), 22 percent of children in the United States live in families whose income falls below the federal poverty level. These children are at increased risk for learning and behavioral problems (NCCP, 2015).

## INFLUENCES DURING CHILDHOOD

The basic heredity of a child, plus environmental influences, exerts a powerful influence on development. Throughout the early years, a child continues to learn about people and the world. If relationships with caregivers are positive and nurturing, the child develops a sense of security and finds the world a place for exploring and satisfying curiosity. If the child experiences a chaotic environment and harsh relationships with caregivers, the child learns to distrust other people and tends to fear new experiences or strange places.

## Home

The home environment is of great importance in the young child's development.

- How well does the family provide for the child's physical needs?
- What health practices are followed?
- Is the home atmosphere democratic or authoritarian?
- Do the parents "wait on" the child, or do they allow the child to develop self-reliance gradually?
- Is there an anxious parent who repeatedly warns the child about getting hurt?

The child's home may include an abusive parent. Child abuse is widespread; many abusive parents were themselves abused as children. The abuse may be physical, mental, or emotional. Mental and emotional abuse may be inflicted verbally (e.g., with put-downs or guilt-arousing statements) or by specific actions (isolation, darkness). Physical abuse may be in the form of beatings or sexual activities. The abuser may even threaten to harm the child if this "secret" is revealed to anyone. The abused child has a heavy burden. In addition to physical trauma, the child has to deal with fear, anger, and guilt. And unless they get help, abused children may grow up to become abusive parents.

What is the neighborhood environment? Is it safe or full of hazards for children? Are there opportunities for a wide variety of experiences? Are there relatives and neighbors who care about the child, or is the social climate of the neighborhood hostile? Are the parents from another country? If so, do they require the child to behave in ways appropriate for the home country, but inappropriate in the present community?

## The School Years

When the child enters school, the physical and social environments are greatly extended. If development has proceeded according to schedule, the child is ready for this expansion of experience. If the physical or social environment of early life inhibited some aspect of development, then the child may not be ready to benefit fully from school. Early school experiences may be so unsatisfying that they inhibit development of one or more dimensions. Elementary school students show marked differences in development and in behavior patterns; these differences reflect both hereditary and environmental influences.

- Some children readily adapt to being with a group of their own age; others hang back, afraid to join the group.
- Some see the teacher as absolute authority, to be obeyed without question; others show rebellion toward authority.
- Some students work independently; others depend on the teacher for assistance with every task.
- Some are bubbling with ideas and participate fully in every activity; others sit quietly and participate only when urged.

These differences are not accidental. They are the result of both heredity and early influences on patterns of behavior.

# CHANGING INFLUENCES DURING LIFE

Early learning continues to influence behavior throughout life, often without the individual's awareness. On the other hand, one can learn to recognize certain early influences on behavior and, where desirable, modify the behavior patterns that have resulted. *As children we do not choose our heredity, our home environment, or our developmental influences. However, as we mature into adults, we can become self-directing.*

- The adult can recognize an undesirable behavior pattern and choose to change it.
- An adult can seek to understand the basis for a particular behavior and, with such understanding, resist or eliminate that early influence.
- An adult can leave an unhealthy situation and seek a more favorable environment.

These options are not available to a child, who is trapped in a specific living situation. As adults, we can choose not to remain trapped in past patterns but to change our behaviors, habits, and living conditions.

## Modifying Early Learnings

Prejudice is one example of early learning that can influence a person's behavior throughout life unless the individual chooses to examine behavior patterns and their apparent origins. Prejudice is usually learned early in life from those people around us. In its most common form, prejudice consists of negative feelings toward people from a different race or subculture. If parents and their friends speak in unkind terms about members of another race, the child may learn to exhibit hostility or disrespect toward members of another race. As adults, however, we can change these early learnings. We can reexamine our attitudes in light of new knowledge and personal experience. Often, we find that our prejudice does not hold up against rational examination. *As adults, we can modify early learnings and take control of our own behavior, attitudes, and beliefs.*

An example of unexamined prejudice is the behavior of people who belong to one of the "hate groups." The leaders of such groups depend on "us versus them" thinking to arouse strong feelings and mobilize people to behave as the leaders wish them to behave. Televised reports of demonstrations show people who are controlled by their emotions, rather than by clear thinking. And those emotions probably have their roots in early learning that has not been reexamined during adulthood. People who blindly accept the hate policies of a group, or even of a government, are allowing others to do their thinking, determine their beliefs, and control their behavior. *Throughout adult life, one should continuously evaluate and modify beliefs and value systems.*

## Interests

Interests also influence behavior. They determine where we direct our attention. They even enter into the decisions we make, the activities we pursue, the occupations we choose, and the types of recreation we select for our leisure time. People who have many interests

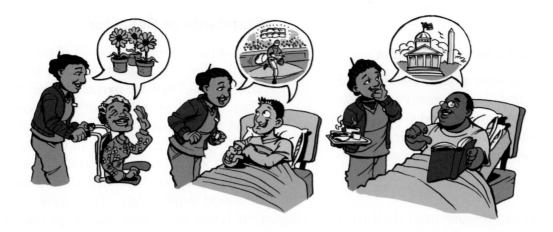

FIGURE 4-3 **Having a variety of interests will help you relate effectively with different people.**

are well prepared for forming effective relationships with a variety of people. Those whose only activities are work, television, and social media do not have much to offer others in the way of interesting companionship. Developing a variety of interests is one way to become a more interesting person, find greater satisfaction in living, and form satisfying relationships.

**For Discussion and Reflection**

What are your interests? What activities do you enjoy? Do these interests and activities provide topics of conversation or other ways to interact with others?

## Value Systems

A value system is the degree of importance we attach (largely unconsciously) to various beliefs, ideas, or material things. Each person's values have a strong influence on behavior. Our daily choices provide evidence of our values.

- Did you give up watching a movie in order to do an assignment for today? Then you placed a higher value on some aspect of being a student—responsibility, achievement, or perhaps duty—than you did on recreation, at least in this instance.

- Did you return the extra dollar you received as change at the grocery store? Then you placed a higher value on honesty than on "getting the best of the other person."

- Did you cheat on that last test in order to improve your grade? Then you placed a higher value on a grade than on honesty or true learning.

The value system includes many things: character traits such as honesty and truthfulness, personal achievement, the symbols of achievement, love and friendship, material possessions, religion, recreation, work, and family living. Each person's values begin to form early in life, influenced by the rewards or punishments that followed specific types of behavior. Throughout life, the value system exerts a powerful influence on behavior, particularly when there is a choice to be made. Your enrollment in this educational program indicates that you value education enough to attend classes and do your assignments.

## Standards of Behavior

Standards of behavior consist of our own personal rules and regulations, our own "dos" and "don'ts," that are part of our self-concept. There is a close relationship between one's value system and one's standards of behavior. Both are learned early in life and continually modified according to life experiences.

Standards of behavior should never be modified impulsively. Teenagers are often subjected to pressure from their friends to abandon home teachings and adopt the group's code of behavior. This can be a difficult decision for a young person, since peer acceptance is very important during adolescence.

There is a difference between current standards and those of the previous generation. Standards of behavior are a frequent source of misunderstanding between parents and adolescents. There are also wide differences in standards of behavior from one subculture to another. Standards of behavior, including sexual behavior, vary between socioeconomic levels, cultural groups, and generations.

Taking time to consciously examine your own beliefs and standards of behavior will help you make your own choices as an adult rather than simply deferring to "the way you were brought up" or "what everyone else is doing." You may decide that you wish to maintain some or all of the standards of behavior you were taught as a child, or you may not. Either way, you benefit from making a conscious choice.

## Sleep and Nutrition

Our behavior is also influenced by whether we get sufficient sleep and appropriate nutrition. The need for sleep is discussed in greater detail in Chapter 5. In short, insufficient sleep weakens the immune system, affects mood, and inhibits our ability to think clearly. You have likely noticed that you (or your family members) tend to be more short-tempered or accident-prone when you have not had enough sleep. Similarly, eating nutritious food without artificial colors or preservatives has been found to have a positive behavioral effect, particularly in children.

## ASSUMING RESPONSIBILITY FOR BEHAVIOR

You should now be aware that human personality is the result of many ingredients. It is continuously molded by the environment and by life experiences. It is always subject to further change as a result of future life situations.

As children, our early learnings were determined by circumstances beyond our control. As adults, we have a choice.

- We can continue to live without consciously directing our lives, or we can take control.
- We can foster certain aspects of our personalities and play down other aspects.
- We can learn to make sound decisions.
- We can learn to recognize ineffective behaviors that may prevent us from reaching our goals.

Thus, we can become relatively self-directing instead of living by patterns of thought and behavior established during childhood. Even more important, as adults we can think through various issues, decide what our values are, set our own standards of behavior, and accept or reject the values and standards proposed to us by others.

## THE HEALTH CARE PROFESSIONAL AND THE PATIENT

As a health care professional, you will find great satisfaction in your work if you make a conscious and continuous effort to study behavior—both your own and that of other people. You will meet people from many different backgrounds. With some, it will be easy to establish a pleasant relationship, one in which the patient believes that *you understand* and that *you are sincerely concerned*. Such a relationship is called **rapport**.

With some patients, you will find it more difficult to communicate. Perhaps the patient's behavior makes you uncomfortable. Perhaps you just do not find the patient "interesting" as a person. As long as this climate exists between you and the patient, rapport will not be established.

Any patient who has been labeled "difficult" needs special attention from the health team. The behaviors that cause the patient to be labeled "difficult" may actually be signs that the patient's needs are not being met. But, on the other hand, the pleasant, agreeable patient may be covering up true feelings and may have just as much need for understanding and concern. In other words, as a health care professional, you will need to apply interpersonal skills to *establish rapport with each patient* as an individual. Some patients will be more of a challenge than others, but all need your understanding and sincere interest if you are to make a positive contribution to their health care.

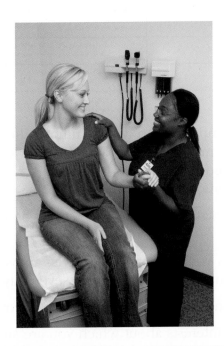

**FIGURE 4-4  As a health care professional, you will need to apply interpersonal skills to *establish rapport with each patient as an individual.***

## ACTIVITIES

The following exercises are designed to give you an opportunity to apply some of the ideas discussed in Chapter 4.

1. Using the following format, develop your family genetic chart as a guide to the possible contributions of heredity to your present and future health. Add additional lines as needed to list all members of your extended family. Add any cousins who have significant health problems or congenital conditions. Because the purpose of this activity is to explore your heredity, include only relatives to whom you are biologically related (i.e., not step or adoptive relatives).

| Relation | Current Age or Age at Death | Cause of Death | Health Problems |
|---|---|---|---|
| Father | | | |
| Grandfather | | | |
| Grandmother | NA | NA | NA |
| Uncles | 60 | Heart attack | Pain in chest |
| Aunts | 53 | intestine Cancer | Rectal bleeding Abdominal discomfort |
| Mother | | | |
| Grandfather | | | |
| Grandmother | | | |
| Uncles | | | |
| Aunts | | | |
| Sisters | | | |
| Brothers | | | |

2. List 10 things that are important to you. Number them from 1 to 10 in order of importance—with 1 being most important and 10 being least important. Describe a decision that may be influenced by this order of values. Are you spending your time on the things you listed as most important?

3. List five of your interests. State how each interest will be helpful to you as a health care professional.

4. Review the list of interests you made for the activity above. Estimate the amount of time you have spent on each interest during the past seven days.

   a. Place a star by those interests to which you have devoted as much as five hours.

   b. Place an "X" by those interests about which you are sufficiently informed to carry on a conversation with someone who is knowledgeable on that subject.

    c.  Evaluate your interests in terms of variety, keeping in mind that it is not really one of your interests *unless you devote time to it and are informed about it.*

    d.  Select one activity for increasing the variety of your interests. Plan how you will learn about this activity and develop the skills of that activity during the next six months.

5.  If one of your parents died at age 42 of a disorder that is known to be genetic, would you choose to have genetic testing to determine if you have the gene for that disorder (yes or no)?

    a.  Write a brief explanation for your answer.

    b.  If the test result is positive, what is the likely effect of that information on your life?

6.  Consider the following scenarios and describe what each child is learning:

    a.  Alex is a 15-month-old who is developing his walking, running, and climbing skills as he actively explores the environment. When Alex falls, his parents say "Uh-oh," and Alex gets up and resumes his activities. He now reacts to a fall by saying "Uh-oh" himself.

    b.  The mother of Joey, a 20-month-old toddler, frequently calls out to her child, "Don't run. Don't climb on that. You'll fall and hurt yourself." When Joey does fall, he starts to cry and his mother picks him up, often saying angrily, "You know you shouldn't do that!"

## REFERENCES AND SUGGESTED READINGS

Burt, S. A., & Klump, K. L. (2012). Etiological distinctions between aggressive and non-aggressive antisocial behavior: Results from a nuclear twin family model. *Journal of Abnormal Child Psychology, 40*(7), 1059–1071.

Lewis, G. J., Haworth, C. A., & Plomin, R. (2014). Identical genetic influences underpin behavior problems in adolescence and basic traits of personality. *Journal of Child Psychology and Psychiatry, and Allied Disciplines, 55*(8), 865–875. doi:10.1111/jcpp.12156.

National Center for Children in Poverty. (2015). *Child poverty.* Retrieved from http://www.nccp.org /topics/childpoverty.html.

National Human Genome Research Institute. (2015). *All about the human genome project.* Retrieved from http://www.genome.gov/10001772.

Slane, J., Burt, S., & Klump, K. (2012). Bulimic behaviors and alcohol use: Shared genetic influences. *Behavior Genetics, 42*(4), 603–613. doi:10.1007/s10519-012-9525-2.

6. Evaluate your interests in terms of variety, keeping in mind that it is not really one of your interests unless you devote time to it and enjoy experiences doing it.

7. Select one activity that increases the variety of your interests. Plan how you will learn about this activity and develop the skills of that activity during the next six months.

8. If one of your parents died at age 72 of a disorder that is known to be genetic, would you choose to have genetic testing to determine if you have the gene for that disorder, yes or no?

   a. Write a brief explanation for your answer.

   b. If the test result is positive, what is the likely effect of that information on your life?

9. Consider the following scenarios and describe what each child is learning.

   a. Alex is a 15-month-old who is developing his walking, running, and climbing skills as he actively explores the environment. When Alex falls, he quickly gets up and Alex gets up and resumes his activities. He now reacts to a fall by saying "Up" to himself.

   b. The mother of Devon, a 18-month-old toddler, frequently calls out to her child, "Don't run. Don't climb on that. You'll fall and hurt yourself." When Devon does fall, he starts to cry and his mother picks him up, often saying something like "I know you shouldn't do that."

## REFERENCES AND SUGGESTED READINGS

Burt, S. A., & Klump, K. L. (2013). Parental overt conflict as between appositive and non-appositive, and non-behaviors: Results from a monozygotic twins model. *Journal of Abnormal Child Psychology*, 1057–1075.

Lewis, G., Ellsworth, C. A., & Bogdan, R. (2014). Licensed genetic influence on behavior between twins to relationships and basic traits of personality. *Journal of Child Psychology and Psychiatry*, 54(6), 549–579. doi:10.1111/jcpp.12356.

National Center for Children in Poverty. (2015). *Child poverty*. Retrieved from http://www.nccp.org/topic/childpoverty.html.

National Human Genome Research Institute. (2015). *Behind the human genome project*. Retrieved from http://www.genome.gov/10001772.

Shawn, J., Ren, S., & Klump, K. (2013). Defining behaviors and related the causal genetic influence on *Behavior Genetics*, 43. doi:10.1007/s10519-013-9759-5.

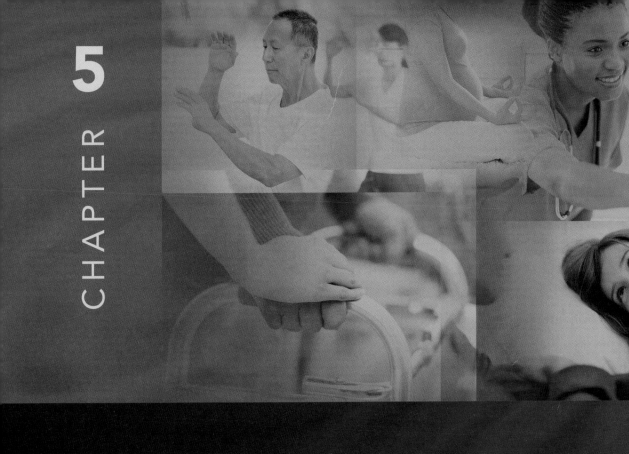

# CHAPTER 5

# Physical Needs

## OBJECTIVES

After completing this chapter, you should be able to:

- List the levels of human needs as proposed by Maslow.
- Explain why Maslow stated these needs as a hierarchy.
- Describe influences on the formation of behavior patterns.
- List physical needs that are essential to survival.
- Explain how need-satisfaction influences behavior.

## KEY TERMS

| | | |
|---|---|---|
| Compensation | Hierarchy | REM sleep |
| Consequences | Necrosis | Suffocation |
| Dehydration | | |

All humans share certain basic needs that we are driven to satisfy. However, we are all different in the ways we attempt to satisfy these needs. What satisfies one person does not satisfy another. Most patterns of behavior can be understood as a person's effort to fulfill one or more needs.

Psychologists and sociologists engaged in the study of human behavior have described these needs in various ways. The most useful approach for our purpose is the model provided by psychologist Abraham Maslow. This model is known as Maslow's Hierarchy of Needs. The term **hierarchy** means "arranged in a specific order or rank."

## MASLOW'S HIERARCHY OF NEEDS

Maslow's hierarchy identifies the following needs. Maslow theorized that each level of need must be satisfied before an individual can focus on satisfying of the next level of need.

1. Physiological or survival needs
2. Safety needs
3. Love, affection, and belongingness needs
4. Esteem needs
5. Need for self-actualization

This chapter discusses the physical needs, which include levels 1 and 2. Levels 3, 4, and 5 are discussed in Chapter 6.

## ESSENTIAL PHYSICAL NEEDS

Some physical needs are essential to life; others contribute to comfort and satisfaction. The physical needs that are essential to life are oxygen, water, food, protection, and sleep. These needs are not only essential to the life of the total organism, but also to the survival of individual cells. For example, a body part that does not receive a continuous supply of oxygen and nourishment will die. If this body part is a vital organ, then the individual will also die. If, however, the body part is a finger, the affected finger can be surgically removed and the individual will survive, minus the finger. Death of tissues in a limited area is called **necrosis**. It is usually due to lack of an adequate blood supply that deprives the cells of oxygen and nourishment. As you work in the health field, you may see patients with necrosis of some body part or area.

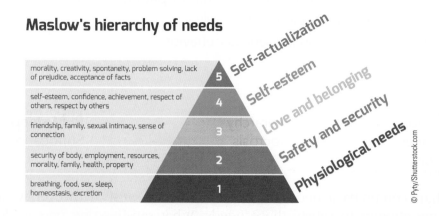

**FIGURE 5-1** Maslow's hierarchy of needs: Maslow theorized that each level of need must be satisfied before an individual can focus on the next level of need.

## Importance of Oxygen

The physical need for oxygen pertains to every cell in the body. Submersion of the face in water for more than a few minutes can result in death due to drowning. Although some people have been resuscitated after about 20 minutes under water, in such cases there is serious risk of permanent brain damage, because the brain needs a continuous supply of oxygen. If deprivation of oxygen is due to the face being covered, as in a cave-in, the death is called a **suffocation**. Accidental drowning or suffocation may be the result of carelessness, failure to use appropriate precautions (e.g., not wearing a life jacket when going out in a boat), or inappropriate sleeping arrangements (in the case of a baby). Because of so many instances of sudden infant death syndrome (SIDS), it is now considered safer to place babies on their backs to protect against suffocation.

## Importance of Water

The body must have adequate water for various functions, on average, eight to ten cups of water each day. Even more water is needed if you work or exercise vigorously or spend time outside during hot weather. Water provides liquid and is the carrier for various nutrients that cannot be digested and absorbed without a liquid medium.

When the body does not receive adequate water each day, chronic **dehydration** develops and certain body functions are affected. When the body loses water, as through diarrhea, persistent vomiting, or high fever, dehydration develops. Severe dehydration leads to an imbalance in body chemistry, a life-threatening condition. In hospitals, intravenous fluids are used for patients who cannot drink enough fluids to prevent dehydration. Persons who are stranded where there is no water available, as in a desert, can survive only a few days. For this reason, survival training includes learning how to extract water from plants and use liquids from other sources to maintain life until rescued.

## Importance of Food

Because of its ability to store food in various tissues and organs, the body can survive without food for longer periods of time than it can survive without oxygen or water. Prolonged lack of food results in stored nutrients being used for basic metabolic processes and for the energy needed for physical activities. Even thinking requires energy! Muscle movement requires a lot of energy. If lack of food continues, tissues shrink and body wasting occurs. When body reserves have been exhausted, death occurs due to starvation.

Regular intake of food, then, is essential for providing the body with the nutrients needed to carry out metabolic processes, build and repair tissues, and produce energy for various activities. The nutrients needed include proteins, fats, carbohydrates, vitamins, minerals, amino acids, and essential fatty acids. Optimal health requires that *all* of these nutrients be included in one's daily diet, since even a slight deficiency of certain nutrients results in less efficient body functions.

Even more significant, a slight deficiency in certain nutrients, especially vitamins, minerals, and amino acids, can lead to symptoms. For example, a prolonged clotting time or a tendency to bruise easily may indicate a serious health problem or may simply indicate that the individual needs additional vitamin C or vitamin K. A deficiency of magnesium can result in a cardiac arrhythmia that may be misdiagnosed as a heart disorder. There is currently a trend in health care to acknowledge the relationship of certain nutrients to specific body functions. Health care professionals should become informed about nutrients in order to protect their own personal health and that of their families. Sometimes it may be appropriate to suggest dietary changes to a friend or patient or recommend a consultation with a nutritionist.

## Importance of Protection

In its broadest sense, protection includes the safety and security of having a home that protects one from the elements, using safety precautions to avoid accidents, having a lifestyle that includes healthful eating and drinking clean water, avoiding exposure to extremes of heat and cold, and avoiding substances that can harm the body.

Commonsense measures, such as avoiding times and places where one might be attacked and practicing safe driving, can decrease the likelihood of a serious accident or traumatic experience. Small children, especially, need protection against a variety of hazards in the community and in the home. It is a responsibility of adults to "child-proof" the home, so that children do not have access to household cleaners, medicines, and other harmful substances. Adults have a responsibility to provide safe and healthful lifestyles for themselves and their children.

To illustrate the importance of safety, consider the following 2013 data from the Center for Disease Control:

- Unintentional injuries were the leading cause of death for people aged 1–44.
- Unintentional falls were the leading cause of non-fatal injuries requiring a visit to hospital emergency rooms for all age groups combined.
- Accidental poisoning, motor vehicle accidents, and falls were the three leading causes of death for all age groups combined.

Not all accidents can be avoided. However, maintaining safety in homes, schools, and workplaces can prevent many injuries.

## Importance of Sleep

Sleep is essential to life and health, but people are more inclined to deprive themselves of sleep than of water, food, and air. The body's demand for sleep can be resisted, or even ignored, more easily than hunger, thirst, and the need for air. Of the various aspects of lifestyle that are *essential* to health, recent research indicates that sleep ranks third, behind diet and exercise.

Although individual needs for sleep vary, the average person needs one hour of sleep for every two hours of wakefulness. Sleep needs are biologically determined; a person who needs 10 hours of sleep is not "lazy" and will be healthier if that need is respected. On the other hand, persons who claim to need

**For Discussion and Reflection**

Think about your usual sleep pattern. How many hours do you sleep on week-nights? On Saturday nights? On Sunday nights? If you are sleeping less than eight hours each night, list reasons that you stay up too late to get a full night's sleep or get up before you have had eight hours of sleep.

only a few hours of sleep per night place their health at risk. Researchers believe that loss of sleep contributes to accidents, decreases efficiency, and increases a person's tendency toward anger and violence.

The National Institute of Health recommends the following amounts of sleep:

- 10 hours per night for school-aged children
- 9–10 hours per night for teens
- 7–8 hours per night for adults

However, in a 2009 survey, less than a third of high school students reported getting at least eight hours of sleep per night. In 2006-2007, almost a third of adults reported sleeping fewer than six hours per night. (CDC, Sleep, 2015). Chronic sleep deprivation can affect a person's emotions, behavior, and performance at school or work.

## THE SLEEP CYCLE

Sleep consists of two phases that alternate throughout the sleep period: **REM sleep** and non-REM sleep. The latter phase is a period when most body processes slow down, the muscles are relaxed, and the eyes are relatively still. This phase includes four stages of progressively deeper sleep. Following a complete cycle of the four stages, the REM (rapid eye movement) phase begins. In this phase, there is an increase in mental activity, dreaming occurs concurrently with bursts of rapid eye movement, breathing is irregular, and pulse and blood pressure rise and fall. In normal young adults, the first non-REM phase lasts about 90 minutes and is followed by about 15 minutes of REM sleep. The frequency and duration of REM sleep periods increase during the final hours of sleep, especially between the sixth and eighth hours.

The dreaming that occurs during REM sleep is thought to be a major factor in stress management. The entire sleep period is a time when the brain cleanses itself of the day's accumulated sensory input and prepares for the next day's mental activity; it is also the time when the brain replenishes its stock of neurotransmitters. Although people vary in the amount of sleep they need to awaken rested and refreshed, less than eight hours of sleep deprives the body of some periods of REM sleep. Research conducted in sleep laboratories has revealed that deprivation of REM sleep has the same effects as sleep deprivation.

### Effects of Sleep Deprivation

After the loss of one night of sleep, a person has poor concentration and coordination; usually irritability is increased. Anyone who is deprived of sleep for several days will experience hallucinations and exhibit psychotic behavior.

Sleep deprivation is an increasing problem in American society. The temptations of late-night television and the lure of the Internet are causing large numbers of people to get as little as two or three hours of sleep per night.

Some health care professionals work a double shift; those who regularly work the night shift may experience 24- to 30-hour periods without sleep before or after their days off. These people should make a special effort to ensure adequate sleep and rest, for both personal health and avoidance of errors due to fatigue and lack of sleep.

## SATISFACTION OF PHYSICAL NEEDS

The physical needs have an important characteristic that sets them apart from psychological needs—*they can be satisfied in only one way.* An abundant supply of oxygen cannot make up for a lack of food. Abundant food stored within body tissues cannot provide survival for the worker who has just been buried in a cave-in and has no supply of oxygen. The need for sleep can be satisfied only by sleeping; though eating may enable one to delay going to sleep, food cannot satisfy the body's need for sleep. *Each essential physical need can be met only by a specific substance or condition.* Neither substitution nor **compensation** is possible. In contrast, people often use compensation or substitution to address social and emotion needs when they are not able to meet the actual need directly. Social and emotional needs will be explored in the upcoming chapters.

## COMFORT AND SAFETY NEEDS

There are also physical needs that are highly desirable but not essential to life. These needs are related to comfort and a sense of well-being. Labor-saving devices, soundly built homes, running water, comfortable clothing, and automatic heat seem like essential needs to those who are accustomed to them. Though some of these comforts are not essential for survival, they do meet safety needs and contribute to health and well-being.

The satisfaction of sexual needs falls into two categories: emotional needs and physical needs. Intimacy can contribute to a sense of belonging—an especially important need of adolescents. Sexual activity was formerly considered an adult activity, but currently many young people—adolescents and children—are sexually active. This is an issue for families and individuals to address in terms of beliefs and standards of behavior. The issue of *responsibility,* however, extends beyond the family to the larger community because of health issues and the risk of pregnancies that produce children who are unwanted or whose parents cannot or will not provide for them.

Anyone who is sexually active, regardless of age, should practice safe sex. For young people who are not prepared to assume the adult responsibilities of parenting (which includes financial support), prevention of pregnancy requires the use of protection. For everyone who is sexually active but is not in a stable, one-partner relationship, responsibility means protecting oneself against sexually transmitted diseases. Safe sex, then, has two very important purposes: (1) avoidance of an unwanted pregnancy and (2) prevention of a sexually transmitted disease.

## PHYSICAL NEEDS AND BEHAVIOR

Each person has specific ways for trying to meet needs. The baby cries when hungry but is dependent on others to provide nourishment. Throughout childhood each of us learned which behaviors were successful or unsuccessful in meeting our needs within the home and in the subculture. *The child tends to repeat any behavior that results in satisfaction of a need and to abandon behaviors that do not get results.* Behavior patterns are established on the basis of **consequences**—what happens following a specific behavior.

If you find yourself or someone else repeating a particular pattern of behavior, try to identify the consequence (outcome) that reinforces the behavior. A typical example is a young child whining for candy at the store. If the parent first says "no" but later buys the candy to stop the child's whining, the parent has reinforced the behavior of whining. The child has learned that whining gets her what she wants.

## Cultural Influences

A city person purchases food at the grocery store but is dependent upon a complex system of marketing and distribution to keep a supply available. A rural person may purchase only staples and depend on a garden and livestock to provide most of the family's food. A rural family living at a subsistence level may depend upon hunting or fishing for food. A family living in poverty in a large city may depend upon the welfare department for food. Patterns of behavior used to meet these needs are learned in childhood and influenced by the customs and practices of the family, neighborhood, and community. Patterns of behavior are also influenced by individual factors, such as the desire to obtain the comforts of life and the value placed on conforming to group standards.

### For Discussion and Reflection

1. If you have children, have you ever "given in" to negative behavior as described? If you do not have children, think of ways you have seen adults complain or threaten to get what they want from others.
2. When someone receives what they want as a result of a negative behavior, how likely are they to continue using negative behaviors in the future?

## UNDERSTANDING BEHAVIOR IN TERMS OF PHYSICAL NEEDS

There are certain physical needs that people must meet in order to survive. There are other needs that make people more comfortable or free them from routine tasks so they may do other things that are more satisfying. In having these needs, people are alike. In the specific ways they meet these needs, people are different. Each person behaves in ways that have been learned by imitating members of one's subculture and from personal experiences. Each person tends to repeat the behavior that has been successful in satisfying a particular need. This repetition becomes established as a behavior pattern.

Most people meet their needs in ways acceptable within the laws, customs, and religious beliefs of their group. Some people choose or are forced by circumstances to violate the laws or customs of the group in order to satisfy their needs. These people may be meeting their needs in the only way they know. Here, too, the health care professional's philosophy of individual worth can be applied to understanding, rather than judging, a patient.

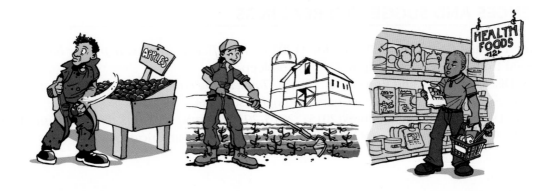

**FIGURE 5-2** Our life situation influences behavior patterns for meeting basic needs.

## ACTIVITIES

1. Think of some early influences in your life that shaped the patterns of behavior you now use to meet your physical needs. Do your patterns reflect dependence on others? Or self-reliance? How would these patterns be affected if you should become disabled? Visualize yourself in such a situation. How might your reaction to this forced change be reflected in your behavior?

2. If you have ever experienced any of the following, describe how it affected you physically, mentally, and emotionally:

   a. Difficulty in getting air for several minutes

   b. No water (or any other beverage) for eight hours

   c. No way to obtain food for two days

   d. Exposure to severe weather, without any way to get to shelter for several hours

   e. Deprivation of sleep for 36 hours

3. Think of a situation in your community where someone drowned. Using all the information available to your class, discuss the circumstances and identify actions someone (including the victim) could have taken in advance to prevent this drowning.

4. If you average less than eight hours of sleep each night, list changes in your habits or lifestyle that would enable you to get more sleep.

5. Participate in a class discussion about the importance of safe sex from the standpoint of:

   a. Adolescent boys

   b. Adolescent girls

   c. Parents of a girl between the ages of 10 and 18

   d. Parents of a boy between the ages of 10 and 18

6. Consider the implications of safe sex for you personally.

7. Consider the implications of safe sex for you as a health care professional.

## REFERENCES AND SUGGESTED READINGS

Centers for Disease Control and Prevention. (2015). *Insufficient sleep is a public health problem.* Retrieved from http://www.cdc.gov/features/dssleep/.

Centers for Disease Control and Prevention. (2015). *Ten leading causes of death and injury.* Retrieved from http://www.cdc.gov/injury/wisqars/leadingcauses.html.

United States Department of Agriculture. (2015). *2015-2020 dietary guidelines for Americans.* Retrieved from http://www.cnpp.usda.gov/2015-2020-dietary-guidelines-americans.

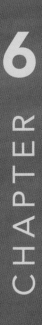

# CHAPTER 6

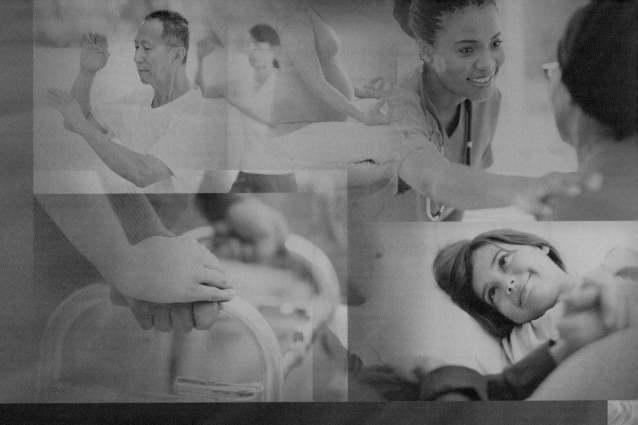

# Self-Esteem and Social Needs

## OBJECTIVES

After completing this chapter, you should be able to:

- Explain social needs.
- Compare self-concept and self-esteem.
- Explain the influence of success and failure experiences on self-concept and self-esteem.
- Describe the relationship between "success expectation" and "performance."
- Describe the problem-solving process.
- Recognize behaviors that may represent an effort to meet the need for approval, acceptance, or appreciation.
- Express approval, caring, or appreciation appropriately.

## KEY TERMS

| | | |
|---|---|---|
| Appraisal | Compensation | Martyr complex |
| Aptitudes | Conformity | Sympathy |
| Autonomy | Empathy | |

Remember Maslow's hierarchy of needs? In Chapter 5, we discussed physical needs, which included levels 1 and 2 of the hierarchy. This chapter discusses level 3, love and belongingness; level 4, esteem needs; and level 5, self-actualization. These social and psychological needs are just as important to comfort and happiness as physical needs, though they are less obvious. As we discussed in Chapter 5, most human behavior is an attempt to meet a need. However, people use a variety of behaviors to meet their social and psychological needs, based on their own unique blend of heredity, environmental influences, previous experiences, and personal preferences.

## SOCIAL/EMOTIONAL NEEDS

For the most part, physical needs can be met either alone or in the company of others. However, sharing with others is more satisfying than meeting these needs alone. You enjoy your dinner more if you have pleasant company than if you eat alone or with someone you dislike. When physical needs and social needs are met simultaneously, you are more likely to experience enjoyment and a sense of well-being.

### Types of Social/Emotional Needs

There are many different kinds of social/emotional needs: psychological, emotional, intellectual, spiritual, and recreational. These terms overlap, because each term refers to groups of needs that are closely related.

Some social needs can be partially met alone, but relationships with other people are necessary for full satisfaction. For example, the person who enjoys studying a subject can partially meet intellectual needs alone. Greater satisfaction might be experienced, however, if there are opportunities to discuss the subject with others who share the same interest. *Satisfying relationships with other people lead to full satisfaction of the social/emotional needs.*

Some social/emotional needs are related to the self; other needs are related to contact with other people. Each of us needs to feel important as a person, to have a sense of achievement,

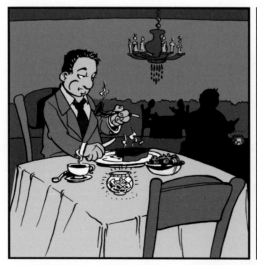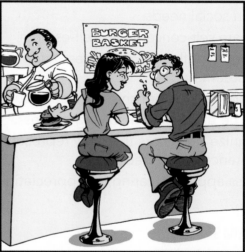

**FIGURE 6-1 Basic physical needs can be met alone, while social needs are met by interacting with others.**

and to feel worthy. We also need to feel that we are important to others, that other people approve of us, and that we are accepted as a member of the group. These two sets of needs are closely tied together, for feelings and beliefs about oneself affect acceptance by others.

## Compensation

You have learned that each of the physical needs can be met only in a specific way. With the social/emotional needs, a type of substitution known as **compensation** is possible. It is important to remember, however, that *compensation does not satisfy a basic need;* it is a device that provides temporary relief from the discomfort felt when a basic social/emotional need is not being met.

Do you know a person who habitually talks loudly, tends to brag, is a showoff, or dresses in flashy clothes? Is this person popular? Is this person accepted by the group? Probably not, for these are attention-seeking behaviors. For some people it is better to be noticed, even disapprovingly, than to be ignored. Behavior that gets attention can relieve the inner discomfort of being ignored. Attention-seeking behavior is an example of compensation. This behavior temporarily relieves inner discomfort and gains attention from the group. Obtaining approval meets a basic need; getting attention compensates for not gaining approval. People who compensate are usually unaware that they are getting temporary relief from inner discomfort instead of the full satisfaction that comes only from meeting basic social/emotional needs.

# THE SELF-CONCEPT

Each of us has an image of "self." We think of ourselves as a certain kind of person, possessing specific characteristics. Self-concept may be thought of as all the things a person thinks are true about the self. It is a mental image of "me." A particular person's self-concept may be realistic or unrealistic.

## Behavior as an Indicator of the Self-Concept

The person with a realistic self-concept thinks of the self in terms that are consistent with behavior. Usually, behavior is an accurate indicator of a person's self-concept. Joe's behavior indicates that he is not honest, but if Joe's self-concept includes honesty as an attribute, then his behavior and his self-concept are not consistent. Which reflects the real Joe?

Behavior is not always an accurate indicator of a person's true characteristics. Behavior may not be consistent with a person's beliefs and values. Suppose a person in the health field talks about the philosophy of individual worth and treats all patients courteously and with impartial efficiency, yet actually has strong prejudice against members of certain groups. This prejudice may not be revealed in day-to-day behavior but would be reflected in an important decision. Such a person's *public* self—the self that is revealed to others—is inconsistent with the *private* self—the self that is known only to the individual.

## A Realistic Self-Concept

The person who has a realistic self-concept is able to be honest about the real self. Such a person's behavior accurately reflects the person's own beliefs, values, and standards.

The person whose self-concept is unrealistic is not ready to set goals for personal growth until the self-concept has been revised. "What is" must be acknowledged before considering "what can be." An unrealistic self-concept may be either idealized or self-derogatory.

For example, Crystal has great difficulty with high school subjects, but thinks of herself as a person who can do anything she attempts. Her ambition is to be a scientist. Crystal's *idealized self-concept* may trap her into setting goals that she cannot achieve. In contrast, Crystal's friend, Erica, is an excellent student but lacks self-confidence. Erica has an older sister who is a good student, is very pretty, and sings extremely well. Erica does not seem to have any artistic talent. She is average in appearance. Because she has always compared herself unfavorably with her sister, Erica thinks of herself as a second-rate person, yet she has tremendous potential and can probably succeed in any field of study she undertakes. Erica has a derogatory *self-concept,* meaning that she is overly critical of herself and does not fully recognize her abilities and talents. Unless Erica revises her self-perception, she may settle for goals less challenging than those she could achieve.

## Building a Realistic Self-Concept

A realistic self-concept requires conscious and thoughtful consideration of "what is." By honestly appraising your strengths and weaknesses, identifying your interests, and clarifying your values, you will get in touch with the "real you." This is the starting point for planning ways to develop your potential and gaining greater satisfaction from living.

## Formation of the Self-Concept

The self-concept begins to form at a very early age and is well established by about age 6. It can be modified later in life, but only with conscious effort over a period of time. The self-concept is greatly affected by all life experiences, but it is most susceptible to the influence of other people *during the early formative years and during adolescence.* The young child's relationships with other people establish the early pattern. Is the child considered a person with rights and feelings? Many adults demand expressions of courtesy from a child, yet fail to use courteous behavior toward the child.

A positive self-concept develops if the young child has positive experiences and positive verbal interactions with the important adults of his or her social environment:

*"You are sweet."*

*"I love you."*

*"You are so strong."*

*"You are special."*

*"It's fun being with you."*

*"I like for you to ask questions."*

A busy adult may forget to tell a child that he is loved and is important. A child needs to hear such positive statements in order to think of "me" as one who is loved and is important to other people. Children also need positive nonverbal messages: hugs and kisses, a squeeze of the hand, a pat on the shoulder, and other appropriate forms of touch. The most important message is conveyed through time spent with the child, time in which the child is the primary focus of a parent's attention. Working parents should plan for quality time with the child each day—reading, playing, walking, and talking.

The form of discipline used with a child also has an extensive influence on the child's self-concept. If Greg is repeatedly told that he is a bad boy, he will begin to think of himself as being bad. Why should Greg try to be good if he has learned to think of himself as "bad" and believes that "everyone expects me to be bad"?

During adolescence, the peer group exerts a powerful influence on self-concept. Teens experience pressure to conform to the group's standards and values. Adolescents may label those who do not conform. A teenager must have a strong self-concept to resist those pressures, to stand up for personal beliefs and values, and at the same time gain acceptance from the peer group.

In these and many other ways, the people around a young child mold the developing child's self-concept. In the following sections, we will explore two aspects of personality development: self-reliance (a strong, capable person) or dependence (a weak, incompetent person who relies on others). Obviously, the tendency to remain dependent on others, versus the tendency to become progressively more self-reliant, influences a person's self-concept.

## Learning Independence

One of the most important aspects of development during childhood and adolescence is a gradual increase in independence, with less and less dependence on others. The need for self-reliance is an inborn force. Many infant behaviors reflect the need for this type of development: efforts at self-feeding, attempts to help with dressing and undressing, and attempts to "do it myself!" A child's angry reaction when an adult interferes in something the child is trying to do reflects this need for independence.

**Autonomy versus Dependence** The struggle between self-reliance and dependence on others continues throughout life. Each of us has a need for **autonomy**, the ability to function independently without outside control. No one ever achieves complete autonomy. We are social beings, and in many ways our welfare depends upon our being able to function as a member of the group. The mature person has learned to live harmoniously with his fellow man, functioning autonomously in many ways and accepting that dependence on others for some things is a matter of necessity.

Autonomy must be achieved over a period of time, by gradually learning to be self-reliant in the simple tasks of daily living (e.g., dressing and eating) and then progressing to self-reliance in more complex situations. It is impossible to be dependent on others throughout childhood and adolescence and then suddenly, at age 18 or 21, become a self-directing, autonomous adult. Effective parenting provides for the gradual development of independence throughout childhood by encouraging the child to do simple tasks. It also requires being available when help is requested or frustration becomes more than the child can handle.

### For Discussion and Reflection

If you are a parent, how have you encouraged your child to develop independence by doing tasks for him- or herself? If you are not a parent, recall a task your own parents encouraged you to do independently.

This struggle for a compromise between autonomy and dependence reaches its peak during adolescence. The young person struggling for autonomy rebels against dependence on others. The parents may resent the young person's insisting on greater independence than they believe the child can handle. Young people who do not successfully resolve this conflict may carry the struggle for autonomy into adulthood, usually as rebellion toward any form of authority, such as the teacher or the "boss." You may find it interesting to study examples of rebellious behavior in terms of the struggle for autonomy.

The self-concept can be modified in adulthood, either by experiences that change one's perception of self or by a conscious approach to self-study. A realistic self-concept is based on thinking of oneself as a worthy person with a high level of capability for some activities, but not for others. You need to *accept yourself as a worthy person* before you will be able to make a constructive **appraisal** of your strengths and weaknesses.

## SELF-ESTEEM

Self-esteem refers to one's *feelings about self at a given moment* or period of time. Self-esteem is closely related to self-concept, but is not the same. Although self-concept is established during the early years and is relatively permanent, self-esteem is quite changeable and is affected by life experiences. A person's self-esteem may be high in the morning; then, some negative experience may plunge that person's self-esteem to a very low point. For most people, a period of low self-esteem is short-lived. If a negative experience, such as being unemployed, extends over a period of weeks, then self-esteem may remain low throughout that period. Effectively dealing with a life problem usually restores self-esteem to a high level. Good life experiences tend to maintain self-esteem at a high level, whereas negative experiences can lower a person's self-esteem.

## INFLUENCE OF OTHERS ON ONE'S SENSE OF SELF

Other people have a strong influence on one's sense of self, beginning with the interactions of adults and the newborn baby. A sense of self-and-others begins to develop during infancy. The struggle for autonomy, "self" as separate from others, begins during the toddler stage, continues throughout childhood, and becomes intense during adolescence. During the infant and toddler periods, family members and caretakers influence the early sense of self. The child's exposure to the world widens with entry into preschool programs and school itself; from that time on, teachers and others make significant contributions to the formative sense of self. These early interactions help establish the child's self-concept, which then acts as a sort of filter for the effects of later experiences and relationships.

The struggle for self-identity, a clarification of the "Who am I?" question, intensifies during adolescence and early adulthood. Dating and marriage introduce another influence, so powerful that it may lead to modification of some aspect of the self-concept. Any intimate relationship can have a powerful effect on one's self-concept, as well as day-by-day effects on self-esteem.

### For Discussion and Reflection

Have you had a teacher, coach, relative, or friend who inspired you or helped you recognize your own strengths? What did this person do or say that contributed to your self-concept?

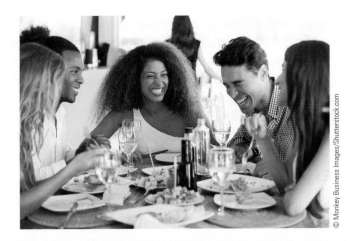

**FIGURE 6-2 Interactions with other people can have a negative or positive effect on self-esteem.**

You should now become more aware of the role other persons play in determining how you feel about yourself at a particular time. Your interactions with some people almost always make you feel good. Some people say and do things that make you feel good about yourself. Other people tend to have the opposite effect: they make put-down statements, are often critical, play the one-upmanship game, or otherwise have a diminishing effect on your sense of self. If there are many such people in your daily life, you are probably struggling to maintain a positive level of self-esteem. In order to correct the situation, you have certain choices:

1. Avoid such people.

2. Be assertive about not accepting negative statements.

3. Refuse to participate in their emotional games.

4. Learn ways to respond to communications that have a negative effect on you.

Obviously, the first choice is not available to you if members of your family or your co-workers have a negative effect on you. In that case, you can begin to learn how to deal with such people through various activities, such as reading about effective relationships and participating in assertiveness training and communication skills.

In summary, positive relationships can help one to develop a strong self-concept and maintain high self-esteem most of the time. Negative relationships can have a destructive effect on self-concept and may result in a chronic state of low self-esteem.

## EFFECTS OF SUCCESS AND FAILURE

Have you ever had a task so difficult that you did not believe you could complete it? Perhaps it was a reading assignment that just did not make sense when you read it. Perhaps it was a written assignment, and you did not know how to proceed.

What was your approach to this task that appeared so hopeless? Did you pitch in, try your best, and find that you could do it, after all? How did you feel about your accomplishment? You should have felt good, for you overcame obstacles and successfully completed a difficult task.

Each successful experience should be consciously recognized as a success. Each success should help you believe in *yourself as a person who can overcome obstacles.*

On the other hand, you may have found a particular task just as hard as you expected and were unable to complete it. No doubt you still have some negative feelings about this experience. Perhaps you were angry at yourself for not finishing it. Perhaps you were angry with the person who assigned the task to you. In either case, your self-confidence was threatened. You were discouraged and probably approached the next difficult task with greater self-doubt.

## Meaning of Failure Expectation

Discouragement and a sense of failure can be quite damaging to self-confidence, especially if experienced frequently. But this is only part of the problem. When failure occurs too frequently, there is a tendency to develop "failure expectation." Each failure adds to self-doubt; self-doubt creates failure expectation; failure expectation interferes with performance. Thus, there is increased probability that the next task will result in another failure. If this cycle becomes well established, the individual may need professional help to break the pattern and believe in the possibility of future successful performances.

## Success Expectation

For most people, however, the problem is lack of self-confidence rather than an established failure expectation. Self-confidence might be thought of as "success expectation." The key to

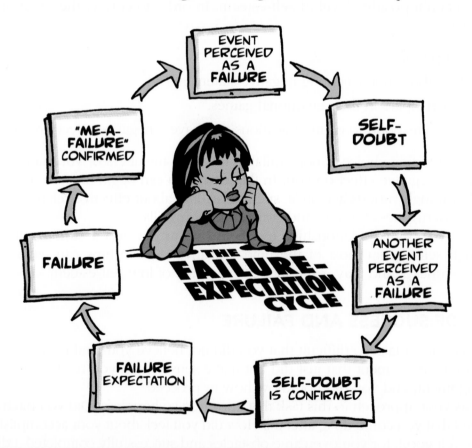

**FIGURE 6-3 Expecting failure can create a negative cycle, or failure expectation.**

building self-confidence is conscious recognition of each successful experience, with awareness that life includes both successful experiences and disappointing experiences.

Success expectation is an attitude that affects the way you attack a task. Your approach, to a great extent, will determine the outcome. Two personal traits that are helpful in the performance of any task are persistence and determination. Successful performance may be dependent upon time—some tasks require a slow, careful performance, whereas others should be performed quickly. Successful performance as a health care professional requires that you choose the appropriate method of performance in a wide variety of situations.

Confidence comes from having a reasonable balance of successes and failures. Perhaps you have such a balance, but give undue attention to failure experiences and do not consciously acknowledge your successes.

Everyone has some failures and some disappointments in spite of a conscientious effort to do well. It is possible to use such experiences as opportunities to identify factors that may have contributed to a poor outcome:

- Did I begin the task without proper preparation?
- Did I attempt to do the task too rapidly? Did I give enough attention to details (or technique)?
- Did I allow too little time for the task?
- Did I use efficient work habits? If not, what work habits might have been more effective?
- Did I use the appropriate method for this task? If not, what method would have been better?
- Did I give up too soon?
- Did I have control over the outcome, or was the outcome controlled by someone else? If the outcome was controlled by someone else, then the failure is not yours. Habitually blaming others, however, can prevent you from taking responsibility for your actions, and therefore inhibit learning from experience.

Successful experiences in life make it easier to accept the occasional failures that all of us have. If you can maintain a reasonable balance between successes and failures and experience satisfaction after each success, then your self-esteem will likely be high most of the time, and any periods of low self-esteem will be brief.

## SUCCESS

Do you think of "success" as making a lot of money, gaining power, having a late-model car, or perhaps even becoming a movie star? Only a few people get to the top, and some of those who do get to the top in their field find that their "success" does not provide happiness.

### Influence of Success

Each of us has many opportunities for success if we recognize daily accomplishments and grant ourselves the right to feel good about them. Each time a job is done well, you should feel inner satisfaction. If others notice and express approval, this should add to your enjoyment. But even when you do not gain approval from others, you should feel good when you know, deep inside, that you did a job well.

If you recognize and acknowledge daily successes, each one will build your self-confidence and prepare you for succeeding in the next task you undertake. Each success diminishes the probability that self-doubt will interfere with success in future undertakings.

## As a Student

As a student, you will have many opportunities to experience success. New information, new insights, new understandings, and new skills can give you a sense of accomplishment. Take pride in each achievement, seeing it as another step toward becoming a health care professional. Remember, however, that none of us can experience success in every task. There are times when we do not do as well as we would like. From the disappointments, however, we can learn what to avoid in the next similar situation. Thus, "failures" can be used constructively as learning experiences, instead of being allowed to create destructive self-doubt.

## As a Health Care Professional

When you have become a full-fledged health care professional, recognize your successes each day and gain satisfaction from them. Regard your "nonsuccesses" as learning experiences that will help you perform more effectively in the future. Set goals for developing those traits that are fundamental to self-confidence: persistence, determination, and adaptability. Learn to use a systematic, problem-solving approach. Develop efficient work habits. As successes increase, disappointments will be less damaging to your self-esteem. Thus, you can build belief in yourself as a competent person.

## FINDING SELF-APPROVAL

### Modifying Habits

In order to build self-confidence, you must be realistic. You have many, many personal traits. Some are so highly developed that they characterize you as a person; in trying to describe you, someone would mention those traits. Other traits are not so prominent, but can be developed if you give your attention to them. Some traits are favorable; others are unfavorable. Try to identify the traits that will help you as a person and as a health care professional and strive to develop those traits to a high degree. Also, identify those traits that hold you back and work to minimize or eliminate those traits from your behavior patterns.

It takes persistence to replace an undesirable habit with a more desirable one. The following steps can help:

* Identify the habit you want to change.

* Identify the function, or purpose, that the habit serves. Does it help you relax? Reward yourself? Avoid an undesirable task?

- Select a replacement behavior that serves the same function as the bad habit without the negative effects.

- Develop a plan or routine for when you will use the replacement behavior.

- Start small, but be consistent. For example, if beginning an exercise routine, start with just five or ten minutes, but do it every day.

- As your new behavior becomes a habit, add to it if appropriate. For example, gradually lengthen your exercise session.

**For Discussion and Reflection**

Have you ever worked to change a bad habit? Were you successful? If so, what strategies helped you change your habit?

## Developing Problem-Solving Skills

You can also deal with problems more effectively by using a systematic method. The following steps to choosing successful behavior can be applied to a variety of situations:

1. Identify the problem. Think it through. Discuss it with someone who might help you understand it or to see the problem in a new light. Write out a statement of the problem.

2. Collect information and/or ideas that might help you understand the problem better.

3. Consider all available information, then look at your statement of the problem. Reconsider what the problem is and rewrite the statement, if necessary.

**NOTE** At this point, your perception of the problem may have changed completely. You may eventually see the problem as being entirely different from what you initially thought.

4. Write down every imaginable solution. In a second column beside each possible solution, write out the possible consequences of trying that solution.

5. Select the solution that seems most likely to lead to the desired outcome and carry out the actions required.

6. Evaluate the outcome. If the result was not satisfactory, try another solution that appears likely to succeed.

It requires practice to become skillful in using a problem-solving approach, but if you apply it to daily problems, you will soon become skillful in thinking through these steps. In other words, thinking through a problem may become a work habit. Skill in problem solving enables a person to choose a specific behavior for a desired result.

## Setting Goals

Your true interests and **aptitudes** influence the success you are likely to experience and the satisfaction you are likely to gain from certain types of activities. Each of us tends to do best those things that we enjoy doing. Also, we learn more easily and perform best those activities for which we have an aptitude. A realistic appraisal of "what is" provides the foundation for setting goals, or "what may be."

Goals that are in accordance with your true interests and aptitudes are more likely to be achieved than goals set for you by someone else. If your goals offer a challenge, then reaching them will provide much satisfaction—the feeling of having overcome obstacles and of being a person who can achieve goals. This is self-approval. When goals are too high for your aptitudes or readiness, then you may experience disappointment, failure, and self-doubt. Goals that are too low are easily reached, do not challenge you to develop your potential, and provide only limited satisfaction.

It is desirable to have both short-range and long-range goals. Short-range goals are the stepping-stones that lead to long-range goals. If Carissa wants to study medicine and is qualified to do so, her high school curriculum and college courses will be a series of short-range goals leading to the long-range goal of becoming a physician. If there are financial problems, Carissa may use a health occupations course as a short-term goal, obtaining job skills that enable her to work part-time while attending college. Thus, Carissa may eventually reach her long-range goal through a series of intermediate goals. Intermediate goals provide inner satisfaction and a sense of achievement that can help one persist in striving for the long-range goal.

## THE IMPORTANCE OF ACCEPTANCE

You have learned that social/emotional needs can be met fully only through satisfying relationships with other people. Satisfaction of social/emotional needs requires both self-approval and approval and acceptance by others. The person who has achieved self-approval finds it easier to gain approval and acceptance by others. On the other hand, acceptance by others makes us feel more comfortable with ourselves. So these two needs are closely tied together; the person who can grow in self-approval can become increasingly acceptable to others and vice versa.

Each of us needs to believe that others accept us as a worthwhile person. To satisfy this need, we must see and hear expressions of approval from time to time, in order to remain

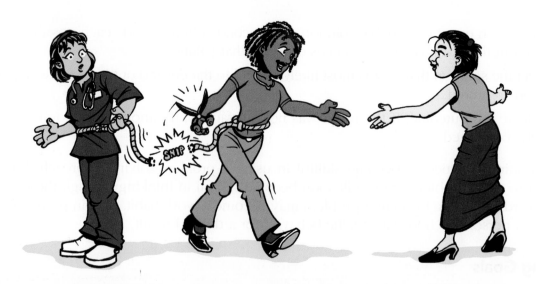

**FIGURE 6-4** A relationship deteriorates when it no longer satisfies the social needs of one or both parties.

convinced of this acceptance. We also need to believe that others understand our viewpoint, our feelings, and our problems. Obviously, satisfying the need for acceptance requires receiving indications of approval and caring from other people.

Friendships develop and are maintained on the basis of whether or not two people meet each other's needs. Ideally, a relationship between two people involves a balance of give-and-take. This ideal can be met only if the behavior of each person helps the other to satisfy basic social/emotional needs. In some relationships, the balance of give-and-take appears to be one-sided. One person exerts much effort to please the other and seems to get little in return. If the relationship continues over a long period without change in this balance, both parties are satisfying certain needs. Self-sacrificing behavior is sometimes referred to as the "**martyr complex**," meaning that the individual actually derives satisfaction from being taken advantage of by another person.

> ### For Discussion and Reflection
>
> Have you or someone you know experienced a relationship (either as a friend or as a romantic partner) in which one person seemed to repeatedly take advantage of the other? If this pattern continued for a period of time, what needs do you think each person in the relationship was meeting?

To a great extent, we can understand our behavior and that of others in terms of basic needs—behaviors that satisfy a basic need, and behaviors that compensate for not being able to satisfy a basic need. Usually, a person puts up with certain circumstances or with the behavior of others because some need is being met. Perhaps compensation is taking place. Perhaps the need is unhealthy, as illustrated by martyr behavior. If no need is being met, the individual will usually engage in behavior that either changes the situation or provides escape.

## THE IMPORTANCE OF APPROVAL FROM OTHERS

Have you ever expected to be praised for something you did, but instead you were criticized? How did it make you feel? How did you behave? How did you feel about the person who was critical instead of approving? This person, in failing to give approval, deprived you of a basic need. Each of us has had such experiences. The one who failed to give us our earned approval may have been a parent, friend, classmate, teacher, or boss. The hurt associated with such experiences is proportional to the importance we attach to the other person.

Now consider the other side of the coin. Have you ever had a friend show you something new, yet you failed to express approval? Has a friend ever won an honor, but for some reason you could not bring yourself to offer congratulations? If so, you were depriving this person of approval. Why did you withhold your approval?

### Hunger for Approval

Being deprived of approval early in life can create a hunger for approval that never seems satisfied. Do you know someone who "looks for compliments"? How do you feel about this person? Seeking compliments usually indicates a strong need for expressions of approval. The next time you observe such behavior, will you recognize the need for approval? Assuming it is deserved, will you express your approval freely and sincerely? If so, you will be helping that person meet an important need. You will be contributing to that person's inner comfort, but the cost to you is only the effort it takes to state your sincere approval.

## Failure to Offer Approval

Some people fail to notice others. Some are indifferent to a job well done, but very ready to react to a job or a person not meeting their approval. Some people may notice that a job has been well done, but make no comment. Some, for reasons of their own, deliberately avoid saying nice things to others. The habit of not expressing approval can be easily overcome, once you are aware that approval is a need we all have. Deliberately withholding approval is another matter, however. To understand this trait may be more difficult because it indicates negative feelings toward others and, probably, toward oneself.

## Appropriate Use of Approval

Approval should be given freely for everyday tasks—not just for the big tasks that come only occasionally. The child who voluntarily does a task at home deserves expressions of approval. The student who does an assignment well deserves approval. The person who serves a tasty meal deserves approval. Each of us has opportunities throughout the day to express sincere approval to others. It only requires that we form the habit of noticing others and expressing approval when it has been earned.

When will you have your next opportunity to express approval to someone? Perhaps your young son washes his hands for dinner without being told. Perhaps a patient shows the first interest in grooming since an operation. Perhaps the teacher presents an especially interesting class. All of these people need approval too!

This is not a recommendation that you rush around paying compliments freely. Insincerity is worse than silence. The desirable behavior is *noticing others and unselfishly expressing approval when it has been earned*. This is an easy way to meet your own needs while also helping someone else satisfy a basic need. Giving approval to others can be quite enjoyable.

# CONFORMITY

**Conformity** means acting in accordance with the behaviors, beliefs, and values of a specific group. Conformity expectations of group members may extend to lifestyle choices, including manner of dress, foods, sexual behavior, and relationships with the group's authority figures. In groups that emphasize conformity, individuality is not valued and may be perceived as rebellion against the group's beliefs. The person who "dares to be different" may be excluded from the group; if allowed to remain within the group, that person may be viewed with suspicion and watched closely for evidence of unacceptable behavior.

Being overly concerned about conformity places one at risk of allowing others to make decisions that mature people make for themselves. A person who readily accepts the opinions of others, without becoming informed and giving thought to the situation, depends upon conformity as a means of gaining acceptance.

## Importance of Acceptance during Adolescence

Have you ever arrived at a party and found you were dressed differently from most of those present? Perhaps you dressed casually and the others "dressed up." If among friends, you were probably not overly uncomfortable. But if you were trying to gain acceptance by the members of this group, discovering that you dressed inappropriately may have made you very uncomfortable.

During adolescence the need for acceptance by the peer group is very strong, and conformity is almost necessary to gain acceptance. Parents are often distressed to find that their teenager is more concerned about the opinions of friends than about their parents' beliefs. Some people never outgrow depending on conformity to win the acceptance of the group to which they wish to belong.

Lauren has just entered high school. She and her classmates notice that many girls in the sophomore class have various body piercings: eyebrows, nose, tongue, "belly button," and two or more in the ears. Lauren wears stud earrings, but now she and many of her classmates see additional piercings as the means for acceptance into the high school culture. When Lauren asks her parents for permission (and money) for additional piercings, they refuse. Lauren uses the argument, "Everybody is doing it." Her parents respond, "That doesn't make it sensible." Over the next several weeks, Lauren is uncomfortable as many of her friends acquire additional piercings; she even feels "left out" as she witnesses the attention and admiration generated from members of the peer group as each new piercing is displayed. Lauren has not yet learned that acceptance does not require conformity to each new fad.

## Group Standards and Conformity

Some of the policies of your health care preparatory program may seem unreasonable to you, but they are probably based on sound reasons. The ethics of the health professions are based on high principles and establish what is "appropriate" behavior for health care professionals. As a health care professional, you will be expected to conform to the standards and practices of the health care field. There will be some minor differences in policies and procedures from one clinical facility to another, but emphasis on appropriate dress, ethical behavior, and high standards of performance extends throughout the entire field of health care.

There are many situations where conformity is desirable, perhaps necessary. Military service, for example, requires conformity to rules, regulations, procedures, dress codes, and almost all aspects of daily life. Many other situations require conformity to a particular group's expectations in order to gain acceptance. This need for conformity in certain situations is reflected in the familiar expression, "When in Rome, do as the Romans do." In all situations, however, it is important to maintain your integrity and your own high principles.

If you find yourself in a group whose standards are not acceptable to you, you must either change your belief, convince the group that their standards should change, or find another group whose standards reflect your own. In other words, use good judgment in deciding when to conform to a group's standards and when to go by your own standards, even at the risk of disapproval.

## THE NEED TO BELIEVE THAT OTHERS CARE

Another social/emotional need that requires appropriate responses from other people is the need to believe that other people care. The extent to which we believe that a particular person does care about us has an influence on how we feel about that person. To put it another way, the more important a particular person is to us, the more strongly we need to believe that person cares about our feelings. Expressions of caring promote strong ties between people.

## Sympathy

As a health care professional, you will be hearing the terms **sympathy** and **empathy**. Perhaps you think of sympathy as "feeling sorry for someone." Actually, few people want or expect pity from others, and some would react to expressions of pity with anger. But most people, when sick or experiencing some type of difficulty, need to believe that their loved ones and friends care, share their feelings, and regret that they are having a bad experience. Sympathy, then, implies sharing and feeling with another, while retaining one's own point of view.

## Empathy

Empathy is similar to *some* of the meanings of sympathy, but it is not the same. Empathy means identifying with another person in such a way that we see another person's situation from her point of view, rather than from our own perspective.

As a health care professional you will be exposed to many situations in which an effort to feel empathy for the patient and the family—*to see the situation as they see it*—will help you understand their behavior. Most patients do not want others to feel sorry for them. They *do* want others to care about them, to understand what they are experiencing, and to care about their feelings and beliefs.

# THE NEED FOR APPRECIATION

Each of us needs to believe that someone appreciates us. We especially need to feel appreciated by those who are important to us. Appreciation may mean "to be grateful," by saying "thank you," or "to have respect," as shown by the statement, "She has great appreciation for modern art."

Expressing appreciation might indicate either of these meanings and might even imply approval or caring as well. For example, a child's first attempt to help with a household task will be unsuccessful by adult standards, yet the child may be proud of the effort. The adult reaction will affect future efforts. For a positive effect, the parent could show gratitude for the attempt to be helpful, could show respect for the child's effort, or could show caring and pleasure with the child's intent to help. All of these should be shown sincerely, even though the result of the child's performance may not meet adult standards.

Expressions of approval, appreciation, and caring provide a sense of satisfaction. The absence of any such expressions can have as negative an effect as open criticism or disapproval. If a task has been attempted but not performed well, sincere *approval* cannot be given; yet it is quite likely that an expression of *appreciation* would be appropriate. If suggestions for improvement are needed, these suggestions are less likely to appear as criticism if they are preceded by an expression of appreciation, caring, and understanding. Thus, there are some situations where approval should be expressed, but indications of appreciation or caring are not necessary. At other times, approval is not needed or has not been earned, but appreciation could be shown. Sometimes neither approval nor appreciation can be expressed, yet an expression of caring would be appropriate.

Our social/emotional needs are interrelated. The person who is aware of social/emotional needs and their importance in interpersonal relations will recognize opportunities to contribute to the satisfaction of another's needs. The person who is unaware may blunder through life, contributing little to the needs of others and lacking personal satisfaction from meeting social/emotional needs.

## SOCIAL/EMOTIONAL NEEDS AND BEHAVIOR

Perhaps you are now more aware of the complexity of human behavior. One person seeks approval by strict conformity to a group's standards of behavior, another by getting good grades, another by acquiring symbols of success, another by doing favors for people, still another by being the life of the party. Some people find effective patterns of behavior that lead to self-approval and acceptance by others. Some people compensate with behavior that temporarily relieves their inner discomfort but fails to satisfy basic social/emotional needs.

All behavior is caused; it does not just happen. However, it is seldom possible to pinpoint one particular cause of a specific action. The causes of behavior are numerous and complex. Some of these causes lie in the situation in which the behavior occurs; other causes are within the individual, as a result of past experiences and their continuing influence on behavior. Many behaviors are goal-oriented; that is, they represent an individual's efforts to achieve some goal, such as satisfying the need for acceptance. We can increase our understanding and tolerance for behavior of others by being more aware of possible contributing causes, some apparent and others hidden. It is also helpful to study behavior in terms of its effectiveness— the degree to which it satisfies some basic need.

## BEHAVIOR AND THE HEALTH CARE PROFESSIONAL

For health care professionals, being aware of the social/emotional needs of others can mean the difference between effective and ineffective relations with patients and their families. People under the physical and psychological stress of illness are more likely to cope with their illness successfully if caregivers help them meet social and emotional needs, as well as physical needs.

As a health care professional, you can be more effective if you are also a student of human behavior. You know that there is no ready answer to the "why" of any one person's behavior. You know that basic needs, both physical and social/emotional, continue during illness. However, the need for relieving distress and releasing emotions such as fear may temporarily push the need for approval or acceptance into the background. On the other hand, some patients try to cover up their own emotional distress to win acceptance from health care professionals by being pleasant and cooperative.

As you observe people in apparently similar situations reacting in very different ways, you are seeing evidence of individual differences. Patients differ in their behavior used to cope with stress, in the strength of different needs, in relative importance given to specific needs, and in the capacity to find behavior patterns to meet their needs in a particular situation.

## ACTIVITIES

1. Briefly describe a time you have experienced each of the following situations:

   a. You attempted a task but gave up without completing it.

   b. You attempted a difficult task and finished it.

   c. You expected someone to praise your performance, but no one commented.

   d. Someone complimented you on how well you did something. It was a routine job that you do regularly without giving it much thought.

2. Review each of the above situations. Describe how each experience made you feel about yourself.

3. Select a problem you now have and apply the problem-solving method. Write out several possible solutions; beside each, list the probable results. Select the solution you think will have the most desirable outcome. Try this solution. After one week, review the problem, your action, and the outcome. Evaluate your use of the problem-solving method. Did you select the best action? Do you now think another action would have had a better result?

4. Describe how you could use sympathy and empathy with the following:

   a.  Your relations with patients and their families

   b.  Your relations with coworkers

   c.  Your personal life

5. Imagine that in your work as a health care professional, you have seen several patients who have infections that resulted from body piercings and one who developed hepatitis C after getting a tattoo. Today, your 15-year-old son announces that he wants to have his girlfriend's name tattooed on his forearm, "where everyone will see it." You know that many of his classmates already have a tattoo. Using your awareness of the importance of conformity and peer approval during adolescence, how will you handle this request?

## REFERENCES AND SUGGESTED READINGS

Canfield, Jack. (2015). *The success principles: how to get from where you are to where you want to be.* New York: HarperCollins.

Goltz, H., & Brown, T. (2014). Are children's psychological self-concepts predictive of their self-reported activity preferences and leisure participation? *Australian Occupational Therapy Journal, 61*(3), 177–186. doi:10.1111/1440-1630.12101.

Koruklu, N. (2015). Personality and social problem-solving: The mediating role of self-esteem. *Educational Sciences: Theory and Practice, 15*(2), 481–487.

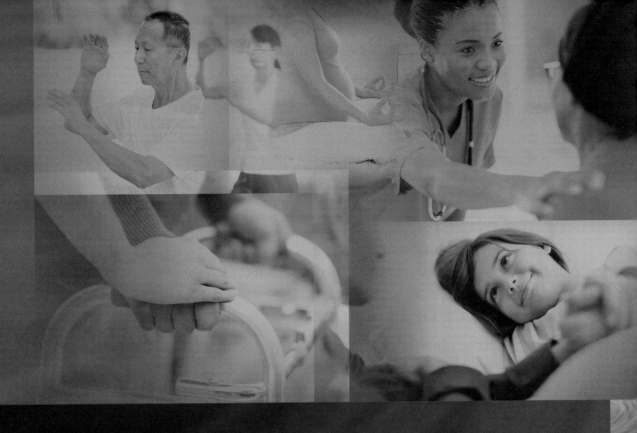

# CHAPTER 7

# Emotions and Behavior

## OBJECTIVES

After completing this chapter, you should be able to:

- Describe the physiological effects of emotional arousal.
- Define stress, distress, and stressor.
- Explain how emotional patterns are formed.
- Identify ways to use emotions constructively.
- Practice using "I-statements."

## KEY TERMS

| | | |
|---|---|---|
| Adrenalin | Mental chatter | Stress |
| Altruism | Noradrenalin | Stressors |
| Compassion | Physiological | Suppression |
| Cynicism | Repressed | |
| Hostility | Resentment | |

## MEANING OF EMOTIONS

*Emotions* are the inner feelings that all of us have. They are responses to life situations, varying in type and intensity according to the experience of the moment. Many different terms are used to describe emotions. Some of these terms describe the *type* of feeling; other terms imply the *intensity* of the feeling.

*Emotions are neither good nor bad.* We all experience these inner feelings according to what is happening to us and how we perceive the experience. To think of any emotion as good or bad, in a moral sense, is as pointless as considering hunger to be morally good or bad. Both positive and negative emotions are natural reactions to life experiences. However, as adults, we are responsible for expressing and managing our emotions in a healthy way.

## IMPORTANCE OF EMOTIONS

Emotions have physical and mental effects. Indirectly, emotions determine the amount of satisfaction we get from life, the degree of success we have in solving life problems, the satisfaction we find in relations with other people, and, ultimately, our *physical* and *mental* well-being throughout life.

The relationship between negative emotions and physical health is now well established by research. Anger, when experienced frequently, tends to evolve into **resentment** (chronic, low-level anger), **hostility** (an angry attitude toward a specific person or group), or **cynicism** (an attitude of contempt or distrust of others). Thus, anger can influence the personality.

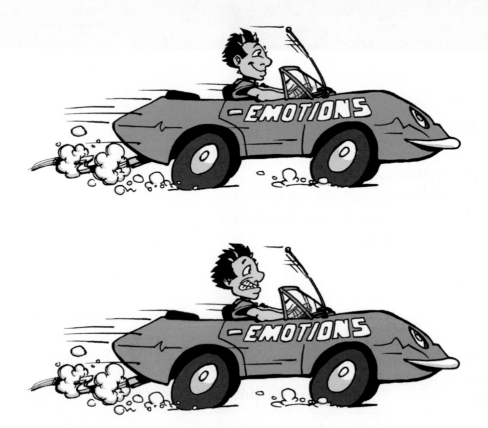

**FIGURE 7-1** To manage emotions effectively, it is important to remain in control.

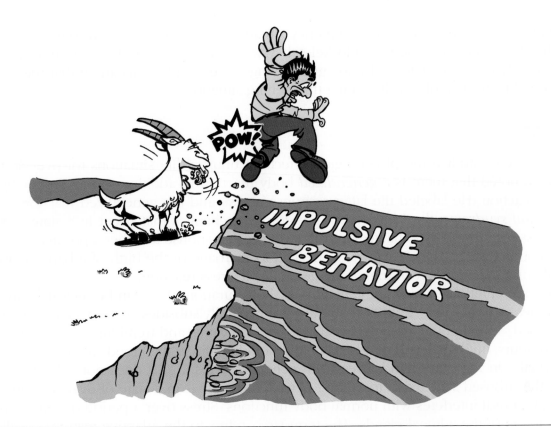

**FIGURE 7-2 Unmanaged emotions can propel us toward undesirable behavior.**

Since our emotions have powerful mental and physical effects, it is important that we learn to use emotions effectively, rather than allow emotions to control our behavior. The person who has learned to express feelings in socially acceptable ways is competent in dealing with life situations—both good and bad. A person who has not learned to use emotions constructively is likely to lose control when feelings become strong. The sudden eruption of powerful feelings may result in impulsive behavior that is ineffective in dealing with a situation. Appropriate expression of emotions in any job situation influences relations with coworkers, supervisors, and patients/clients.

## PHYSIOLOGICAL EFFECTS OF EMOTIONS

Emotions influence physical functioning, with particular effect on the autonomic nervous system, which influences the functioning of internal organs. Through this indirect influence, the emotional state can stimulate certain organs and inhibit the activity of others. If the emotion is strong, the effect is of short duration. If it is a long-term emotion, as in chronic anxiety, internal processes are kept in a state of "semi-emergency alert." Over a period of time, this long-term **physiological** situation can lead to actual physical changes.

Studies of body reactions to situations that arouse fear or anger show that the adrenal glands discharge large amounts of **adrenalin** and the sympathetic nervous system produces **noradrenalin**. These two hormones speed up the circulation of blood, accelerate blood clotting, dilate the blood vessels that serve the skeletal muscles, and increase the respiratory rate. The purpose of these changes is to prepare the body for unusual activity—that is, a "fight or flight" state—to deal with the emergency situation. While the body's resources are being mobilized to strengthen the musculoskeletal system, other areas of the body have a diminished supply of blood. These physiological changes are adaptive, meaning that they enable the individual to deal physically with a threatening situation.

## STRESS

Dr. Hans Selye studied the physiological effects of unusual life situations for over 30 years. Dr. Selye noted that there is a *generalized* body reaction in addition to the alarm ("fight or flight") reaction. He labeled the latter response **stress** and the generalized reaction *general adaptation syndrome*, the sum total of physiological changes that occur in a state of stress. The stress response is essential to survival; it occurs in response to either a positive or a negative emotional state. Thus, a happy event such as marriage or the birth of a baby, as well as an unhappy experience, can trigger the generalized stress reaction.

Extreme emotional states are generally of short duration; they can be measured in terms of minutes or hours. The "fight or flight" arousal generally subsides as soon as the emergency has passed, although the aftereffects, such as sweaty palms and trembling, may continue for several hours, until the levels of adrenalin and noradrenalin in the bloodstream have returned to normal. On the other hand, stress (the generalized response) does not subside quickly; when this aroused state exists for a long period, the body is in a state of distress. The physiological arousal interferes with normal body functions. Stress over a period of years can lead to depletion of the adrenal glands. The term *stress* refers to the adaptive response itself. The outside influences that create a state of arousal are **stressors**.

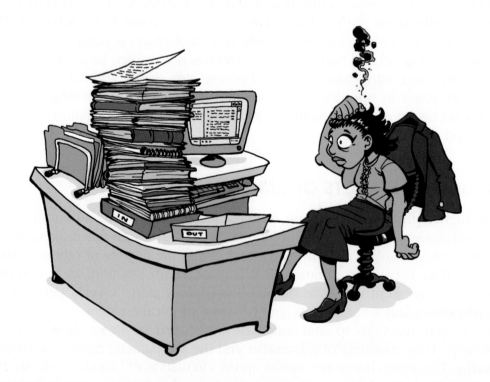

**FIGURE 7-3 A heavy workload can cause significant stress.**

Dr. Selye's research led to the discovery that the stress reaction includes increased body resistance to outside agents such as infectious organisms. This is the basis for immunity to specific diseases (i.e., production of antibodies). During a period of increased resistance to a specific stressor, resistance to other stressors is decreased. For example, working long hours, eating improperly, and not getting sufficient sleep and recreation add up to stress. A person with such a lifestyle is likely to have lowered resistance and, therefore, to be more susceptible to infection.

The person whose stress reaction is due to invasion by a specific infectious agent, such as the measles virus, has the physiological response specific to that infectious agent (e.g., in case of measles, fever, rash, runny nose). At that time, the measles victim has lowered resistance to other organisms, such as the bacteria or viruses that cause pneumonia. While the body mobilizes its resources to deal with the measles virus, only limited resources are available to deal with other threats to health.

Unfortunately, resistance to psychological stressors does not automatically develop, as is the case with immunity to some infectious organisms. Nor does the stress reaction subside as quickly or as completely after a psychological threat is no longer a part of the immediate life situation. Because of mental/emotional/physiological interactions, we can experience stress by remembering a past event, by anticipating some undesirable future event, or even by imagining that something has happened or is happening. When one's thoughts are directed to an undesirable event (e.g., failing a course, being fired, being overworked), the emotional reaction to this *mental activity* triggers the adaptive response.

Another major source of stress for many people is **mental chatter**. This almost continuous stream of thoughts and memories is most likely to occur when an individual is performing routine tasks (i.e., ironing, raking leaves) that do not require concentrated thought or during quiet times when trying to relax. Mental chatter contributes to insomnia, since the physiological reaction to thoughts can lead to increasing wakefulness. Mental chatter, as used in this discussion, is ongoing, not fully under conscious control, and not purposeful. It is different from conscious use of mental processes for thinking, planning, evaluating, analyzing, and remembering.

Mental chatter that deals with past events may include an embarrassing situation, a failure or an unsatisfactory performance, a disappointment, a lost opportunity for a smart response, or an extensive review of a conversation. But past events cannot be changed; only the present and the future can be altered. This habit of frequently recalling past events that aroused a negative emotion results in a state of chronic stress that can lead to permanent physiological changes—the basis for psychosomatic (*psycho* = mind; *soma* = body) illness.

Mental chatter can also focus on future possible events, rather than memories of past events. These thoughts may involve rehearsal of an expected conversation, something "bad" that could happen to oneself or to a loved one, a loss, or the possibility of abandonment. If worrying about possible future events is habitual, the individual maintains a state of anxiety, and a state of stress exists.

### For Discussion and Reflection

What times of day or during what activities do you experience mental chatter? What types of thoughts or memories go through your mind throughout the day when you are driving, cooking, or completing other routine tasks?

Mental chatter can also include remembering good things that happened or anticipating some type of good experience. Mental chatter concerned with "good" things is satisfying, rather than stress-inducing. Everyone experiences mental chatter, but people vary in the extent to which they react emotionally. Stress management requires learning to control mental chatter so that it does not arouse negative emotions or interfere with sleep.

## POSITIVE EMOTIONS

The positive emotions, primarily joy and love, contribute to our feeling good. Words such as *elation* and *ecstasy* describe extremely high states of joy, whereas *pleasure* and *satisfaction* imply a less intense state of joy. Love is a complex emotion; there are various types of love and the intensity varies according to type, the object of the love, and circumstances of the moment.

These two emotions are essential to the state we call "happiness." Some degree of joy is experienced whenever good things happen, when life is relatively free of difficulties, and when we are aware of loving others and being loved. Yet happiness is possible even when our life situations include problems, some degree of stress, and times of negative feelings. The experience of happiness is dependent upon one's ability to focus on positive aspects of life and minimize negative feelings by dealing competently with the challenges of daily living.

### Love

Love is an important positive emotion. Strong feelings of warmth for another person might be thought of as *love*, with milder feelings of the same type being termed *friendliness*. *Affection* implies a feeling less intense than love, but stronger than friendliness. Love implies caring about someone else, being concerned enough to help, understand, and respect the person loved. The capacity for feeling love influences one's outlook on life and attitudes toward people and has a powerful effect on physical and mental health.

**Kinds of Love** There are many kinds of love: the love of a mother for her child; the child's love, at first self-centered and then extended to others; love for one's playmates; love for material things associated with pleasant memories; love for friends with whom life experiences have been shared; love for unfortunate ones wherever they might be; and love for a patient and his family who are all struggling with their stressful situation. Spiritual love is different still and varies according to one's concept of the Divine. Each kind of love is expressed in specific ways. Newspaper accounts of some family's misfortune often result in a flood of contributions from strangers, illustrating the capacity of many people to express love for strangers who are less fortunate than themselves. This type of love is an example of **compassion**.

**Learning to Love** Love is essential to an infant's normal development. Throughout childhood, one gradually learns to extend love to others: parents, siblings, other family members, caretakers, and eventually a widening circle of friends and associates. This learning is basic to the development of such traits as generosity, **altruism**, respect, and courtesy toward others.

During adolescence, romantic love becomes a primary concern, which may extend throughout adulthood. Mature love is a special type of love that evolves through a long-term adult relationship. Each of these types of love can flourish only if the individual's early experiences fostered the development of self-love.

**Self-Love** Self-love is basic to the experience of love. Without self-love, a person is not able to truly love others. Self-love is not selfish, nor is it egotistic. It is an awareness of "self" as a worthwhile, lovable being who deserves to be cared for. A religious person may experience self-love through the belief, "I am a child of God." Loving oneself and believing oneself to be lovable are fundamental to a positive self-concept, the best protection one can have against threats to self-esteem as various difficulties of life are experienced.

Self-love enables a person to experience joy and happiness. It also contributes to health and well-being, in part because those who have self-love care enough about themselves to practice habits of safety and health maintenance. They do not abuse their bodies with toxic substances, such as alcohol, nicotine, or other addictive drugs. They eat right, exercise appropriately, get enough sleep, wear seat belts in the car, and do not drive recklessly or otherwise place themselves at needless risk. In other words, a person who has self-love takes responsibility for "self" in all aspects of living.

**Unconditional Love** Love should be *unconditional,* which means that it is not subject to being withheld whenever one is displeased. Conditional love has an "if/then" basis: *if* you do (or do not do) such and so, *then* I will love you. All too often, conditional love is used as a manipulative tool to control another person. This is destructive to a relationship, but is especially damaging when used by parents to control a child. Conditional love teaches, "You're only lovable when you do as I say." This style of parenting can lead to a negative self-concept, the belief that one is only lovable when meeting the demands of another.

Unconditional love, then, not only provides a growing child with a strong, positive self-concept, it also prepares the individual for a more healthful future life. Unconditional love does not mean that one must put up with undesirable behavior from others. It is important to differentiate between the person and that person's behavior. It is also important to realize that you can *love* someone even when you do not *like* them. Unconditional love is available at all times; it survives the ups and downs of a relationship.

Love for a child also includes teaching appropriate behaviors at each stage of development; boundaries must be set in terms of what is acceptable behavior and what is not. Setting boundaries—making it clear that one will not tolerate a specific behavior—is a way of clarifying a relationship; it is not a matter of withholding love.

## NEGATIVE EMOTIONS

Negative emotions are uncomfortable. The intensity of each emotion can range from mild to very strong, causing one to feel a vague restlessness, a feeling of dissatisfaction, or a state of intense agitation. Negative emotions such as anger, fear, guilt, or sadness may occur as a response to the behavior of another person, a specific event or piece of information, or mental chatter. These emotions result in stress and physiological changes.

## Anger

Anger is aroused by obstacles, threats, or otherwise offensive situations. It is usually short-term and directed at a specific object or person, but can be generalized as anger at the world or society. *Hate* may be thought of as intense anger felt toward a specific person or group. *Annoyance* is used to describe a mild form of anger. *Rage* describes intense anger and implies that the anger is expressed through violent physical activity. *Hostility* is a mild form of anger/hate directed to a specific person or group. *Resentment* is chronic anger, which can be a powerful influence on one's behavior.

Anger is the emotional response to one's perception of a situation. The perception usually involves feeling wronged, neglected, cheated, deprived, ignored, or exploited. If the anger is not resolved, it becomes resentment. Many resentments have their origins in childhood, with a parent or sibling as the object of the resentment. Both anger and resentment can arise from feeling powerless to change a situation or to fight back. Anger may be aroused by an unsuccessful effort to control another person, or by awareness of being controlled or manipulated by another person. When anger is shared by a large number of people and control is held by a faceless group ("administration" or "the owners" or "government"), the anger of powerlessness can erupt as rebellion.

As individuals, we may generate our own anger. Some psychologists believe that anger is often secondary to some other emotion. A parent feels fear when a child cannot be found; once the child's safety is assured, anger is directed at the child for having "caused" the situation. Anger may be secondary to other primary feelings, such as embarrassment or disappointment. When one experiences anger toward a friend or family member, it is advisable to consider whether or not the anger is due to some need of our own not being met. If the anger is due to some type of problem/situation, it is better to state that one is experiencing anger, and then suggest that an effort to solve the problem or situation be undertaken by all parties involved. If the anger is not used constructively, it may develop into smoldering resentment, hostility, or even hatred. **Suppression** of these feelings is likely to result eventually in an explosive verbal outpouring or even destructive physical actions.

One unfortunate example of destructive anger is domestic violence. Violence against another person is an inappropriate expression of anger. Domestic violence involves directing anger toward one's spouse or child, usually through physical assault; it also includes verbal assault and any menacing actions that arouse fear in the victim.

The problem of child abuse has received increasing attention over the past two decades. Studies of child abusers reveal that many were themselves abused as children. This is a tragic example of how inappropriate adult behavior influences the child's future patterns for emotional expression. The child who grows up in a home where violent behavior occurs perceives this pattern of family interaction as "normal." Unless that perception is changed through education and counseling, the pattern of violent behavior within the family will continue through succeeding generations.

## Fear

Fear is aroused by the threat of physical harm or danger to one's sense of security. Fear of physical harm is usually short-lived; the danger passes or the person copes with the dangerous situation. *Terror* and *panic* are terms for describing intense fear; the person who is in a state of terror or panic may flee the situation or may be immobilized by the intensity of the emotional reaction.

Fear is a natural reaction to threat or danger. It mobilizes the body for action—for fighting or fleeing a threatening situation. The body releases adrenalin, which increases the flow of blood, raises the rate of respiration, and stimulates muscle tone. If physical activity does not occur, this readiness for action may be released through "the shakes." Perhaps you have been involved in a dangerous situation, remaining calm until the danger was over and then finding yourself shaking all over or "weak in the knees." Many examples of heroic action involve physical exertion that the individual could not repeat after the excitement had subsided. The outpouring of adrenalin resulted in physical strength far beyond the person's usual abilities.

Fear can also be a reaction to mental chatter. *Worry* is fear based on thoughts about a *possible* event, such as losing one's job, losing a loved one, losing some type of property, or displeasing someone. *Anxiety* involves a higher intensity of fear than worry; it is likely to be a chronic pattern of emotional response to mental chatter. *Apprehension* and *dread* describe fear based on thoughts about some pending event that one perceives as threatening.

Fear is healthful when it is a reaction to a threatening event or situation. When self-generated through mental chatter, fear is pointless and destructive, unless it is used to plan ways to deal effectively with an expected situation. If one is apprehensive about a speech to be delivered on Monday, the best way to deal with the fear is to prepare well, practice the speech until completely comfortable with it, mentally picture oneself delivering the speech effectively, then remember to take several deep breaths before starting to deliver the speech. In the process of preparing for an effective delivery, self-confidence will replace apprehension.

## Grief

Grief is the emotional response to loss. It can range in intensity from momentary disappointment to deep sorrow that completely absorbs the individual. *Grief* describes intense feelings; *sorrow* implies grief without indicating intensity; *sadness* implies grieving of moderate intensity; *disappointment* implies a mild form of grief. While fear and anger tend to arouse one physically, grief has the opposite effect. A person who is grieving may find it difficult to perform simple tasks. The body seems to reserve energy at this time for the individual to work through the grief. It is highly desirable, even healthful, to consciously grant oneself time to grieve when loss has been experienced.

## Guilt

Guilt, as discussed here, refers to self-blaming, rather than to any legal/criminal aspects. A clinical psychology professor once referred to guilt as the "most useless emotion there is." We can feel guilty about many things: something we did or said in the past, something we now wish we had done but did not do at the proper time, words we could have spoken but didn't.

*It is impossible to change the past, so it is pointless to wallow in guilt about what cannot be changed.* Some things can be remedied by doing now what could have been done in the past. Another remedy is forgiveness—of self and others. But forgiveness is not easy; self-forgiveness is especially difficult for people who have been controlled by guilt. Those who try to control others, especially family members or lovers, may use guilt as a manipulative tool.

Striving for self-understanding and learning effective interpersonal skills are one's best protection against the damaging effects of guilt. Anyone who realizes his or her behavior is strongly influenced by guilt feelings, or that someone is controlling him or her through guilt, will find professional counseling helpful.

## FORMATION OF EMOTIONAL PATTERNS

Emotional patterns are learned through the satisfaction or distress that accompanies various life experiences. Each person's capacity to feel specific emotions may be hereditary, as indicated by the fact that newborn infants show marked differences in their responses to distress. In spite of this hereditary factor, differences in adult emotional patterns are primarily the result of learning.

The people of a baby's world—the social environment—determine to a great degree whether the baby's experiences are pleasing or distressing. Throughout infancy, childhood, and adolescence the formation of emotional patterns is influenced by the emotional expressions and behaviors of others, especially primary caregivers and family members. Later in life, the balance of successes and failures in daily living has great influence on emotional expression. Also, the reactions of other people influence the tendency to show one's feelings or attempt to hide them. Patterns for expressing feelings develop within a framework of various influences on behavior: heredity, environment, basic needs, the consequences of behavior that follow specific life experiences, and interactions with other people.

Family patterns of emotional expression influence the formation of a child's emotional patterns. Ideally, the child receives loving care from both parents and other family members, thereby learning love and trust. In these days of single-parent and two-wage-earner homes, the primary caregivers may be the staff of a childcare facility, rather than a parent. The demands of a full-time job plus homemaking responsibilities limit the amount of time and energy a parent has for parenting. And so, the child may be exposed to a hectic schedule, rushed to the child care center in the morning and picked up later in the day by an exhausted parent. At times, the balance of emotional expression may be more negative than positive. The behaviors of the adults are the behaviors the child will learn. In addition, the behaviors of childcare personnel and their beliefs about the expression of feelings are important influences on the child's developing emotional patterns.

Although these patterns are learned early in life, they are influenced later through exposure to widening circles of relatives, friends, schoolmates, coworkers, and various peer groups. As you study the remainder of this unit, be aware of your own patterns for expressing each emotion.

### For Discussion and Reflection

As you remember specific behaviors you saw in your home as a child, what emotions were likely being expressed? As a child, did you adopt the same behavior? What changes have you made in expressing emotions since your childhood?

## INDIVIDUAL DIFFERENCES IN EMOTIONAL PATTERNS

Everyone experiences negative and positive feelings. The tendency to respond to a certain type of situation with a specific emotion, the intensity of our emotional responses, the ways in which we express our feelings, the balance between positive and negative feelings, and the duration of a particular emotion are all characteristic of each person as an individual. People differ, then, in regard to the inner experience (feeling) and in the outward expression (behavior) of emotions.

Sometimes we suppress, or choose not to express, an emotion while in the situation that arouses it, then express it later; this is especially common with anger. If an emotion is extremely intense, and/or the situation that aroused the feeling is painful or unacceptable, then the emotion may be **repressed**. The memory of a traumatic event and the feelings associated with that event may both be repressed, meaning that they are not available to conscious memory. Therapy can help a person access repressed memories/feelings.

## Intensity and Frequency

Some people have the capacity for very strong feelings, whereas others seem to feel less intensely. Some people react frequently with strong emotion, even to daily annoyances such as traffic slowdowns. Other people react with strong emotion only to situations in which an intense emotional reaction is justified. Some people hide their feelings, which can result in a chronic state of stress.

## Temperament

The type of emotion (positive or negative) that a person feels most of the time is known as *temperament*. An optimistic person is one whose feelings are primarily positive; a pessimistic person is one whose feelings are primarily negative. Temperament is indicated by the way emotions are expressed: words and tone of voice, facial expression and other nonverbal behavior, and actions.

Most of us prefer the company of people who usually reflect positive emotions. Sometimes people with a pessimistic outlook find mutual satisfaction in each other, which brings to mind the saying, "Misery loves company." Some people do not show their feelings readily; their appearance is somewhat the same whether they are feeling good or bad inside. This lack of expressiveness may indicate suppression of emotion, rather than lack of feeling. It is difficult to know how such people feel, and therefore difficult to adapt your own behavior appropriately.

## Mood Swings

Another difference in individual emotional reactions is the tendency to have mood swings. Each of us has times when we are "blue"; each of us has times when we feel especially good for no apparent reason. This swing from up to down is normal. Some people, however, swing from one extreme to another or remain "down" for long periods and "up" for long periods. Extreme mood swings and/or a prolonged mood at one extreme or the other may indicate a need for professional counsel. Those whose mood swings are within normal range can learn to make full use of the times when they feel good and develop techniques for coping with periods when they feel "low."

The tendency to have long "down" periods can indicate that a person is clinically depressed. Extreme mood swings, down periods alternating with periods of high energy and productivity, may indicate that a person has bipolar disorder. The line between "normal" mood swings and those indicative of a mood disorder is not clear-cut. If the mood swings are serious enough to interfere with work, study, or family relations, then the individual should seek medical

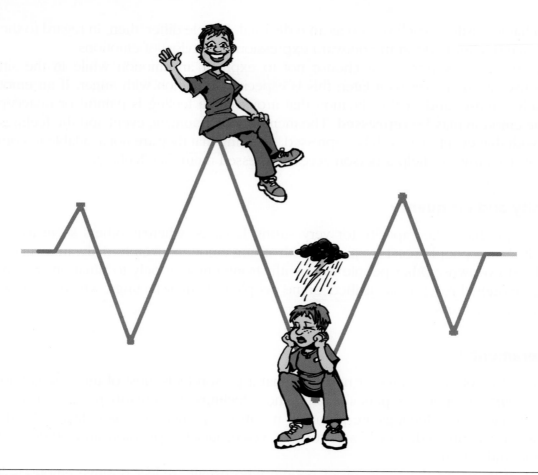

**FIGURE 7-4** Everyone experiences emotional "ups" and "downs."

evaluation. If destructive or threatening behavior occurs, the individual should have a psychiatric evaluation as soon as possible.

## GENDER DIFFERENCES IN EMOTIONS

In the past, it was generally believed that women tended to be more "emotional" than men. At one time, women may have felt that society frowned upon their showing negative emotions such as anger. Research suggests that these stereotypes do not hold true today. In a 2004 study, researchers found that men and women surveyed reported similar numbers of emotional experiences, including the experience of anger. However, men reported a higher number of positive emotional experiences, while women reported more negative ones. Though men and women reported similar rates of experiencing anger, women's anger tended to last longer, and women were more likely to feel that their anger was appropriate to the situation (Simon & Nath, 2004).

While cultural stereotypes about men and women's emotions may be unfounded, researchers continue to identify differences in the way emotions affect brain chemistry and health in men and women. For example, in a study of patients over age 65, researchers found that symptoms of depression measurably affected the cardiac function of the male patients. The same symptoms did not have a measurable cardiac effect among female patients (Chen et al., 2010). Another study found differences in the way men's and women's brain chemistry changes as they age (Kovacs et al., 2010). New information about gender differences continues to develop. As a health care professional, you should be aware of which gender differences are based on evidence and which are based upon opinions or stereotypes.

> **For Discussion and Reflection**
>
> In your experience, do you see differences in the ways men and women show emotions? If so, describe the differences you have observed.

## USING EMOTIONS CONSTRUCTIVELY

### Accentuating the Positive

Happiness is determined by how we react to both pleasant and unpleasant experiences in life. Some people use their unhappy experiences for endless conversational material. Others give only short notice to unhappy experiences, rapidly turning their attention to activities that give them satisfaction.

Each of us is free to choose between a negative and a positive outlook. We cannot eliminate all of life's disappointments, but we can refuse to let negative emotions dominate our lives. It is important, however, to consider each negative experience in terms of any lesson that can be learned. By learning from negative experiences, we become more competent for coping with life events.

### Open and Honest Communication

Owning your feelings involves stating how a situation is affecting you. Suppose you have a supervisor who frequently changes the schedule for no apparent reason. Some of your coworkers rearrange their personal plans in order to work the changed hours, but criticize the supervisor to other coworkers and the family. One person confronts the supervisor in anger and refuses to accept the changed hours. Still another worker says nothing about the change, but takes sick leave on the day for which the hours were changed. Each of these three approaches has disadvantages. None is likely to alter the supervisor's habit of changing hours on short notice. A cooperative approach is preferable; but first, the supervisor must become aware that there is a problem.

Suppose you approach the supervisor at an appropriate time and calmly state, "I have a problem when my hours are changed. I have to make different arrangements for care of my children." You have made statements of fact, using "I" to describe the effect of the schedule changes. This is "open and honest" communication. No accusation has been made; no blame has been laid on the supervisor. The climate is right for a discussion of the problem and a cooperative approach to finding a solution.

Perhaps there is a good reason for the change in hours. It is easier to accept an undesirable situation if you know that it exists because of unavoidable circumstances, rather than because of someone's poor planning. Perhaps the supervisor was not aware of your childcare needs and therefore was unaware of the inconvenience created by a change in schedule. Regardless of how the supervisor responds, you would have diffused any anger that was felt; it will not erupt

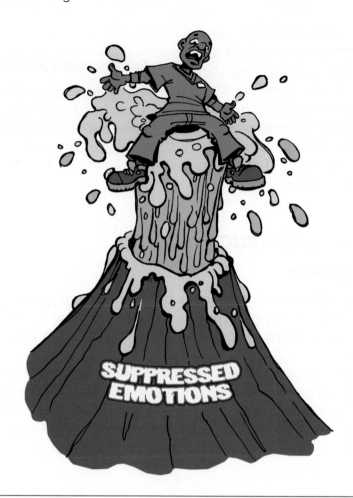

**FIGURE 7-5 Suppressed emotions can lead to a blow-up.**

later in an uncontrolled outburst of feeling. Even more important, the anger will not be displaced onto patients, coworkers, or members of the family who did nothing to cause the anger.

This approach is called an "I-statement," meaning that *feelings* are expressed in a statement beginning with "I" rather than a "you-statement" that accuses or blames the other person. Compare the suggested "I-statement" with an accusative statement: "You are always changing the hours! You are forcing me to change my babysitting arrangement! Why can't you make up a schedule and stick to it?" These statements would result in an angry supervisor. Certainly being on the defensive would not put the supervisor in a problem-solving frame of mind.

"I-statements" are valuable as a means of expressing both positive and negative feelings. This technique can lead to improved interpersonal relations. Consider the possible effect of the following statements:

- "You always keep me waiting."
- "I really get angry when I have to wait."
- "I was disappointed when I arrived and you were not here yet."
- "You are 15 minutes late."

Obviously, the "you-statements" put the other person on the defensive, may create angry feelings toward you, or may arouse feelings of guilt. On the other hand, the "I-statements" simply state how you feel. The other person cannot deny you your feelings. There is no basis for argument. And you have expressed the feeling verbally and are no longer burdened with anger.

Open and honest communication of positive feelings will greatly improve relations with others. All of us like to hear good things. Open and honest communication is especially important as a means of dealing with negative emotions. The following sections deal with approaches to handling specific negative emotional states.

## Dealing with Anger

Negative emotions must be dealt with constructively, or they will have destructive effects. When inner tension builds up from anger, this tension needs release. If a patient makes you angry, you cannot throw a bedpan or physically attack the patient. It is not desirable to "blow up" at your supervisor; nor is it fair for you to bottle up your anger until you get home, and then let it loose on your family. (This is called "displaced anger.") Perhaps the tension built up from your anger can help you mow the grass, repair that broken gate, or whip up a cake. In other words, use energy generated by anger in some type of constructive physical activity. While you are in the situation, use "I-statements" as appropriate or ask questions that will help you understand the other person's views or the circumstances. As you gain understanding, your anger may subside.

Once you are out of the situation in which you became angry, try to understand the reason for your anger. Is the reaction related to old resentments? Do you display a pattern of becoming angry with this person or in this type of situation? Were you frustrated in your efforts to meet some need? Did you have expectations that the other person failed to meet? Were you treated unfairly (in your opinion)?

If you still feel anger, there are several techniques for safely diffusing the feelings.

- Talk with someone who knows how to listen. Just talking about the situation—the facts and also your feelings—can provide effective release.

- If you cannot talk to someone about it, set up a recorder, visualize it as the person at whom you are angry, and tell it exactly how you feel. Then, listen to a playback. Continue until your anger has been released. (Don't forget to erase the recording!)

- Another technique for working off feelings is to "punch out" a pillow, preferably a large, firm one. The physical activity provides for release of energy generated by the anger.

- Physical activity, such as riding a bike, walking, or dancing, can also release energy and calm anger. Once you are calm, you can make a rational decision about whether you need to discuss the situation with others or seek a solution.

Many therapists consider that the most effective technique for dealing with anger is forgiveness. It is difficult to forgive someone who has hurt you or cheated you. Yet the anger you carry with you is actually harming *you*—your health and well-being—rather than the one who is the object of your anger. Learning to forgive may be one of life's most difficult lessons. But the power of another person to harm you psychologically is diminished when you are able to forgive. Forgiveness of those who are deceased is just as important as forgiveness of those who are still living.

Self-forgiveness is especially important. It is only human to make mistakes. We all have regrets about things we did or didn't do, about what we said or didn't say. Some matters can be corrected by making amends toward the other person. If the other person is deceased, then the only recourse is self-forgiveness. It is desirable that we learn from the past, however, so that new regrets do not accumulate.

## Dealing with Fear

To deal with fear effectively, we must first acknowledge the fear. We all encounter situations that arouse mild fear: a test, an oral report, returning to care for the patient who was critical of you yesterday, reporting to the supervisor that you broke a piece of equipment. In some situations the fear is justified, and the only recourse is to deal with the situation as effectively as possible. Sometimes mentally rehearsing the event in advance as a successful experience prepares you to deal with the situation with less fear.

Sometimes a person's fear is out of proportion to the expected event; fear tends to magnify the dreaded aspects of the situation. Fear can interfere with realistic thinking about a problem, but the problem-solving approach often reveals that there is an acceptable solution. Once a solution is apparent, fear tends to decrease.

**Phobias**  Some people have an intense fear, known as a phobia, regarding something that most people do not find fearful (i.e., heights, being closed up in a small space such as an elevator, flying in an airplane). These fears are "abnormal" when they interfere with daily activities or cause the individual to take extreme measures to avoid the feared experience. Psychotherapy often results in the identification of some past traumatic event that the person had repressed, so that it was not available to conscious memory. In severe cases, the phobia requires a process of systematic desensitization, which may be done by various licensed mental health practitioners.

**Post-Traumatic Stress Disorder**  A more serious example of fear-related memory is known as post-traumatic stress disorder (PTSD). This is manifested by panic attacks, in which the individual relives a traumatic experience through sudden flashbacks or nightmares. This disorder came to the attention of the public after many Vietnam veterans had difficulty adapting to civilian life following discharge from military service. PTSD can have a severe disabling effect if left untreated.

PTSD is experienced by many people who have been involved in a serious accident or experience a frightening event such as a flood, hurricane, or tornado. For several weeks or months after such an experience, the individual may relive the experience when trying to go to sleep, or wake up suddenly in a cold sweat with rapid heartbeat, clammy skin, and uncontrollable shaking—a panic attack. Usually this tendency passes after several weeks, as physical healing occurs. If not, the individual should have professional counseling; it requires skilled professional intervention to desensitize survivors of traumatic events and free them from recurrent panic attacks.

## Dealing with Grief

Grief is an emotion that lasts over a period of time. It may take weeks or months to work through the intense feelings and readjust one's life pattern. Whenever a loss occurs, permit yourself to grieve. When feelings of guilt are associated with grief, professional counseling may be needed to work through both emotions; such a combination is difficult to handle alone.

# EMOTIONS AND BEHAVIOR

Emotions do exist, and they do affect us physically, psychologically, and mentally. To deny these feelings is a form of suppression. Suppressed emotions will have their effects sooner or later, through "blowing up" in an uncontrolled display of emotion, illness, poor coping mechanisms, or poor interpersonal relations.

Self-control is a constructive way of using emotions, rather than not showing emotions. Self-control is a learned behavioral pattern for expressing feelings in socially acceptable ways while dealing with a situation intelligently. The following guidelines can be used to increase self-control:

- Express your feelings at the time they are experienced; if for some reason that is not appropriate, express the feelings as soon as possible in a "safe" setting.

- Own your feelings; use "I-statements" rather than accusative "you-statements" in your interactions with other people.

- Acknowledge (do not deny to yourself or others) that you experienced a particular emotion in a specific situation.

- Ask yourself, "Is this situation important enough to me to justify these feelings?" If the answer is "No," turn your attention to other matters. If "Yes," then deal with the situation effectively, perhaps using some of the guidelines that follow.

- Work with others to clarify a problem and find a solution acceptable to all—a "win-win" situation.

- If you begin to experience anger, ask questions about the situation, then *listen* to the answers; better understanding of the other person's point of view may dissipate your anger.

- When you become aware of fear or apprehension, ask yourself whether or not you are in *real* danger. If the answer is "Yes," take appropriate action; if "No," analyze the basis for your feelings and take preventive action if needed.

- Use problem solving to deal with a situation—present or future—so that you feel competent to find a solution and no longer need to feel apprehensive.

- Take responsibility for your feelings and your behavior; avoid blaming others for "causing" your feelings.

- Avoid negative mental chatter. If your thoughts involve future possible events and you become anxious, realize that mental chatter, not a real event, is the source of your anxiety.

- If you have a particular phobia, seek professional help so you can free yourself from this unrealistic fear. Once you have exposed the basis for your phobia, it no longer has the power to control your behavior.

- Use and enjoy humor; be willing to laugh at yourself for getting upset over something trivial. Defuse a tense situation, as appropriate, with a humorous comment or anecdote.

- If you are still "worked up" after a situation that aroused strong emotions, use the energy for some type of constructive physical activity, such as mowing the grass, working out, running, or walking.

- Allow yourself to grieve for any loss you have experienced.

- Become aware of the events of your daily life that give you pleasure and allow time at the end of the day to enjoy thoughts of these good experiences.
- Love yourself. Take credit for your strengths, your competence, your willingness to grow; forgive yourself for being less than perfect.

The foregoing suggestions are intended to help you understand yourself and your emotions better. As you become more open and honest with yourself and others about your feelings, you will have a favorable effect on others. As you learn to replace impulsive emotional behavior with actions based on reasoning, you will be free to control situations more effectively. As you develop greater sensitivity to the feelings of others, you are more likely to react appropriately to their behavior.

Emotions are somewhat like a chain reaction. Hostile behavior by one person tends to bring out hostility in others. Aggressive behavior by one person brings about defensive behavior in others. When someone else expresses a negative emotion, do not allow that behavior to arouse a negative emotion in you. Instead, maintain a positive feeling and show your concern with such statements as, "I sense that you are angry" or "I sense that you are really feeling down today." This approach is called "reflecting," meaning that you act as a mirror for the person's feelings. Reflecting indicates that you are "tuned in" to what that person is experiencing, that you care, and that you are giving that person your full attention.

Although you can choose how to express your feelings most of the time, you cannot *control* the feelings or behavior of another person. However, your behavior can *influence* another person's behavior. It requires practice to develop sensitivity to the feelings of others. We can best adapt our own behavior and respond effectively to another person only if we are aware of the other person's emotional state.

As you work with patients and their families, strive to understand their feelings. Notice behavior that may indicate fear, anger, or grief. Avoid adding to such feelings by your own behavior. Take a little more time with the fearful patient, giving effective reassurances as best you can. Acknowledge the grieving person's right to sorrow, recognizing that this emotion needs expression and cannot be worked through quickly. Grant your patient the right to be angry in certain situations; instead of becoming defensive, listen. Then try to resolve the problem that aroused the patient's anger.

Through continuing effort, you can become a health care professional who practices the *art of human relations* along with the technical skills of your field.

## ACTIVITIES

1. Consider how you are affected by anger and how you usually express it:
   a. Can you think clearly when you are angry?
   b. Do you usually express your anger *verbally* by:

      saying something you later regret?

      calling the other person a "dirty name"?

      raising your voice? shouting or screaming?

      threatening to do something the other person would not like?

    c.  Do you usually express your anger *physically* by:

        throwing things or kicking something?

        slamming a door?

        attacking the other person with your fists?

        slapping the other person?

    d.  Do you try to express your anger, but burst into tears?

    e.  Do you usually leave a situation when you become angry?

    f.  Do you manage to appear completely calm even though you are seething with anger inside?

    g.  Do you express your anger later, "taking it out" on someone other than the person at whom you are angry?

    h.  Do you believe that other people or events *cause* your anger?

2.  Consider how you are affected by sadness and how you usually express it:

    a.  Can you think clearly when you are unhappy?

    b.  Can you concentrate when you are unhappy?

    c.  Is it difficult to do things you know you should do?

    d.  Is it difficult to make decisions?

    e.  Have you ever made a decision while feeling sad, then later realized you did not use good judgment?

    f.  Do you believe another person or some situation is the cause of your unhappiness?

3.  Do you tend to feel anger toward those you believe caused your unhappiness? What are some alternatives to holding this anger?

4.  Your spouse or significant other has just come home and states that he or she and a colleague "really got into it today." You sense his or her anger and want to talk about what happened. Instead, he or she changes clothes and goes out for a five-mile jog. What do you think of this behavior?

5.  Mary Ann is 17 years old. Her mother died the day before her 17th birthday. Mary Ann occasionally states, somewhat proudly, "I didn't even cry." You know that she and her mother were very close. What do you think of Mary Ann's behavior?

6.  You are assigned to Mr. J. today. You enter his room and say "Good morning" in your most cheerful voice. Mr. J. answers in an angry tone, "What's good about it?" What would be an effective response? What are some possible reasons for Mr. J. responding in such a way? How would you feel about Mr. J.?

7.  Mrs. K. is scheduled for heart surgery. She is cheerful, never has a complaint, and tries to be helpful to the other patients. Your coworker says, "Mrs. K. is certainly unusual. She is not at all worried about her surgery." Do you agree with your coworker? Explain your answer.

8. Your supervisor calls you to the office and angrily says, "I'm changing the hours. You will have to work Saturday and Sunday." You have no plans, but it is your turn to have a weekend off. You become angry and say you will not work, even if it means being fired. Later that day you learn that two members of the staff are sick and one has been called out of town because of family problems. Describe the supervisor's probable emotional state when she called you into the office. List five ways you could have responded that might have prevented the unpleasant scene.

9. Consider each of the following statements. Be prepared to discuss each in terms of possible effects on the listener's emotional patterns:

   a. "You must not cry. You're a big boy now!"

   b. "If you do that again, I'll shut you in the closet."

   c. "You're a bad boy!"

   d. "It's bad to hate someone. You must love everyone."

   e. "My friend had that same operation you're going to have. She had a terrible time and hasn't been the same since the operation."

   f. "Oh, you don't have a thing to worry about" (to a patient scheduled for surgery).

   g. "Shame on you! I expect you to get all A's."

   h. "How dare you stomp your foot! You're a little girl; you must be sweet."

10. Your child usually goes to his room whenever his older brother teases him. What does this mean, in terms of his pattern for expressing feelings? Now that you've noted his behavior, what should you do?

## REFERENCES AND SUGGESTED READINGS

Chapman, Alexander & Gratz, Kim. (2015). *The dialectical behavior therapy skills workbook for anger: using DBT mindfulness and emotion regulation skills to manage anger.* Oakland, CA: New Harbinger.

Chen, His-Chung et al. (2010, March). Gender differences in the relationship between depression and cardiac autonomic function among community elderly. *International Journal of Geriatric Psychiatry, 25*(3), 314–322.

Kovács, Zsolt et al. (2010, April). Gender- and age-dependent changes in nucleoside levels in the cerebral cortex and white matter of the human brain. *Brain Research Bulletin, 81*(6), 579–584.

Selye, Hans. (1987). Stress without distress. *Psychological Bulletin, 131*(6), 925–972.

Simon, Robin, & Nath, Leda. (2004, March). Gender and emotion in the United States: Do men and women differ in self-reports of feelings and expressive behavior? *American Journal of Sociology, 109*(5), 1137–1176.

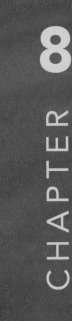

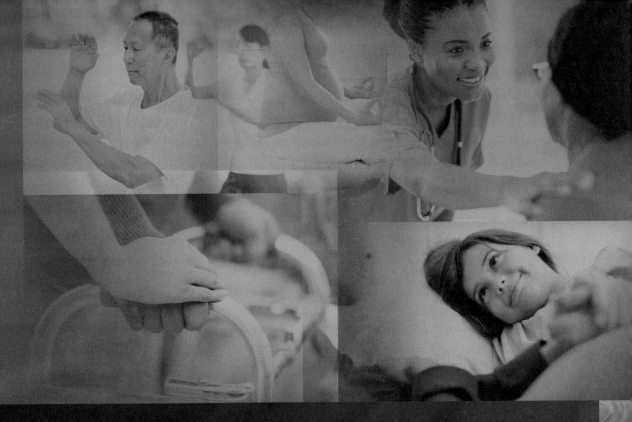

# Adjustment and Patterns of Behavior

## OBJECTIVES

After completing this chapter, you should be able to:

- Contrast characteristics of a person who is well adjusted with characteristics of a person who is poorly adjusted.
- Explain why poor adjustment can be a vicious cycle.
- Discuss strategies for improving adjustment and for adapting to a new situation.
- Describe how one's emotional patterns influence adjustment.

## KEY TERMS

Adjustment

Burnout

Hassle

Vicious cycle

**Adjustment** refers to how well an individual has learned to deal with life situations. Each person's adjustment is variable, depending upon circumstances. A person may be well adjusted most of the time, but poorly adjusted during a period when there is a serious problem. Some people are poorly adjusted most of the time. They have not learned to deal with ordinary life situations effectively.

## GOOD ADJUSTMENT

A person who is well adjusted deals effectively with problems and finds satisfaction in living. A well-adjusted person has developed the habits and skills needed to solve common problems and has developed patterns of behavior that satisfy basic needs. This type of person is well prepared to weather a crisis and reestablish good adjustment within a reasonable period of time.

## POOR ADJUSTMENT

A person who is poorly adjusted is not living a full life. Such a person feels dissatisfied much of the time. Actually, the poorly adjusted person may not have any more problems than a well-adjusted person. *The difference is that the poorly adjusted person has not learned to cope with obstacles or effectively deal with everyday problems of living.*

The biggest obstacle for the poorly adjusted person is the poor adjustment itself. The habits, attitudes, emotional reactions, and behavior patterns that are a part of poor adjustment create additional problems for the individual. Poor adjustment is a **vicious cycle**. Ineffective behavior often creates additional problems that the individual handles with more ineffective behavior. For that reason, poor adjustment can be modified only if the individual learns to deal with life situations more effectively.

## EFFECTIVE BEHAVIOR VERSUS INEFFECTIVE BEHAVIOR

The key to adjustment is learning to recognize ineffective behavior and replacing it with another behavior that gets better results. The person who is willing to change can improve adjustment. The person who is unwilling or unable to change behavior patterns will not improve adjustment.

Change is a test of one's ability to adjust. If familiar habits are used in new situations, the results may be quite different from results in the old situation. Change is an opportunity for growth that calls for conscious evaluation of habitual behavior. Ineffective habits should be discarded and new, more effective ones established. To acquire new friends, to fit into a new community, to succeed in a new job, and to do well in a course of study all require that some old habits be discarded and that some new ones be developed.

Larissa and Kay are two high school juniors enrolled in the health occupations course. Both are new in the school, faced with a new and unfamiliar setting. Kay wants desperately to be popular; when her new classmates ignore her, she feels resentment. She becomes critical of the class leaders, looking for opportunities to make uncomplimentary remarks about them. Her classmates soon tire of her negativity. They do not understand that Kay gets some relief from inner discomfort by criticizing those she envies. Kay is using ineffective behavior. Criticizing others makes her feel better momentarily, but it interferes with her forming new friendships.

In the meantime, Larissa decides to broaden her interests. She becomes more active in school affairs, helping with the newspaper and joining several clubs. Each new activity leads to new friends for Larissa. She is also learning new skills and acquiring new outlooks through these various activities. Larissa is using effective behavior to improve her adjustment. She took action to adapt to her new situation and that action proved to be effective. Larissa's goal was to become comfortable in the new situation and broaden her range of interests; gaining many new friends was only one of several benefits.

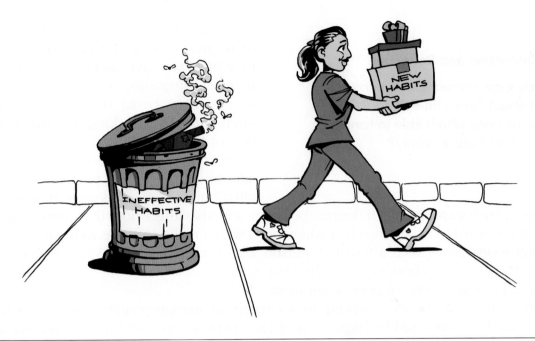

**FIGURE 8-1 Improving your adjustment requires giving up ineffective habits.**

Julian is a student in the surgical technician program. He knows the procedures must be performed correctly, but his performance often includes errors. The instructor has talked with Julian about his performance. Every error and every problem, according to Julian, was the fault of someone else: the circulating nurse, another student, whoever set up the tray or pack, some member of the surgical team. Julian does not learn from his mistakes or from the instructor/student conference, because he is unable or unwilling to admit that he can make a mistake. He has not learned to take responsibility for his actions, and he denies the consequences of his errors by claiming "It wasn't my fault." Unless Julian changes this pattern of behavior, he will have problems throughout life. He will not be acceptable as a health care professional because he would not be a safe practitioner.

## EMOTIONS AND ADJUSTMENT

Emotions are a major influence on one's adjustment. A person who experiences positive emotions several times a day is likely to have better adjustment than one who frequently experiences negative emotions. Sometimes the emotion one experiences is a matter of choice. For example, you drop your keys as you try to unlock the car door. You feel annoyed as you pick them up and try again to fit the key into the lock. Somehow the keys slip out of your fingers and fall to the ground a second time. At this point, you can utter a string of four-letter words to express your anger and exasperation. Or, you could pick the keys up again, laughingly comment that you seem to have butterfingers today, then pay close attention to getting the key into the lock successfully.

Everyone's daily experiences include some difficulties and some positive experiences. At the end of the day, one person remembers a number of these "good experiences" and gives little thought to the things that did not go well. Another person may finish the day feeling angry about several problem situations that occurred, and have little or no conscious

**For Discussion and Reflection**

Do you know someone who becomes upset about "every little thing"? Do you know someone who is able to handle almost any situation calmly?

awareness of any good experiences. Each of us may *choose* the type of experience to which we give most of our attention. In most situations, we may either choose to be angry or to deal with a situation unemotionally, working toward a resolution of the difficulty.

Fear is also a powerful influence on adjustment. A person who lives in fear of what "might happen" is expecting bad things to happen. Such expectations influence behavior and also affect how that person perceives events. It is normal to experience fear when faced with a real threat; the well-adjusted person reacts appropriately to such a threat. A person who is chronically anxious, however, is living with fear that arises from negative thinking, rather than any real threat. Habitual negative thinking represents a state of poor adjustment.

Sadness also may be experienced appropriately or inappropriately. Each of us has life experiences that arouse sad feelings. Each of us is exposed to world news revealing terrible things happening, events that we are powerless to change. Someone who is truly grieved by conditions in a third-world country might join the Peace Corps and devote two or more years to try to improve those conditions. Many people address their prayers to such situations; persons who meditate may focus a daily meditation on peaceful resolution of a specific problem, wherever it exists. Others might feel real empathy for the victims of some distant tragedy and send a contribution to an organization that is providing help. Others may feel a brief period of sadness and then shift their attention to their own affairs. These reactions indicate healthful use of sadness.

A person who chooses to focus on tragic events may remain in a sad state, indulge in "Ain't it awful" talk, yet take no action to correct the situation. This focus of attention on tragic events allows sadness to interfere with adjustment. As with anger and fear, a person can *choose* the extent to which sadness is allowed to affect one's feelings overall.

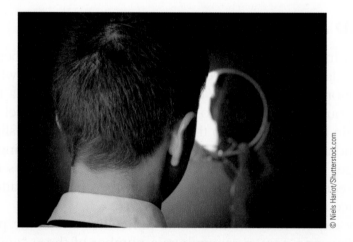

© Niels Hariot/Shutterstock.com

**FIGURE 8-2 When you look in the mirror, do you see a person who finds satisfaction in life, or one who focuses on negative experiences?**

## DAILY HASSLES

**Hassle** denotes "any event that causes you to feel irritated, annoyed, frustrated, fearful, or angry." How one copes with "daily hassles," or minor frustrations, is a reflection of one's adjustment. However, one's usual state of adjustment is also a factor in how well one copes with "daily hassles":

My kids' rooms are a mess.

I can't find the keys.

Traffic was awful.

I had a flat tire.

Hassles like these are inevitable, but we can choose whether to take them in stride or to become upset about each one.

Box 8-1, "Hassles in My Life," is designed to help you identify hassles in your life. Box 8-2, "Satisfactions in My Life," permits you to identify the "good" things that occur. You choose which type of events receive most of your attention, and therefore which type of emotions dominate your daily life.

---

### BOX 8-1

### Hassles in My Life

**Instructions:** In the following list circle (1) for each event you experienced yesterday and (2) for each event you experienced during the past week or month. Substitute appropriate words (e.g., "my glasses" for "keys") to adapt a statement to your situation. If a statement just does not apply to you, leave it blank.

| | | |
|---|---|---|
| **1.** I couldn't find my keys. | 1 | 2 |
| **2.** My neighbor's dog barked all night. | 1 | 2 |
| **3.** My sister called to talk about her problems. | 1 | 2 |
| **4.** There's no way I can pay all my bills this month. | 1 | 2 |
| **5.** My spouse is thrilled with our new sound system; I'm not, because our charge card is now "maxed out." | 1 | 2 |
| **6.** I had to make a difficult decision. | 1 | 2 |
| **7.** My coworkers take extended breaks and I end up doing more than my share of the work. | 1 | 2 |
| **8.** One of my clients was especially unpleasant, even though I had given him extra time. | 1 | 2 |
| **9.** I am having a plumbing problem (again!). | 1 | 2 |
| **10.** I'm having a really bad hair day. | 1 | 2 |

*(Continues...)*

*(Box 8-1 Continued)*

| | | | |
|---|---|---|---|
| **11.** | I tossed and turned all night. (I went to bed really sleepy, then couldn't go to sleep; or, I woke up at 2 a.m. and couldn't get back to sleep.) | 1 | 2 |
| **12.** | My car wouldn't start. | 1 | 2 |
| **13.** | I locked my keys in the car. | 1 | 2 |
| **14.** | Traffic was terrible this morning. | 1 | 2 |
| **15.** | The news is full of crime reports; I just don't feel safe anymore. | 1 | 2 |
| **16.** | There's a rumor that administration plans to "downsize" the patient care staff. | 1 | 2 |
| **17.** | Even on my day off, I just couldn't relax. | 1 | 2 |
| **18.** | Someone (insert name or title) took advantage of me; I'm afraid to confront him or her. | 1 | 2 |
| **19.** | Someone (insert name) smokes too much; I'm afraid he or she will develop lung cancer. | 1 | 2 |
| **20.** | It's harder and harder to please my spouse; he or she complained all through breakfast this morning. | 1 | 2 |

Total your score for each column. Note that items 1–14 deal primarily with anger and frustration; items 15–20 are more closely related to fear and anxiety.

Now follow the same procedure with Box 8-2 to identify some "good" experiences in your life.

## BOX 8-2

### Satisfactions in My Life

**Instructions:** In the following list circle (1) for each event you experienced yesterday and (2) for those you experienced during the past week or month. Substitute appropriate words to adapt statements to your situation. If a statement does not apply to you, leave it blank.

| | | | |
|---|---|---|---|
| **1.** | I had a good night's sleep. | 1 | 2 |
| **2.** | My supervisor complimented me on my work. | 1 | 2 |
| **3.** | I am scheduled to be off on my birthday. | 1 | 2 |
| **4.** | I found a good buy on my family's favorite food. | 1 | 2 |
| **5.** | I enjoyed talking with a new coworker during break. | 1 | 2 |
| **6.** | One of my patients said, "You are the best!" | 1 | 2 |
| **7.** | When I reconciled my checkbook with my bank statement, I found a $50 deposit I had failed to enter. | 1 | 2 |
| **8.** | My energy level has been up lately. | 1 | 2 |

*(Continues...)*

*(Box 8-2 Continued)*

| | | |
|---|---|---|
| **9.** I stopped smoking. | 1 | 2 |
| **10.** I ate less fat (sugar, snacks, caffeine). | 1 | 2 |
| **11.** I exercised for 20 minutes. | 1 | 2 |
| **12.** I managed my time so that I had free time in the evening. | 1 | 2 |
| **13.** I included some recreation in my schedule. | 1 | 2 |
| **14.** I spent time with friends and really enjoyed it. | 1 | 2 |
| **15.** I confronted (insert name) about (insert issue) and, to my surprise, we had a very satisfying discussion. | 1 | 2 |
| **16.** I weighed myself this morning; I have lost 3 pounds. | 1 | 2 |
| **17.** I was able to relax and enjoy my day off. | 1 | 2 |
| **18.** My neighbor got rid of his barking dog. | 1 | 2 |
| **19.** My sister liked the birthday present I gave her. | 1 | |
| **20.** My child's grades have improved and he or she likes the new teacher. | 1 | 2 |
| **21.** I didn't think I could handle an assignment, but I did and was complimented on my work. | 1 | 2 |
| **22.** I received a favorable work review (grade). | 1 | 2 |

Total the two columns. Now, compare your "hassles" scores with your "satisfaction" scores. Which score is higher? Was it easier to recognize hassles than satisfactions? Or were the satisfactions more recognizable? Do you tend to focus more on your satisfactions or hassles?

## IMPROVING ADJUSTMENT

How can you improve adjustment? The following guidelines can be useful in directing your efforts to improve adjustment. First, focus on one or two of the guidelines until you have made significant progress, then select one or two others. If you attempt to focus on all of the guidelines at the same time, you are likely to become discouraged.

- Find patterns of behavior that satisfy basic needs.
- Assume conscious control of your behavior.
- Use problem solving to find the best possible solution for a problem situation instead of acting impulsively.
- Use emotions constructively. When appropriate, express feelings at the time they are experienced.
- Evaluate your behavior in a specific situation. Was the outcome favorable for you? What other possible behavior on your part would have been appropriate? Is it likely that another behavior would have been more effective?
- Self-evaluate in a constructive sense. Look for ways to improve but avoid feelings of guilt or inadequacy.
- Select appropriate goals in terms of "all that I can be" and plan how you will reach these goals.

If you can achieve reasonably good adjustment in your usual life situation, then you will be prepared for the challenge of adapting to new situations and dealing with the occasional crisis situations that are an unavoidable part of life.

## Maintaining a Healthful Lifestyle

The suggestions just listed for improving your state of adjustment are somewhat broad and require conscious effort over a period of time. Steps for improving your daily habits can be taken immediately, and these daily habits definitely contribute to one's state of adjustment. A diet that consists largely of junk food, the use of addictive substances, lack of balance in work and play, lack of exercise, and inadequate sleep can all interfere with good adjustment. To feel and function at your best, include the following habits in your lifestyle:

- Eat several servings each day of fresh vegetables and fruit, some eaten raw.
- Drink at least eight cups of water each day.
- Exercise regularly.
- Avoid harmful and addictive substances.
- Participate regularly in recreational activities that help you release stress and regenerate your energies.
- Allow adequate time for sleep.

It is tempting to dismiss these habits by saying "With my schedule, I don't have time to cook fresh food, exercise, or sleep a full eight hours." However, most people find that when they make self-care a higher priority than television, social media, or talking and texting on the phone, they are able to make small, positive changes that increase their sense of well-being and their ability to maintain a state of good adjustment.

## The Role of Joy and Laughter

The therapeutic effects of laughter came to the attention of the public and the health community with the publication in 1979 of Norman Cousins's book, *Anatomy of an Illness as Perceived by the Patient*. Cousins described how laughter had helped him recover from a debilitating illness for which there was no known cure. Since Cousins was an internationally famous journalist, his story had such a high level of credibility that it had an impact on health care delivery. Within a year or two, conferences were being held to teach health care professionals about the value of humor and laughter.

Research since that time has revealed that there are physical, mental, and emotional benefits of laughter and joyous experiences. The physical benefits include improved circulation, higher oxygen levels, enhanced immune functions, and increased levels of hormones that influence how one copes with stress. Laughter is now acknowledged as a factor in health, whether for the purpose

**For Discussion and Reflection**

How much time each day do you spend on social media, watching television, or "on your phone"? How much time do you spend each day preparing healthy meals, exercising, and sleeping?

of maintaining health, managing stress, or coping with illness. Some simple techniques for purposely putting more laughter into your day include:

- Look in the mirror at least once a day and tell the image you see there to laugh with you; even that moment of forced laughter will be beneficial.
- At least once a day, remember some funny incident or joyful experience; take a few minutes to laugh or experience joyful feelings.
- Place a keepsake from some fun or joyful experience where you can see it and enjoy a laugh or feelings of joy, even if only for a moment.
- Share funny experiences with other people; when you make them laugh, you also laugh and everyone benefits.
- Choose friends who like to laugh; it is hard to be "down" when you are around people who laugh often.
- Seek out humor that you can share with others.

## Avoiding Burnout

Every health care professional is at risk for developing burnout syndrome. **Burnout** is a state of deterioration that affects an individual physically, mentally, and emotionally. It develops gradually over a period of weeks, months, or years of living or working in a high-stress situation, during which the individual may not eat properly, gets minimal rest, has few opportunities for recreation and self-renewal, experiences much frustration, receives little emotional support from others, and/or ignores signs of illness in order to keep going. Anyone with a tendency to be a "workaholic" is risking burnout. Some common signs of burnout include the following:

- A conscientious worker begins to make errors, take longer to perform tasks, or fail to complete assigned work.
- The worker feels increasing frustration and loss of interest in work.
- The worker may believe that his or her efforts are unappreciated and develop a negative attitude about the job.
- Fulfilling job responsibilities becomes increasingly difficult.
- Coworkers may notice increased irritability or complaints.
- Physical symptoms include fatigue, frequent minor illnesses, gastrointestinal disorders, headaches, or various aches and pains.
- There may be increased consumption of caffeine, tobacco, or alcohol or a tendency to seek relief through drugs, either legal or illegal.

The causes of burnout may lie within the individual—unhealthful life habits, failure to take responsibility for one's own well-being, a dedication to the job that results in too much work and not enough self-care, and failure to use effective stress management strategies. Often the causes of burnout are within the work environment—stressors such as uncomfortable physical conditions, unpleasant working relations, supervisor or management behavior, lack of encouragement and emotional support, and lack of recognition or reward for work done well. In

**For Discussion and Reflection**

Have you experienced the symptoms of burnout described? To what extent did your working conditions contribute to your experience? Your personal habits?

many cases, the causes of burnout may be a combination of personal habits and working conditions.

The best protection is a lifestyle that includes all of the above suggestions for improving adjustment plus the regular use of effective stress management techniques. If the stressors of the work setting affect numerous workers, management should eliminate as many stressful conditions as possible. If work conditions cannot be improved and the worker is not able to deal effectively with the resulting stress, then it is time to seek employment elsewhere!

## Adapting to New Situations

When a change occurs in your life situation—for better or worse—modify some of your patterns of behavior in order to achieve a state of good adjustment in the new situation. If the change is minor, you may adapt with little awareness of stress. If the change is great, however, you may go through a stressful period before you achieve adjustment. You may even be very unhappy at first, wishing that you could return to the old situation. As you successfully adapt, you will gradually begin to feel comfortable in the new situation.

The degree of disruption a change causes in one's usual pattern of living is dependent upon the type of change. Some changes you are likely to encounter include job changes, moving to a new neighborhood, a change of supervisors, a new administration in your place of employment, and changes in operational procedures and policies. A major change all of us have to face at some time is the loss of relatives and friends.

In general, adapting to change requires acceptance of the new situation and a conscious effort to adapt. If the change involves new tasks and new people:

1. Study the situation carefully.
2. Observe the behavior of others.
3. Learn the policies and regulations of the new situation.
4. Consciously adopt behaviors that are appropriate for that situation.

If you find that the new situation requires you to follow procedures that are unsafe (for you or your patients) or are unethical, you have a conflict: you can lower your standards and console yourself with the thought, "I'm just doing what everybody else is doing"; you can use appropriate procedures to try to change practices, a risky approach for a new employee; or you can leave the situation.

There is also the possibility that the new situation has more rigorous standards than your previous position. In that case, you have a challenge: to improve your performance in order to be acceptable to your new coworkers and supervisors. Willingness to learn and to improve performance will earn favorable evaluations for you; rebelling against the higher standards will mark you as an unsatisfactory employee.

A behavior that interferes with adapting to a new situation is clinging to the old situation. Comparing the old situation to the new, especially when you indicate your preference for the old, reveals that you do not yet accept the present situation. One sure way to antagonize new

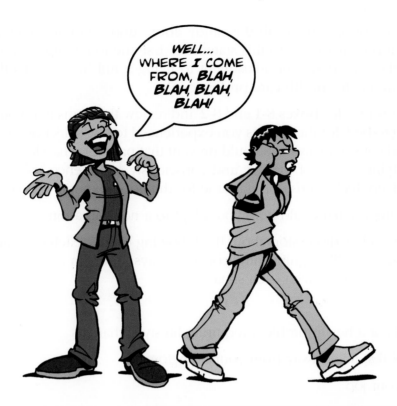

**FIGURE 8-3** Holding on to old situations indicates poor adjustment to the present situation.

coworkers is to tell them repeatedly how you did things on your previous job. This behavior indicates poor adjustment to one's present job situation.

## Adapting to the Role of Health Care Professional

You are already aware that becoming a health care professional requires certain modifications in behavior. Perhaps you have had a job in which you were allowed to do many different tasks and accept as much responsibility as you were able to handle. As a health care professional you will have a well-defined role. You may find it annoying to have limitations placed on your role, especially if others perform tasks you believe you can do. Performance within one's defined role is necessary within the health field; to exceed that role may endanger a patient and also may have legal implications. You are already aware of the change you must make in giving health care suggestions to your friends. Refrain from any advice or actions that appear to be efforts to diagnose or prescribe. Essentially, adjustment to being a health care professional requires knowing one's role and performing within it, while also accepting and abiding by the code of ethics appropriate to that role.

## ACTIVITIES

1. Describe observable behaviors that may indicate poor adjustment. Do you display any of these behaviors?

2. Describe observable behaviors that indicate a person is relatively well adjusted. Do you display any of these behaviors?

3. Your classmate says, "I think all this study about understanding yourself is a waste of time." Write a brief response to this statement. Use the following as a basis for your reasoning: (a) the importance of adjustment to living a full life and (b) the importance of self-understanding for health care professionals.

4. Refer to your scores for Boxes 8-1 and 8-2 and review the items that you marked. Tonight before going to bed, list the hassles you experienced today; select one particularly annoying event and consider ways you could prevent that particular hassle from recurring. Now, list the satisfying events of the day and consciously experience "good feelings." As you drift off to sleep, feel a sense of gratitude for the good experiences you had today.

5. Describe strategies that could help you adapt to a new situation.

6. Participate in a class discussion about the following events, each of which has the potential to change one's life significantly; consider ways a person could experience personal growth through dealing with each situation.

    a. Divorce

    b. Diagnosis of a health problem requiring lifestyle changes

    c. Moving 1,000 miles away from your hometown

    d. Loss of your job

    e. Extensive changes in your job responsibilities

## REFERENCES AND SUGGESTED READINGS

Cann, A., & Kuiper, N. A. (2014). Research on the role of humor in well-being and health. *Europe's Journal of Psychology, 10*(3), 412–428. doi:10.5964/ejop.v10i3.818.

Cousins, Norman. (1979). *Anatomy of an illness as perceived by the patient*. New York: W. W. Norton.

Ferrara, C. M., Nobrega, C., & Dulfan, F. (2013). Obesity, diet, and physical activity behaviors of students in health-related professions. *College Student Journal, 47*(3), 560–565.

McCreaddie, M., & Payne, S. (2014). Humour in health-care interactions: a risk worth taking. *Health Expectations, 17*(3), 332–344. doi:10.1111/j.1369-7625.2011.00758.x.

# SECTION III

# Behavior and Problems in Living

Life does not always flow smoothly. There are many problems in daily living. Anyone with a health need has new problems in addition to those of the usual life situation. Health care professionals must be aware that many patients are reacting to threat and, possibly, overwhelming problems. The patient needs acceptance, understanding, and caring from those who provide health care.

Section III is designed to help you understand some types of behavior likely to result from threat. By learning to cope effectively with personal threat and its effects, the health care professional prepares to understand and accept the behavior of others who are reacting in their own way to threats in their life situations.

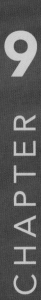

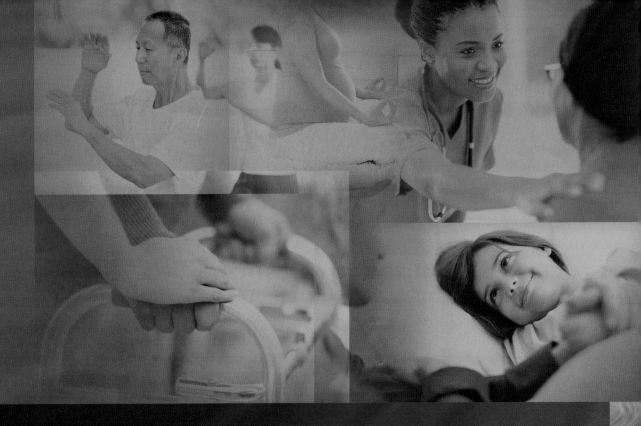

# Common Threats to Adjustment

## OBJECTIVES

After completing this chapter, you should be able to:

- Describe how different stages of life present new challenges to a person's adjustment.
- Explain the significance of peer pressure on adolescents.
- Discuss how learning problems can make school difficult for a student.
- Compare and contrast healthy and unhealthy family relationships.
- Describe cultural stressors that can occur in each of these life stages: childhood, adolescence, adulthood.
- List strategies parents can use to improve a child's behavior.

## KEY TERMS

Attention deficit
　disorder (ADD)
Attention deficit
　hyperactivity
　disorder (ADHD)

Autism spectrum
　disorders
Coping skills
Developmental disorders
Discrimination

Dyslexia
Family dynamics
Resilience
Separation anxiety
Sexism

The adjustment of any one person can be very poor, very good, or anywhere in between. Each person has a relative state of adjustment that characterizes that person most of the time. Adjustment, however, is always subject to change. Life experiences require changes in behavior to adapt to new situations and cope with new problems. Our state of adjustment can always be threatened by difficult situations.

A state of good adjustment *most of the time* is the best protection a person can have against the difficulties of life. By developing skills that help us deal effectively with our daily life problems, we prepare ourselves for dealing with big problems.

## CHANGE AS A THREAT TO ADJUSTMENT

Most people are reasonably well adjusted to their usual life situation. They are able to deal with routine problems, and they get along fairly well with family and friends. Then a change occurs. Perhaps the change appears rather ordinary—a move to a new neighborhood, a change of schools, even a change of jobs. We adapt to "ordinary" changes with slight modifications in our behavior. Perhaps the change is major, such as going away to college or leaving a protective home to enter military service. When major changes occur, we may have to learn new patterns of behavior.

Any type of change is a threat to one's adjustment. Since change is inevitable, learning to adapt our behaviors to new situations will help us maintain a state of good adjustment.

## LIFE STAGES AND CHANGE

As human beings, we are designed to grow, change, and develop throughout our lives. Each stage of life brings new opportunities but also presents new challenges. Sometimes these normal changes threaten our adjustment and require us to learn new behaviors or **coping skills** if we are to remain well-adjusted.

### Early Childhood

Children develop most rapidly during the first few years of their lives. They develop gross motor skills such as walking, running, and jumping and fine motor skills such as holding a pencil or fork. They learn to use language to communicate their wants and needs, and they practice basic social skills such as table manners and sharing.

Children are constantly learning about the world around them. They feel secure when they know what to expect from others, but they often find new people and places frightening. A predictable routine provides security, while chaos or unexpected changes can cause anxiety. Changes in family schedule, bedtime routine, or child care professional should be introduced gently and gradually.

Infants and preschoolers may experience **separation anxiety** when they enter a new day care or school. For days or even weeks, they may cry, claim to be sick, or beg to go home. Some elementary-school students experience anxiety when coming to a new school or returning after a long vacation. To resolve separation anxiety, parents, care professionals, and health professionals should work together to help the child get used to the new situation and should be understanding of the child's feelings without giving in to demands to go home.

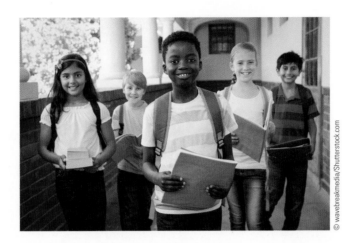

**FIGURE 9-1** For children who have developed physical, intellectual, and social skills during the early years, facing new situations becomes easier as they progress through elementary school.

## Middle Childhood

For children who have developed physical, intellectual, and social skills during the early years, facing new situations becomes easier as they enter and progress through elementary school. Each year brings a new class, new friends, and new experiences. These changes pose only a minor threat to adjustment.

For students who lack basic skills or are developmentally delayed, entering school can create new fears and problems. For many students, difficulties in school can be traced to a lack of school readiness skills. Poor social skills may lead to conflicts with classmates, while delayed intellectual development can create a pattern of school failure. Daily situations such as school assignments and interacting with peers can pose major threats to a child who is already poorly adjusted. The earlier parents, educators, and health care professionals can intervene to help such children develop needed skills, the more likely the child will be successful.

## Adolescence

As young people enter the teen years, they struggle to establish an identity separate from that of their parents. Adolescents are inclined to worry about appearance, self-worth as a person, the future, and—very important—the opinions of others. Relationships with peers become extremely important. Teens need to feel accepted and a part of the group; disappointment or rejection by members of their peer group can pose a major threat to a teen's adjustment. Peer pressure—the feeling of having to go along with the group in order to be accepted—can influence teens' choices about clothing, about using tobacco and alcohol, or about sexual relationships. Mood swings and variable adjustment are typical of the adolescent period.

Romantic relationships form an important part of many teens' lives. Because many young people choose to become sexually active during the teen years, sexual relationships and pressures can create additional stress. Teens may worry about pregnancy or sexually transmitted diseases. Health care professionals may find that teens turn to them with questions the teens are uncomfortable asking a parent.

The teenager who has a positive self-concept and relatively good adjustment is likely to adapt to the challenges of the adolescent period. If one enters adolescence with a negative

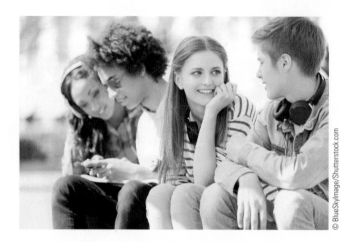

**FIGURE 9-2 Relationships with peers are extremely important to teens.**

self-concept, poor interpersonal skills, ineffective behavior patterns, and/or inability to adapt to change, the problem may become more intense. If adolescence proceeds at a favorable pace, childhood patterns are gradually replaced by more mature patterns of behavior. If such growth does not occur, then childish patterns of behavior may continue into adulthood.

## Young Adulthood

Young adults face many changes as they establish their independence from their parents. Common changes include completing high school and beginning college or a job, setting up a home of one's own, marrying, and starting a family. Each of these changes brings new experiences and responsibilities. Young people who have already developed good coping skills will usually adapt to each of these changes. However, young adults with a pattern of school and family problems may see similar problems develop in their jobs or their own families unless they learn more effective ways of coping. Young adults' decisions about careers, having children, and whether to marry or divorce will influence the rest of their lives.

## Middle Adulthood

Middle-aged adults may become painfully aware of the passing of time. They may not have reached their earlier ambitions or found satisfaction in their jobs and may wonder whether it is too late to start again. Middle-aged adults who have achieved their earlier goals may find that life seems empty or lacking in challenge. Children are growing up and leaving home, leaving parents with an "empty nest." Parents who devoted their early years to their families may now feel unneeded. Physical changes, especially in women, can affect one's moods and emotions. A man's physician may tell him to give up some activities, to slow down. Many adults have difficulty accepting these signs of disappearing youth. The popular term "midlife crisis" describes an adult who is having trouble adjusting to the changes of middle age.

## Older Adulthood

Older adulthood brings many frightening changes. Losses of friends and relatives require frequent funeral attendance. Employers may encourage older adults to retire before they are ready to withdraw from work that has been a major part of life for many years. The widow or widower may find it necessary to change homes. Sometimes family and friends rush an elderly person, just bereaved of a life partner, into a decision to give up the home and move in with one of the children or into a long-term care facility. Such radical changes should not be made until the widow or widower has worked through the grief process (one to three years).

> **For Discussion and Reflection**
>
> Consider your own journey through several of the life stages described. What changes did each stage bring? Did you find it easy or difficult to adjust to these changes?

Older adults may face a number of fears: losing their independence, not having enough money, becoming physically or financially dependent upon others, becoming ill, or dying. The uncertainties of these years can affect attitudes, feelings, relationships, and total behavior. Many elderly persons view the future as dismal, offering only the prospect of increasing losses and, eventually, death.

On the other hand, some older adults experience this portion of life as "the golden years." For those who are financially secure, remain in reasonably good health, and enjoy close ties to friends and family, the later years can be rewarding. These adults enjoy opportunities such as retirement, travel, socializing, and spending time with grandchildren. As with every other age, effective coping skills and supportive relationships help a person deal with life changes and maintain a good state of adjustment.

## SOCIAL AND CULTURAL STRESSORS

As an individual grows up and grows older, he or she must also cope with the pressures of society. Stressors such as peer pressure, drugs, and **discrimination** can become serious threats to a person's adjustment.

### Stressors of Childhood

Many children feel tremendous pressure to do well in school and/or sports and to be accepted by peers. For some children, success in these areas seems to come naturally. For slow learners, shy children, or those with behavioral difficulties, school becomes a major source of stress. Some children may also have difficulty fitting in with others and making friends. As a child moves into the older elementary and middle school years, peer relationships become increasingly important.

### Stressors of Adolescence

All the sources of childhood stress continue through adolescence—accompanied by additional sources of stress: the pressure of competition (athletics, extracurricular activities, school politics), pressure to excel (especially if college-bound), the need to belong, the need to be attractive to members of the opposite sex, eagerness to finish driver education and get one's own car. These are the familiar pressures of adolescence.

There is also the threat of school violence. Gangs exist in many schools; by belonging, there is safety in numbers, but one must conform to the gang's practices and beliefs. Initiation rites may include having sex (or committing a rape), shoplifting, car theft, "beating up" someone of a different race or ethnic group, or mugging. The initiate who fulfills this assignment then "belongs" to the gang, but not just as a member; any attempt to leave the gang may result in blackmail—gang members could provide testimony about the crime, resulting in a prison sentence for the would-be defector. Thus, the gang leader has power and control over members of the gang.

Those who are not gang members may live in fear of gang activity or reprisals following any dispute with a gang member. Weapons, once unheard of in a public school, are now prevalent. Some schools have electronic devices to detect weapons; but weapons are present in the parking lot. Assaults do occur, with both teachers and students as victims.

**Peer Pressure** Adolescence is a period when peer approval is extremely important. It is a time of life when family influence is challenged by the peer group because of the individual's need to belong. For that reason, each adolescent must choose between participating in certain practices that are widespread through the student body and the risk of being the outsider. Those who resist may experience pressure from their classmates to get involved, or to "just try it."

**Drugs** Drugs are a major problem, sometimes being sold and used in school restrooms and parking lots. At social events there is peer pressure to use drugs such as marijuana, crack, cocaine, and heroin. "Just say 'No!'" is not easy advice to follow; by saying, "No," the student risks disapproval of the peer group. According to the National Institute of Drug Abuse (2014), the percent of teens using illegal drugs has declined since the 1990s. However, over a fourth of teens surveyed still report using an illegal drug within the past year.

**Sexual Activity** When the adolescent begins to date, there may be pressure almost immediately to engage in sexual activity. This may conflict with beliefs about morality the adolescent has learned in the home and at church. The adolescent experiences an internal conflict: the need for acceptance by the peer group and the need to uphold one's standards and maintain self-esteem. Today's trend toward becoming sexually active during the teens has serious health implications: pregnancy, sexually transmitted diseases, and the emotional effects of abandonment by a partner to whom one has become emotionally attached. In many communities, sex education remains a controversial subject. Providing information on self-protection or distributing prophylactic materials through a school program is emphatically opposed by many adults. A health care professional is very likely to be approached by a teenager who needs information or help in regard to sexual activity.

Fortunately, not every adolescent is exposed to these stressors, but many are exposed to all of them. Numerous stressors experienced by adolescents today did not exist, or were not prevalent, when their parents were in high school. Many parents therefore do not understand or accept the problems today's adolescents face at school. Every adolescent needs to be able to discuss these problems regularly with an adult who understands the problems, encourages the expression of feelings, and helps identify appropriate ways to deal with these difficult situations.

## Stressors of Adulthood

Many of the stressors and serious traumas of childhood and adolescence continue into adulthood. Some that are discussed below also occur during childhood or adolescence. But certain stressors, such as discrimination, rape, and domestic violence, seem more appropriate for discussion within the framework of adulthood.

**Discrimination and Sexism** Members of minority groups in all cultures and throughout time have experienced discrimination. There seems to be an innate human need for perceiving people in "us/them" terms, favoring those who are members of the "us" group. But this tendency does not excuse discrimination that violates the rights of others because of sex, race, nationality, ethnic group, age, or religion. It required many years of campaigning by a group of courageous women before American women finally gained the right to vote. Until about 50 years ago, it was illegal in some states for a Caucasian to marry a person of Asian descent. African Americans have gained many rights as a result of the civil rights movement of the 1960s. Heightened awareness on the part of many Americans and a series of congressional acts have brought about numerous changes.

Federal laws pertaining to equal employment opportunities and prohibiting discrimination on the basis of race, sex, and age have been passed only in the past 40 years. Such laws do make it illegal to continue certain long-standing policies and practices. But laws do not change attitudes or beliefs. Discriminatory practices still exist, in educational settings as well as in the marketplace.

Discrimination may be practiced against anyone because of a specific attribute, such as race, sex, religion, age, weight, or other physical attributes. The most common basis for discrimination, however, is either race (racism) or sex (**sexism**). Other traumas related to sex include harassment, rape, and domestic violence.

**Sexual Harassment** Sexual harassment is one of the most frequently reported complaints in the workplace today. It may also occur in an educational setting. Usually the victim is someone with limited power (student, secretary), whereas the perpetrator (teacher, supervisor, customer) has some degree of power over the victim. The victim of sexual harassment is usually female, but may be male. The harassment may be verbal, may consist of inappropriate touching, or may involve requests or demands for sexual acts. Sometimes the victim perceives the harassment as including the threat of being fired; sometimes the promise of favorable treatment (a good grade, a promotion, a "business" trip) is implied or stated directly. Some women enjoy the attention and use these "offers" as opportunities for self-advancement; some who make that choice later regret it when the male turns his attention to his next victim. The majority of women, however, consider these unwanted sexual advances as harassment and see themselves as victims. The person who believes that he or she is being harassed should consider several questions:

- What can I do about this situation?
- How can I protect myself?
- What options are available to me?
- What is the best way to stop these unwanted advances?

Emotional reactions to sexual harassment include anger, fear, and guilt; the threat to self-esteem is obvious. The male who is accused of sexual harassment usually either denies that it occurred or blames the woman. At one time the female victim of sexual harassment had no recourse. If she reported the incident to a supervisor, she risked being fired, accused of lying, or worse. All too often, the perpetrator would be the supervisor. Today, however, it is possible to take legal action, since sexual harassment is covered by federal laws against discrimination. The woman who chooses to file a complaint should have some type of evidence, other victims who are willing to join the complaint, and/or witnesses who have heard or seen examples of harassment. The complaint probably will not be handled in the woman's favor if it becomes a matter of "her word against his."

The best approach is to stop harassment when the first incident occurs. Using "I-statements," the victim can express feelings and then in a matter-of-fact way establish limits on behavior. If this does not stop the harassment, then the employer's procedure for filing a complaint should be followed. A complaint can be filed with the proper federal agency if the employer does not take action to stop the harassment. If the victim does decide to file a complaint, she should be aware that there is risk of reprisal from the accused, from the employer, or even from colleagues who choose to side with the accused.

## MAJOR CHANGES

In addition to facing developmental changes and societal pressures, people of all ages must occasionally cope with major changes such as new experiences, illness, divorce, or death. These changes may require a person to give up old behaviors and learn new ones. Some changes considered particularly stressful include:

- Change in marital status (marriage, separation, divorce, or reconciliation)
- Change in employment status (being fired, retiring, or starting a new job)
- Death of a spouse, family member, or close friend
- Injury or illness (one's own or that of a family member)

Each of these changes can threaten a person's adjustment for a time while new behaviors are being learned.

### New Experiences

Even when they are positive, new experiences can be stressful. An adult beginning a new job must learn how to function in a new environment and get to know new coworkers. A student who graduates from high school and begins college must adapt to living away from home and assuming a greater amount of responsibility. A new parent may become exhausted and overwhelmed by the demands of caring for a young child. Adapting successfully to a new situation requires patience and often the support of family and friends.

For the person who is not ready for a new experience, a major change can become a crisis. The bride who is not ready to assume the role of a wife may try to cling to her role as a daughter, or even transfer the daughter role to the relationship with her husband. For the new mother who is frightened by the responsibilities of motherhood, the birth of

**For Discussion and Reflection**

What new experiences have you encountered that required you to make major adjustments to your daily habits? Examples include getting married or divorced, having a child, getting a new job, or going back to school.

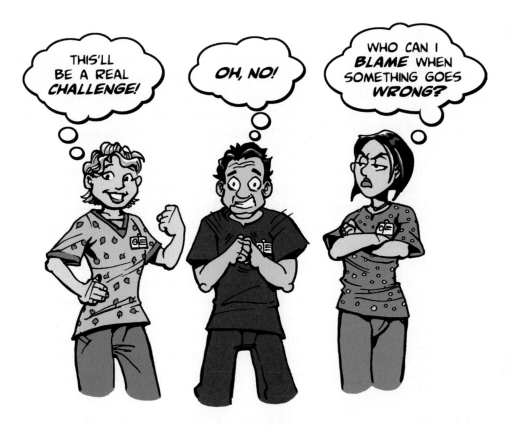

**FIGURE 9-3  How do you approach a new experience?**

her baby is a real crisis. The person who is not ready for the responsibility of being a health care professional may find that the ethics and job requirements of the health care field create a need for adjustments beyond those the individual is willing or able to make. Any crisis in regard to a vocational decision is a serious threat to adjustment. For people who have not learned to adapt to change, every life problem can add to poor adjustment. Any life event can become a crisis that creates anxiety and unhappiness for one who has not learned to deal with change.

## Illness

Illness is always a threat to adjustment. It interferes with the usual pattern of living, is accompanied by discomfort, may involve doubt as to the outcome, and often creates financial problems. Patients and their families react to illness according to the degree of threat it represents. Adjustment is always poorer during illness. Sometimes behavior patterns that are not typical of a person appear during illness. Someone who is usually easy to please, for example, may be very difficult to please during an illness. A person who is usually quite well adjusted may show signs of poor adjustment during the period of illness. The patient may react with anger or fear to feelings of helplessness or being dependent on others. Interestingly, the poorly adjusted person may react with positive feelings if the illness provides an escape from having to deal with daily problems.

The person who is self-reliant and has learned to deal with life problems usually finds illness frustrating. Familiar techniques for solving problems do not cure the illness. Perhaps the patient is accustomed to giving orders; now, the physician, nurse, laboratory assistant, radiology technician, and other personnel seem to be in charge. The shift from being independent to a state of dependency seriously threatens adjustment. The behavior of a patient may be markedly different from that person's usual behavior.

## Divorce

Divorce is almost always a traumatic experience for everyone involved, especially the children. Even if both parents agree that divorce is preferable to continuing the marriage, children are affected emotionally as they see their home and family breaking apart. Their daily life changes in many significant ways. The adults are dealing with their own emotional reactions to the trauma of marital discord. They may be unaware of the child's reactions: anger toward one or both parents, belief that the parent who is moving out "doesn't love me any more," or possibly guilt, believing that he or she is the cause of the family breakup. If the divorce is hostile, there may be a custody battle. Then the child has a serious conflict of loyalties and may witness numerous hostile encounters between the parents. The child experiences emotional turmoil: a mixture of love and hate, anger and grief, guilt about divided loyalty, and negative feelings toward one or both parents.

When either parent remarries, a stepparent enters the picture, further complicating the child's emotional life. If the parent who remarries is the custodial parent, and the new stepparent also has children, the result is a "blended family." A period of turmoil may last for months, because each person must adapt to new family relationships and establish new patterns of interaction. Ideally, these adaptations occur with minimal trauma, and family dynamics eventually become positive. It is unrealistic to expect this to happen immediately after the wedding. Family counseling can assist blended families in making these adaptations.

## Death

The death of a family member or friend can be very traumatic. Children especially need help in understanding death, accepting the permanence of death, dealing with feelings associated with the deceased, and coping with the sense of loss or abandonment. Effective grieving is very important. If grief is not processed, the suppressed emotions can affect future attitudes, emotional expression, and behavior when another loss is experienced. Chapter 16 discusses the effects of grief in greater detail.

# CHRONIC STRESSORS

Change is not the only stressor that can threaten one's adjustment. Some difficult situations develop gradually and persist for a long time. A person with ongoing financial problems, family difficulties, or learning disorders may find it especially difficult to remain well adjusted. Often, difficulty in one of these areas affects an individual's performance in other areas of life. For example, a woman in an unhappy marriage may find it difficult to concentrate at work. A child whose parents fight constantly may misbehave at school. A parent who is struggling to make ends meet may snap at the children. Health care professionals may be able to refer patients to appropriate community agencies for financial help, counseling, or educational evaluation.

## Financial Problems

Financial problems have many causes. Some individuals may be unemployed or lack the skills needed to earn a comfortable living. Others may have a reasonably good income but find themselves faced with overwhelming medical or legal expenses. Many people lack money management skills and find themselves in financial trouble because they do not know how to budget and set priorities. One family could not afford phone service but spent $30 per week on a rent-to-own large-screen TV. A young mother who could barely pay the rent spent about $5 per day on prepackaged lunchbox items for her sons even though they were eligible to receive free lunch at school.

Other individuals face overwhelming credit card debts. Many community agencies offer free financial counseling. Health care professionals should also be aware that out-of-control spending sprees are one symptom of bipolar disorder. For their own protection, individuals diagnosed with this disorder should not have access to checks or credit cards.

## Family Difficulties

Family is an important part of most people's lives. Healthy families provide emotional support, unhealthy or dysfunctional families can create anxiety and distress in a person's life. Put simply, a healthy family is one in which all family members are kind, caring, and respectful toward one another. Effective families function like a team, each person doing his or her part but also helping other members when needed. All families have conflicts and disagreements, but healthy families work to resolve their problems in a way that protects each family member's dignity.

A dysfunctional family may fight often or just not communicate at all. Members of an unhealthy family may not trust one another and may feel that other family members do not respect or care for them. Winning and being "right" become more important than working together. For adults, unhealthy **family dynamics** often lead to separation and divorce. What begins as poor communication and unhealthy dynamics often grows into feelings of unhappiness with the relationship, a lack of love for the spouse, and the desire to be with someone else. Some children in dysfunctional families misbehave or do poorly at school. Some use drugs or alcohol. Still others turn to relatives and friends for support and understanding. Unfortunately, unhealthy family dynamics are often learned and passed on to the next generation.

Being part of an unhealthy family is a tremendous threat to one's adjustment. Unfortunately, many of the families depicted in movies and on television are dysfunctional. Because the media portrays family difficulties as humorous and commonplace, viewers may come to accept fighting, insults, and infidelity as normal. In reality, these behaviors are symptoms of an unhealthy family. Counseling is available in most communities and can help families learn more appropriate ways to interact with one another.

## Learning Problems

In recent years it has become common for parents to seek medical advice when their child has difficulty in school. These difficulties may include poor grades, failure to learn new concepts, trouble completing assignments, or behavior problems. Today attention, learning, and behavioral disorders are most often diagnosed during the elementary school years. However, older students and even adults may suffer from undiagnosed disorders. These disorders can pose a threat to a person's adjustment at any age. Health care professionals should be aware of the signs of some common disorders and should encourage the child's parents or affected adult to seek professional evaluation. Warning signs of learning problems include:

• Slow development in speaking and writing
• Difficulty expressing ideas or understanding directions

- Difficulty with forming letters, writing, and spelling
- Difficulty memorizing and remembering information
- Clumsiness, poor handwriting, or poor coordination
- Difficulty paying attention and completing tasks
- Sloppiness, carelessness, or lack of organization
- Tendency to misinterpret others' behavior and become upset
- Sudden mood changes, frequent frustration

These behaviors may indicate a variety of learning problems. Some of the more common are described in the following sections.

**Attention Deficit Disorder and Attention Deficit Hyperactivity Disorder** **Attention deficit disorder (ADD)** and **attention deficit hyperactivity disorder (ADHD)** describe a pattern of inattentive, impulsive, and hyperactive behaviors. Students with ADD/ADHD may appear disorganized and have difficulty remembering information and completing tasks. They may show aggression and have poor relationships with their peers. Other common behaviors include daydreaming, staring into space, constantly moving or getting up, and blurting out. ADD/ADHD is a medical diagnosis, but health care professionals often seek input from a student's parents and teachers before making a diagnosis. Treatment of ADD/ADHD usually includes behavior modification and medication. Treatments such as hypnotherapy and neurofeedback have also proven successful for some individuals.

**Learning Disorders** When a student's academic achievement is significantly lower than one would expect given the student's level of intelligence, he may have a learning disorder. The three primary types of learning disorders are reading disorders (also called **dyslexia**), mathematics disorders, and writing disorders. A student with a learning disorder isn't "dumb" but has difficulty with a particular subject area. Students with identified learning disorders are entitled by federal law to receive special educational services, so health care professionals should encourage parents to have their child evaluated if a learning disorder is suspected.

## Developmental Disorders

As their name suggests, **developmental disorders** affect an individual's mental or physical development. The two most prevalent developmental disorders in the United States are mental disabilities and autism spectrum disorders. These disorders are usually diagnosed in the preschool or elementary school years.

**Intellectual disabilities** When most people hear the term *intellectual disability*, they imagine a severely handicapped individual. In fact, intellectual disabilities can be mild, moderate, severe, or profound. An intellectual disability is typically identified through tests of intelligence and adaptive behavior skills, or skills needed to care for oneself and function in everyday situations. Mild disabilities may not be identified until the school years, when it becomes clear that a child is learning at a rate slower than that of classmates. In older adults, a mild intellectual disability may never have been formally identified. Like individuals with learning disorders or physical disabilities, intellectually disabled persons are protected against discrimination by federal law.

**Autism Spectrum Disorders** **Autism spectrum disorders** include the disorders which have previously been referred to as classic autism, pervasive developmental order—not otherwise specified (PDD-NOS), and Asperger syndrome. Individuals with these disorders process and respond to information differently than typical individuals, causing difficulty with communication, behavior, and social interactions.

**For Discussion and Reflection**

What experiences have you, a friend, or a relative had with one of the learning or development disorders described? What challenges did the individual have to overcome as a result of the disorder?

Autism affects each individual differently, and the degree to which daily functioning is impaired can be mild to severe. Persons with autism can have low, average, or high levels of intellectual functioning. For example, Sue Rubin is a woman with autism who wrote a documentary about her experiences. Although she is unable to communicate through spoken language, she has an above-average level of intelligence and communicates through writing and the use of assistive communication devices.

Over the past few years, more and more children are being diagnosed with autism spectrum disorders. Treatments include special educational programs, occupational therapy, speech therapy, medication, and modified diet. In 2015, the Centers for Disease Control and Prevention reported that autism spectrum disorders occur at the rate of 1 in 42 boys and 1 in 189 girls.

## Behavior Disorders

While most children misbehave at times, some develop a pattern of problem behaviors that can severely disrupt the school or home environment. Students with oppositional defiant disorder routinely defy the authority of parents or teachers. When told to do something, they may intentionally do the opposite. Students with a conduct disorder may not only disobey parents and teachers but also threaten or harm others, steal, or vandalize school or public property. These students may be treated with behavioral modification, therapy, and/or medication. Whenever possible, families of affected students should also seek counseling, since living with a family member's disorder is stressful. Likewise, many experts believe that family dynamics influence or even create behavior disorders. Improving family interactions can improve the problem behaviors.

**Discipline and Home Environment** While it is important to detect and treat legitimate disorders, families often find that children's behavior and academic performance improve when parents learn more effective discipline techniques. Contrary to popular opinion, *discipline* does not mean *punishment*. Discipline means teaching children the difference between appropriate and inappropriate behaviors and guiding them to choose behavior that is appropriate to the situation. Effective discipline includes the following techniques:

- Develop a warm, caring relationship with children.
- Explain and model socially appropriate behavior.
- Keep rules and expectations clear, simple, and age appropriate.
- Enforce rules calmly and consistently.
- When necessary, punish a child with time out or loss of a privilege, not by hitting or yelling.

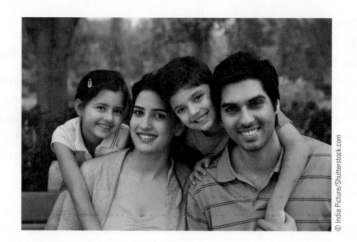

**FIGURE 9-4 Healthy family relationships help children become well-adjusted and able to adapt to new situations.**

In addition, children learn and behave better when they receive good nutrition and when parents monitor television and video games. Exposure to violent TV programs and video games has been linked to aggressive behavior.

Resolving a negative family situation can also improve behavior. One second grader developed a serious problem with aggressive and defiant behavior at school. Upon investigation, it was found that her mother used harsh punishments and often told the girl, "You're no good." Shortly after her father gained custody, the girl began to behave appropriately at school.

## COPING SKILLS AND RESILIENCE

Surprisingly, well-adjusted people are not always those who have led lives free of difficulty or trauma. Ultimately, it is not what happens to us that determines our level of adjustment, but how we cope with it. Good coping skills and resources can help a person regain a good level of adjustment even when faced with difficult circumstances. The following coping skills and resources help individuals deal with problems as they occur:

- Eat a healthful diet and exercise regularly.
- Get a full night's rest.
- Talk to a friend or family member about emotions and problems.
- Set goals and work toward them one step at a time.

A similar concept is **resilience**, the ability to bounce back or recover from problems. Factors associated with resilience include having a positive attitude, believing one has the power to change one's circumstances, and developing strategies to reduce stress. Being part of a support network such as a caring family or a church or community group can also help a person recover from difficulty.

Coping with a difficult situation takes time. During the period of readjustment, a person may find counseling or a support group helpful. These resources are especially important for a person who has experienced a trauma. Chapter 10 examines different types of trauma and the reactions a victim of trauma is likely to experience.

## ACTIVITIES

1. Consider several of your life experiences that involved new situations. Try to recall how you felt during the early days in the new situation. Which of your familiar behaviors were inappropriate in the new situation? What changes did you make in your behavior patterns as you adapted to the new situation?

2. Consider the most uncomfortable experience you have had since entering this health occupations program. Why were you uncomfortable? What was your behavior? List changes in behavior that helped you return to a state of adjustment.

3. List several guidelines for handling the following situations in the future:

   a. A radical change in your life situation

   b. A new job in which many of the techniques used are somewhat different from those you learned as a student

   c. A new job in the health field for which your present learnings provide a foundation, but your job responsibilities require that you learn many new techniques

4. A mother consults you about Joey, a second grader. She tells you that Joey has trouble remembering what his teacher said in class. Homework takes him hours to complete, and he often cries with frustration because he doesn't understand. She says, "One day Joey can do the work, and the next day it's like he's forgotten everything." What might you suggest to her?

5. Sarah, a fourth grader, has developed a behavior problem at school. She blurts out comments in class, hits others, and occasionally steals pencils and other small items. Her parents ask you what they should do to help Sarah. What factors might you consider in discussing Sarah's behavior with her parents?

## REFERENCES AND SUGGESTED READINGS

Centers for Disease Control and Prevention. (2015). *Autism spectrum disorder*. Retrieved from http://www.cdc.gov/ncbddd/autism/data.html.

Centers for Disease Control and Prevention. (2015). *Facts about developmental disabilities*. Retrieved from http://www.cdc.gov/ncbddd/developmentaldisabilities/facts.html.

National Institute of Drug Use. (2014). *Drugfacts: high school and youth trends*. Retrieved from http://www.drugabuse.gov/publications/drugfacts/high-school-youth-trends.

Rubin, Sue (Writer), & Wurzburg, Gerardine (Producer). (2005). *Autism is a world*. [DVD]. United States: CNN.

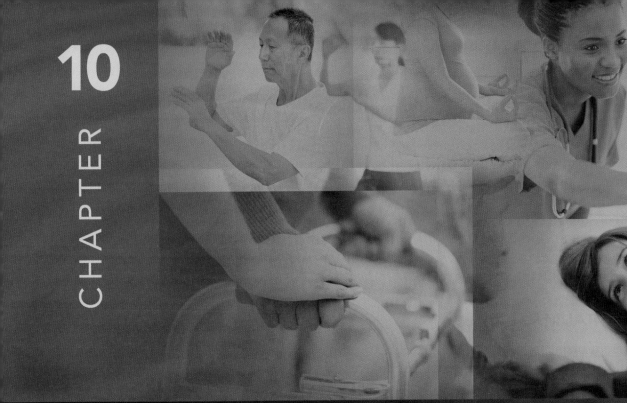

# CHAPTER 10

# Effects of Trauma

## OBJECTIVES

After completing this chapter, you should be able to:

- Discuss why victims of a traumatic experience may need psychological counseling, in addition to treatment for physical injuries.
- Identify normal reactions to a traumatic experience.
- Describe the symptoms of the following psychological disorders: anxiety disorder, panic disorder, post-traumatic stress disorder (PTSD), phobias, and depression.
- List traumatic effects of each of the following: war or terrorism, rape, domestic violence, and child abuse.
- Explain the phrase "blaming the victim."

## KEY TERMS

Abuse
Incest
Neglect

Pedophilia
Perpetrators

Sexually transmitted
   disease (STD)
Trauma-informed care

Chapter 9 describes threats to adjustment that everyone experiences. Some people are fortunate in that they have never experienced severe trauma, but today more and more people, of all ages and from all walks of life, experience some type of trauma. Health care professionals need to be aware that these experiences are serious threats to adjustment and have implications for the physical, mental, and emotional health of victims.

You, as a health care professional, are more likely to encounter victims than perpetrators. You also need to be aware that any given patient may be a victim, even if the patient does not volunteer information to that effect. Any suspicion that you have should be reported to your supervisor and/or the physician for further evaluation and possible legal action. *Follow the policies and procedures of your employing agency; do not attempt to handle such a matter yourself.* Just as important, *do not ignore the indications that aroused your suspicion.*

## WHAT IS TRAUMA?

A trauma is an event that poses a serious threat to one's life or well-being. Trauma includes experiencing, witnessing, or learning of a crime, act of aggression, accident, natural disaster, or act of war. Physical, emotional, and sexual abuse are also considered traumas. Experiencing a trauma poses a serious threat to a person's adjustment. Even people who are normally well-adjusted will develop physical and emotional reactions following a traumatic event.

A traumatized person may require medical attention immediately after the event. In other cases, the person may seek medical advice days or weeks later when secondary symptoms develop. In addition to treating physical injuries, health care professionals should inform patients about normal reactions to trauma and refer them to a mental health professional if these reactions become severe.

## TRAUMATIC EXPERIENCES

While any difficult situation may be perceived as a trauma by the person who experiences it, the following discussion focuses on events that are commonly recognized as traumatic. By understanding the most common types of trauma, health care professionals will be better equipped to assist trauma victims in understanding their own reactions and seeking the help they need.

Victims of a single event, such as a mugging, experience intense emotional reactions in addition to their physical injuries. After the physical injuries have healed, professional counseling may be needed for processing the emotional trauma. Victims of recurrent trauma, such as long-standing **abuse**, need help in escaping their situation; these victims always benefit from professional counseling—to develop new insights and resolve deeply rooted emotional trauma.

### The Perpetrator

In reading the following paragraphs, remember that there are traumatic *events* (e.g., accidents), there are **perpetrators** (i.e., persons who inflict the trauma), and there are *victims* (persons suffering from the event). The perpetrator's behavior may result from behavior patterns learned at home or on the street, cultural patterns, uncontrolled emotional expression, criminal tendencies, or a psychiatric disorder. The perpetrator's behavior may fall within the "normal" range of behavior (i.e., acceptable behavior within that particular culture) or may fall into the category of psychiatric disorder or criminal behavior. Discussion of the "causes" of a perpetrator's behavior is beyond the scope of this book; the study of such behavior falls within the disciplines of sociology, psychology, psychiatry, and criminology.

## Blaming the Victim

The trauma experienced by the victim is magnified when others choose to blame the victim. Those who would defend a rapist are likely to claim the victim "was just asking for it," citing her manner of dress or her presence in a particular location.

This tendency to blame the victim sometimes extends even to those who are the victim of a criminal act or are involved in an accident:

*Why were you out at that time of night?*

*Why did you go to that place? You should have known better!*

*How many times have I told you not to drive so fast?*

Being blamed for what happened adds to a victim's emotional trauma. It is only natural to feel anger when being blamed at a time when one's need is for expressions of caring and emotional support. Although blaming may actually be a friend's or relative's expression of concern, it is inappropriate and not what a victim needs to hear. Also, blaming may be an example of displaced anger, from the cause of the event or the perpetrator, to the victim; this too is inappropriate. The health care professional sometimes has an opportunity to point out to relatives a victim's need for expressions of caring, emotional support, and protection from being blamed.

## Crimes and Accidents

Muggings, carjackings, burglaries, gang beatings, and other types of violence are all too prevalent. Once considered to be dangers characteristic of big cities, these crimes are now commonplace in the suburbs and in small cities and towns. Even more common are automobile accidents, a leading cause of death, especially for males under the age of 25. In addition, thousands of people each year sustain disabling injuries.

Anyone who is the victim of a crime or who survives a serious accident has emotional trauma in addition to any physical injuries sustained. The health care system tends to focus on physical injuries, however. Once victims have been treated in the emergency room or discharged from the hospital, they usually receive follow-up treatment primarily for their physical injuries.

Fear and anger inevitably accompany the physical trauma of crimes and accidents. Some people can process these feelings over time; others need professional counseling to deal with the intensity of the feelings and any disabling effects, such as panic attacks or chronic anxiety. It is appropriate, within the role of some health care professionals, to suggest to victims that they may benefit from counseling to deal with the emotional effects of their traumatic experience.

## Natural Disasters, War, and Terrorism

We often hear news reports of floods, hurricanes, tornadoes, and earthquakes that have taken lives and left many people without homes. A natural disaster can be devastating for both the

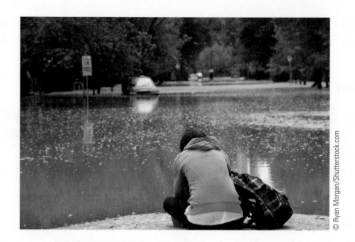

© Ryan Morgan/Shutterstock.com

**FIGURE 10-1** **A natural disaster can be devastating for both the community and the individuals affected.**

community and the individuals affected. Damage to or loss of one's home, school, or workplace threatens one's sense of security and normalcy. An individual who has experienced a natural disaster may experience any of the reactions to trauma described earlier. In addition, some people may develop anxiety or phobias related to the experience. For example, a person who lived through a hurricane or tornado may become distressed during thunderstorms or high winds.

Experiencing or witnessing war or terrorist acts also causes trauma. Individuals often feel overwhelmed by fear, helplessness, and vulnerability. They struggle to understand what has happened and why. Scenes of destruction or suffering may play through a person's mind over and over. For those who lose friends, family, or homes, there is a tremendous sense of grief as well. War and terrorist acts can breed distrust among different nations or ethnic groups, planting the seeds for further aggression in the future.

Military personnel in combat face traumatic situations constantly. For some, the psychological effects are so devastating that they never regain their previous level of adjustment even after returning to civilian life. Many veterans find themselves unable to function after returning home. These veterans suffer from post-traumatic stress disorder.

Natural disasters, war, and terrorism affect not only individuals, but also entire communities. These large-scale traumas provoke many of the same reactions as other traumas. However, a trauma experienced by many has some noteworthy differences. Because many people have been affected, finding someone to talk to about the experience may be easier. Some survivors may find comfort in the feeling that, "We're in this together. I'm not alone." On the other hand, friends and family who are also traumatized may not be able to provide much emotional support. Ongoing media coverage and community discussion become constant reminders of the event.

## Bullying

Many children experience teasing and bullying in the home, on the playground, and at school. The child who is noticeably different (e.g., has a physical handicap or a tendency to stutter) is especially at risk for teasing by the peer group or bullying by larger children. School policies regarding children with behavioral disorders or learning difficulties set these children apart, a practice that often results in a child being labeled and possibly rejected by classmates. Bullying, however, is a more serious problem.

Bullying includes several aggressive behaviors, including name-calling, put-downs, threats, taunting, physical assault, taking or damaging property, and forcing a person to do something he or she does not want to do. A bully may be aggressive or passive. Aggressive bullies may instigate a bullying situation, while passive bullies rarely "start the fight" but join in once an aggressive bully has set the stage. Bullying can be described as follows:

- The behavior is intended to harm or disturb a less powerful victim, one who is smaller, weaker, or unable to defend him- or herself.
- The behavior occurs repeatedly over a period of time.
- The bully chooses a time when winning is almost certain, such as when there is no one present with the authority to intervene.
- The bully often has one or more allies present.

By choosing a weaker victim and surrounding him- or herself with allies, the bully, who lacks real courage, gains a sense of power by overpowering the victim.

Many parents and teachers view bullying as a normal part of growing up and therefore do little to intervene. Boys who fight are often described as "tough" or "standing up for themselves." Some parents of aggressive bullies are secretly proud of their child's tough reputation or blame other children for starting the fight.

Unfortunately, bullying often occurs more in schools than in any other single place. Research suggests that much bullying could be prevented by clear and consistent school discipline policies and close adult supervision on playgrounds before and after school. All students who report bullying should be taken seriously, and their anonymity should be protected.

Children who bully others need both firm discipline and understanding. Bullying behavior is often an indicator that a child comes from an unhealthy family. Researchers suggest that failure to bond with parents in the early years, lack of love, and ineffective discipline increase the likelihood of bullying. Some aggressive children are copying aggressive behavior they have learned from parents. For example, one father told his son, "Don't let anyone walk all over you." While bullying behavior should not be excused on the grounds that a child came from a difficult home, attempting to change the behavior without addressing its cause is unlikely to stop bullying. Many community mental health centers offer family counseling, parenting classes, and anger management sessions that can help bullies and their families learn more acceptable behaviors.

Victims of bullying require help in several areas:

- They need adult intervention to end the bullying or at least avoid bullying situations.
- Victims of bullying often need help to address the low self-esteem and feelings of powerlessness as a result of being repeatedly threatened or overpowered.
- They also need to learn how to protect themselves physically and emotionally in the future.

When bullying is not adequately addressed, the effects can be devastating for the individuals involved and their community. Young people who have been threatened, taunted, and assaulted can develop the attitude, "No one cares about me. Everyone's against me." For some, this attitude leads to depression; for others, it creates a desire to strike back. Investigations into several school shootings in recent years revealed that the shooters had been the targets of bullying or felt rejected by their peers.

Adults may experience bullying in the workplace, the community, or in personal relationships. Anyone who routinely uses intimidation and manipulation to get his or her way at the expense of the rights of others is a bully. Standing up to a bully takes strength and courage. It is important to set limits and let the bully know in no uncertain terms when he or she has crossed the line. The bully must be told that the behavior is unacceptable and will not be tolerated.

With the popularity of the Internet, text messaging, and other technological forms of communication, a new variation of bullying has developed—*cyberbullying*. Cyberbullying has been defined as "willful and repeated harm inflicted through the medium of electronic text" (Patchin & Hinduja, 2006), or more simply, "online cruelty." Examples include spreading vicious rumors, insults, threats, or hate messages through electronic messages. Cyberbullying occurs most often, though not exclusively, among adolescents. Victims of cyberbullying may experience fear, depression, lowered self-esteem, or even become suicidal (Hamm et.al, 2015).

The child who has positive emotional support in the home survives teasing and some degree of bullying without serious damage. The child who does not have opportunities for processing feelings about these experiences is likely to suppress anger and fear, develop a negative self-concept, and have problems with interpersonal relations. These experiences, though not as dramatic as some types of trauma, can have lifelong effects.

## Child Abuse

Child neglect and abuse are serious problems today and can take several forms:

- **Neglect** includes leaving young children unsupervised or failing to provide adequate food, clothing, shelter, hygiene, and medical care.

- Abuse includes harming a child emotionally or physically. Verbal abuse consists of put-downs, cursing, or making repeated comments like "You're no good. I wish you'd never been born. You're going to end up in jail just like your father (or mother)."

- Emotional abuse includes "mind games," manipulation, or using fear to control the child.

- Physical abuse can include inappropriate discipline such as harsh beatings or locking a child in a closet. Any physical assault upon a child can be considered abusive, particularly if marks or bruises are visible afterward.

- Sexual abuse occurs when an adult or older child forces a child to take off his or her clothes or perform any sexual act. While the act itself is physical, the damage to the victim is emotional, mental, and physical.

Both boys and girls can be victims of sexual abuse, but two out of three victims are girls. The perpetrator is most often a close family member, but may be a family friend or authority figure.

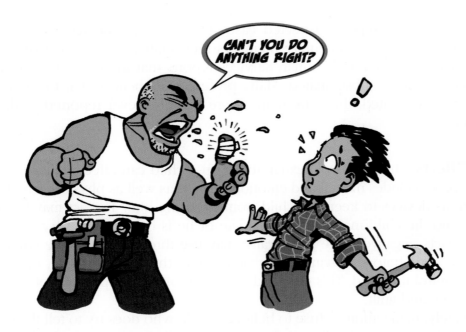

**FIGURE 10-2** **Verbal abuse consists of put-downs, cursing, or repeated negative comments.**

If the perpetrator is a parent or sibling, the sexual encounter is **incest**. If the child is under 13 years old and the perpetrator is 5 to 10 years older than the child, it is **pedophilia**; the abuser is a *pedophile*. Studies of pedophiles indicate that many were themselves sexually abused as children. Because the majority of sexual abusers are male, the pronoun "he" is used for the remainder of this discussion. There are, however, cases of sexual abuse of a male by a female.

With the rise of the Internet, there has been increasing public concern about "sexual predators" who meet young people online and engage them in inappropriate online or in-person sexual activities. The U.S. Department of Justice reported the following findings:

- One in seven youth Internet users had received unwanted sexual solicitations.
- Sexual predators are more likely to target youth who have a past of sexual abuse, who post suggestive photos online, and who participate in online chat rooms.
- Only about 5 percent of predators attempted to deceive the victims by pretending to be other youth. Most predators accurately presented themselves as adult males seeking a sexual encounter.
- Of victims who met the predator in person, 93 percent did so willingly.

Many schools now teach Internet safety guidelines. Parents should also monitor teens' online activity and maintain open communication to encourage teens to discuss any inappropriate online experiences. When teens are unsupervised, lack a supportive and caring family, or have a history of trauma or abuse, they are more vulnerable to sexual predators as well as more likely to engage in other high-risk behaviors.

Health care professionals, teachers, law enforcement officers, and other professionals

**For Discussion and Reflection**

Based on your own knowledge and experiences online, what advice would you give to teens regarding Internet safety?

are legally required to report suspected cases of abuse and neglect to their local Child Protective Services office. Community members and relatives may also make reports. The U.S. Department of Health and Human Services reports that in 2011, 742,000 cases of child abuse and neglect were substantiated. Many professionals believe that for each case that is reported and substantiated, there are many more that are never reported or that would be difficult to prove.

**Traumatic Effects** The effects of sexual abuse on a child can affect adjustment throughout life. Sexual abuse includes mental and emotional abuse as well as physical acts. The perpetrator uses various devices to keep the child from exposing him. The act may be presented as "our secret" and the child made to feel that she or he is being given very special attention. If the child reacts negatively, the perpetrator may use threats to keep the child from telling anyone. Some perpetrators convince their victims that they are to blame, thus using shame and guilt to control the child. This enforced silence results in suppression of intense feelings: anger, fear, grief, and guilt.

Unfortunately, many adults refuse to believe a child who does try to tell them about being sexually abused. It is especially difficult for parents to believe that a respected authority figure, such as a teacher, coach, or member of the clergy, would sexually abuse their child. Many adult survivors of child sexual abuse tell of seeking help from an adult, only to encounter disbelief and accusations of lying. Parents, teachers, ministers, adult friends and neighbors, and especially health care professionals must *listen* when a child tries to tell what some adult did to them. Although the child may not have the vocabulary to describe the event in adult terms, it is important to *let the child tell what happened in his or her own words.* Do not suggest words you think might help the child's description, since that could be construed legally as having "planted the idea in the child's mind."

Sexual abuse can cause physical, mental, and emotional damage:

- Victims grow up with low self-esteem, suppressed anger and fear, feelings of guilt and distrust, and perceptions of the world as a hostile place.
- They may contract a **sexually transmitted disease (STD)** or sustain other physical injuries.
- As adults, many survivors of childhood sexual abuse have difficulty forming an intimate relationship. Many have one relationship after another; others avoid intimacy altogether.

The lifelong effects of child sexual abuse are now acknowledged by the mental health community. Through psychotherapy and techniques such as hypnosis, many adults have been able to bring repressed memories to the conscious level, a necessary step in order for therapy to proceed. Support groups for survivors of abuse and incest have been established in many communities.

While enduring abuse is traumatic for a child, reporting the abuse and ending the situation can be traumatic as well. One 10-year-old girl told her mother that her stepfather had sexually abused her. As a result, the mother took the children and moved out. The abuse had ended, but now the girl faced the trauma of losing her stepfather and stepgrandparents. She had to adjust to a new home, a new neighborhood, and a new school. Some abused children who are "wise to the system" choose not to report being abused because they fear being taken from their parents. Enduring abuse is the price they pay to protect their families and avoid confrontation.

Appropriate action depends on the situation. Criminal charges may be filed against the perpetrator, but adults should not let that possibility prevent them from protecting the child against further molestation. Pedophiles tend to repeat their behavior, so every child within range of a pedophile is at risk.

The sexually abused child enters the adolescent period having already experienced some type of sexual activity. Some behaviors, emotional patterns, attitudes toward sex, levels of trust in others, and interpersonal relations differ from those of their sexually inexperienced classmates. Some children try various forms of escape: alcohol, drugs, food, sleep, or withdrawal. Those who have strong guilty feelings may inflict physical pain on themselves by head banging, beating hard objects with the fists, cutting or mutilating themselves, or even attempting suicide. These behaviors may be exhibited during adolescence or adulthood, years after the sexual abuse stopped or the individual escaped from the abuser.

## Rape

The use of threats or force in order to engage in a sexual act is *rape*. It is a crime and should be reported, even if the perpetrator is a relative, friend, date, or coworker. *Rape is an act of aggression that violates the victim physically and emotionally.* Rapists tend to have a hostile attitude toward women. They may also have an intense need to experience a feeling of power over others. Some rapists want to inflict pain and enjoy the woman's fear. Because the experience satisfies the rapist's need for power and control, he is likely to rape repeatedly and to have more than one victim. The rapist who does not feel powerful enough to force himself on an adult woman may choose a child as victim. Rape is one of a number of acts included in the legal term "sex offender."

The rape victim often is victimized further by family members and/or "the system." If the rapist is a relative, family members may not believe the victim's report; some may actually side with the accused rapist. If the victim reports the rape to police, she may be subjected to dehumanizing procedures by officers who do not understand the significance of rape. Comments made about a rape or a rape victim often show total lack of understanding that *rape is a violent act of aggression.*

In many communities, the concerns of rape survivors, health care professionals, and law enforcement personnel have led to educational efforts to sensitize officials to the needs of a rape victim. Every rape victim should have professional counseling to help her deal with intense emotions and the serious threat to self-esteem. Counseling and a support group can help the victim regain confidence in her ability to go about her daily routine without fear.

## Stalking

The U.S. Department of Justice (2013) estimates that in a 12-month period, 14 out of every 1000 adults are victims of stalking. Stalking may take the form of unwanted letters, phone calls, emails, or gifts, or it may include following or spying on the victim. Posting inappropriate or negative information online or in a public place can also be considered stalking. While many people occasionally find themselves the object of unwanted attention, these behaviors can be considered stalking if they cause victims to fear for the safety of themselves or their family members. The highest rate of stalking occurs among 18- to 24-year-olds.

## Adult Abuse

Adult abuse has received growing media attention. Adult abuse occurs when disabled or elderly adults are neglected or mistreated by adult children, spouses, or other caretakers. For adults with developmental disabilities, the risk of being physically or sexually assaulted may be 4 to 10 times greater than it is for other adults. Disabled women are assaulted, raped, and abused twice as often as nondisabled women. Elderly adults are also at risk for neglect, emotional abuse, and physical abuse. Abusers may include nursing home staff, adult children, spouses, or other relatives. Just as health care professionals have a legal duty to report suspected cases of child abuse, they have an ethical duty to report suspected elder abuse to the authorities.

# DOMESTIC VIOLENCE

Abuse by one's spouse or partner is now recognized as a public health problem in the United States. According to the National Domestic Violence Hotline, one in four females and one in nine males will experience domestic violence at some point in their lives. Spousal abuse is found in all cultures, races, occupations, income levels, and ages.

Spousal abuse can take various forms, including physical aggression (assault), emotional trauma, "mind games," deprivation of needs (including access to money), and isolation from relatives and friends. Employers lose billions of dollars every year because of lost workdays, medical costs, and other problems associated with domestic violence.

## The Abuser Personality

Abusers have two personalities: the public personality, that of "a really nice person," and the private personality, controlling and demanding. Few people would enter knowingly into an abusive relationship. The abuser initially is charming and shows care and concern, so the partner enters the relationship expecting romantic love and warmth. Gradually the abuser begins to make demands that lead up to isolating the victim from family and friends, getting control of the victim's money, controlling the couple's activities (eliminating the victim's activities and interests), requiring explanations for the victim's behavior or comments, demanding a report on any time spent away from the abuser, and making decisions for the victim. These demands are first made within an acceptable, and possibly flattering, context:

- I can't stand to be away from you.
- I want you to spend more time with me.
- You spent all afternoon with your friend when I needed you to be with me.
- I want you to be here while I watch TV.
- I want you to be home when I get back.
- You know how important you are to me.

Initially the abuser makes the victim feel important and loved, but comments such as the above are leading up to controlling not only the relationship, but also all aspects of the victim's life life. The abuser's objective is *power*—total control over the other person.

The following statements illustrate the increasing degree of control:

- What did you and your friend talk about all afternoon?
- What did you do while I was away?
- I'll take care of paying the bills; I handle money better than you do.
- Wear that outfit; you really look great in it.
- Don't wear that to the party.
- What were you and Joe laughing about?
- Why did you stay in the kitchen with Amy so long?
- What did you mean when you said . . . ?

Next, the abuser begins to chip away at the victim's self-esteem:

- Why did you say (. . .)? That was stupid!
- Why can't you be more fun when we party?
- Why can't you be a better parent/spouse?
- You can't do anything right.
- You made me angry (jealous).
- You caused us to run out of money.
- You had me so upset I ran a red light; it's your fault I got this ticket.
- Yes, I drink too much, but it's because you make me so (. . .).
- I didn't get the promotion; you should have been nicer to my boss at the Christmas party.

## Effects on the Victim

Once the victim begins to believe that he or she really is the cause of the couple's problems, the abuser has tremendous power. With low self-esteem and overwhelming feelings of guilt, the victim is less able to evaluate the relationship and definitely less able to leave it. Once the abuser's power is established, the abuse may include physical aggression. The physical abuse may escalate until the victim sustains serious injuries or is killed.

Individuals who grew up in a home where domestic violence was a way of life may simply accept abuse as part of a relationship. At some point, the victim may realize he or she does not have to submit to abuse. The victim may seek escape, but escape may require help from family, friends, or a community agency. Some victims choose to stay in an abusive relationship rather than risk the uncertainties of being alone.

## Escaping Abuse

Most victims of domestic violence need outside help to escape the abusive relationship. Since an abuser takes control of the family's finances, the victim has no financial resources to aid in escape. Sometimes the abuser tries to ensure that the victim remain financially dependent.

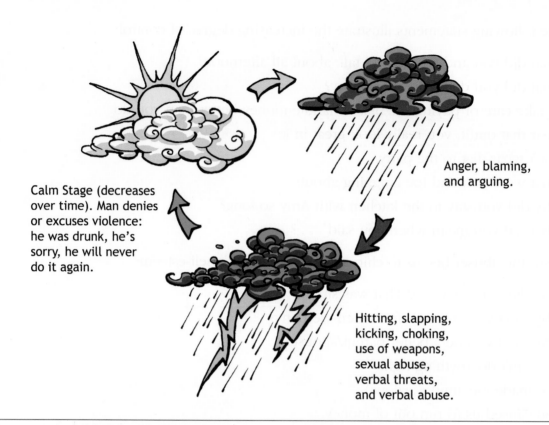

Calm Stage (decreases over time). Man denies or excuses violence: he was drunk, he's sorry, he will never do it again.

Anger, blaming, and arguing.

Hitting, slapping, kicking, choking, use of weapons, sexual abuse, verbal threats, and verbal abuse.

**FIGURE 10-3** **In an abusive relationship, the cycle of abuse intensifies over time as the abuser seeks to gain greater and greater power over the victim.**

Personnel in domestic violence shelters report that many victims who appear ready to become self-reliant actually go back to the abuser. Sometimes it takes several attempts before the victim finally escapes permanently. Many of these victims need several types of help:

- The belief that he or she does not have to submit to abuse
- Financial assistance
- A separate place to live
- Child care
- Job and/or job training
- Child support
- Legal protection

As soon as arrangements are made for physical survival, it is important that the victim receive counseling to counteract the destructive effects of the abusive relationship. The damage to self-esteem may take years to overcome. Processing fear, anger, and guilt may require many months. Without effective counseling, the victim may not be able to trust another partner or establish an intimate relationship based on equality.

## Hopeful Signs

The problem of domestic violence in American society has finally gained legal recognition. In 1995, the U.S. Congress passed the Violence Against Women Act (VAWA). The VAWA was reauthorized in 2000, 2005, and 2013, providing more funding for sexual assault treatment, education, and prevention programs. This is the first federal law that recognizes and attempts to stop violence against women. The VAWA contains a civil rights remedy for victims of violence to file charges through a federal court and seek monetary compensation, court-ordered protection, and costs of legal expenses.

## REACTIONS TO TRAUMA

Normal reactions to a traumatic experience vary by individual. Immediately following the event, an individual may experience any of the following:

- Shock, a feeling of being stunned or dazed.
- Denial, or not accepting what has happened.
- Numbness, or feeling disconnected from the world around them.

Once these initial reactions pass, individuals may experience ongoing symptoms:

- They may become moody, irritable, or anxious.
- They have physical symptoms such as sweating or a rapid heartbeat.
- Sleep and eating patterns can change.
- Individuals may have repeated memories of or dreams about the traumatic event.

These reactions can develop immediately after the traumatic event, or they can be delayed for months or years.

Some people recover quite quickly from trauma, while others suffer for a long time. Friends may tell an individual, "Just get over it, Stop dwelling on the past." But some trauma survivors are not able to return to their prior level of adjustment on their own. Health care professionals can assist these individuals by assuring them that their feelings are normal reactions to trauma and that they aren't "crazy." Counseling or a support group may be particularly helpful for these individuals.

The severity of reactions can also vary. For some individuals, reactions can be so powerful that they appear similar to mental illness. Health care professionals should be familiar with common reactions to trauma so that a traumatized person will receive an appropriate diagnosis and referral for help. The sooner after a trauma a person can talk about the event and receive emotional support, the less likely it is that long-term problems will develop.

### Anxiety

A person experiencing generalized anxiety may worry most of the time, have trouble sleeping, and appear shaky or nervous. A patient with anxiety may say, "Doctor, I need something for my nerves." The anxious person may or may not recognize a connection between the trauma and the anxiety.

**For Discussion and Reflection**

Have you or someone you know experienced a traumatic event? Did you or that individual experience any of the immediate or ongoing effects described?

More specific conditions associated with anxiety include panic disorder, post-traumatic stress disorder, and phobias.

**Panic Disorder**  Some individuals experience recurring, unexpected anxiety or panic attacks. During these attacks, the person can have a pounding heart, chest pain, difficulty breathing, numbness or tingling, and a dizzy or faint feeling. The skin may become pale and cold. A patient may say, "I thought I was dying," or "I thought I was having a heart attack." While a single panic attack does not necessarily indicate panic disorder, recurring panic attacks or fears of having more attacks are signs that a patient needs treatment.

**Post-Traumatic Stress Disorder**  When a person continues to re-experience a trauma for weeks or months after it occurs, he or she may be experiencing post-traumatic stress disorder (PTSD). The term *PTSD* was coined following the Vietnam War when large numbers of soldiers returning from combat were unable to recover from the horrifying situations they had witnessed. Some were unable to function in jobs or in their families, and they felt they had no one to talk to since friends and family back home could not imagine the traumas they had endured. Soldiers in other wars had had similar reactions, referred to as "shell shock" or "battle fatigue" in World War I and World War II. After the Vietnam War, PTSD was recognized as a serious psychological disorder that could result not only from war, but also from almost any trauma.

Symptoms of PTSD include reliving the event through nightmares or flashbacks. The person may have strong reactions to or avoid anything that serves as a reminder of the event. She may be irritable or jumpy, feel in danger, or need to be "on guard" at all times. On the other hand, some people experiencing PTSD may feel numb, have difficulty remembering details of the event, and show a lack of interest in work or leisure activities.

**Phobias**  A phobia is an intense, irrational fear that lasts for six months or more. Phobias may develop in response to a traumatic experience, or they may develop spontaneously. For example, one young girl developed a fear of the dark after her mother's car hit and killed an animal while driving at night. The girl feared that she would see a wounded animal if she looked out the window when it was dark. Some common phobias include fear of snakes, lightning, or speaking in public. A person with a phobia usually avoids the feared situation and experiences extreme anxiety if forced to enter it. Some individuals are unable to leave home because of their phobias. Treatments include therapy, hypnosis, and desensitization, in which the person is gradually exposed to the feared situation while in a state of relaxation. Ultimately, overcoming a phobia involves helping the person lower her anxiety until she is able to enter the feared situation more calmly.

## Depression

Depression is characterized by a feeling of sadness that won't go away. A depressed person may feel tired all the time and show a lack of interest in work, school, or leisure activities. She may have trouble concentrating and making decisions. Low self-esteem or even thoughts of suicide may be present. Additional symptoms of depression include restlessness, trouble sleeping, and sudden changes in appetite or weight. A person experiencing depression may appear to be very emotional, negative, or pessimistic, making comments like, "Nothing seems to matter anymore," or "It doesn't matter what I do. Nothing will help anyway." He or she may withdraw from social activities and avoid interactions with others. Trauma is only one cause of depression; other possible causes include genetics, poor coping skills, or ongoing conditions in a person's life, such as an unhappy relationship.

## THE SURVIVOR ROLE

Each victim reacts to trauma in accordance with her established patterns of behavior. For some, the role of victim provides certain benefits that she does not want to give up, and so "I am a victim" becomes part of the self-concept. Some refuse to work through the emotional effects, choosing instead to hold onto their anger, fear, or hatred. For these individuals, sharing their traumatic experience becomes a way to gain sympathy and support from others. Others find valuable lessons in their traumatic experience and make significant lifestyle changes to improve the quality of their lives.

One woman who was the victim of sexual harassment filed complaints through appropriate channels, with no results. She later filed a lawsuit and eventually received a substantial financial settlement. Instead of simply enjoying her financial gain, she chose to set up a nonprofit organization to provide assistance to others in dealing with sexual harassment. She also serves as a consultant to businesses and provides on-site seminars to help employers establish safeguards against sexual harassment in the workplace. This is an example of how a person can learn from a bad experience and eventually use that learning for a constructive purpose.

## TRAUMA-INFORMED CARE

As a health care professional, you will likely meet many individuals who have experienced some type of trauma. Many health care agencies provide training for their staff in how to address the effects of trauma, both immediate and long term. There are various treatment models for **trauma-informed care**, but most address these common themes (NNHVIP):

- Safety: Developing a plan to keep oneself physically and emotionally safe.
- Managing Emotions: Learning to cope with fear, anger, worry, and other emotions; learning to make decisions rationally; regaining the ability to trust other people.
- Loss: Acknowledging and coping with lost loved ones, relationships, or opportunities.
- Planning for the Future: Developing a positive vision for life in the future and planning achievable step-by-step goals to get there.

Health care professionals should encourage victims and relatives to understand the serious nature of psychological trauma and help them recognize the need for professional assistance. Although the disabling effects of physical trauma are obvious, psychological trauma is less likely to be understood or acknowledged. With encouragement from a health care professional, the victim may accept that he or she needs professional assistance in dealing with the psychological effects of the traumatic experience. With therapy, the victim may regain a healthy state of adjustment within a few weeks or months. Without therapy, the victim may remain in a state of poor adjustment for months or years.

## ACTIVITIES

1. Obtain the name of the agency and the emergency phone number for obtaining help in your community or state for the following situations:

   a. Reporting child abuse

   b. Reporting a rape

   c. Reporting domestic violence

   d. Obtaining emergency shelter for a battered woman

   e. Obtaining legal aid for a battered woman

   f. Filing a complaint about sexual harassment in the workplace (after the employer's established procedures have been followed, without results)

2. Consider any life experience that was emotionally traumatic for you. Did you receive any encouragement and support from friends and relatives? Did any health care personnel who cared for you show concern about the emotional effects of your experience? Do you experience fear, anger, or other strong emotions when you think of that experience? If so, consider the possibility that you could benefit from professional counseling.

3. In reading the sections on domestic violence, did you recognize the behavior of anyone in your family? If so, what would be appropriate actions on your part?

4. Consider the following situations in terms of the trauma experienced by the victim and appropriate action by you as a friend or a health care professional:

   a. A child is brought to the emergency room by both parents, who report that the child fell down the stairs. After determining that the arm is broken, the physician asks you to take the child to the cast room and directs the parents to the waiting room. En route to the cast room, the child whispers to you "I did *NOT* fall down the stairs." What is an appropriate action for you?

   b. Your best friend has been married almost a year. At first you and she continued your custom of having lunch and going to a movie once a week. Then, she began to cancel at the last minute; once, she didn't cancel but failed to meet you. Today, she arrives at the restaurant wearing dark glasses. She says she cannot stay for the movie, as her husband expects her home in an hour. When she adjusts her glasses, you notice bruises on her arm. What are some appropriate statements you could make to her? Or should you just ignore what you have seen?

   c. Your coworker tells you she has a problem and asks if you will meet her after work. She reveals that, as a child, she was sexually abused by her father. She left home as soon as she finished high school and visits her parents (in a nearby city) only on special occasions. She is divorced and has custody of her 10-year-old daughter. Now, her parents are insisting that she allow the daughter to spend one weekend a month with them. The daughter is excited about this, but has told you that Grandpa kissed her on the lips during their last visit. What factors should influence the coworker's decision?

## REFERENCES AND SUGGESTED READINGS

American Psychological Association. (2016). *Understanding and preventing child abuse and neglect.* Retrieved from http://www.apa.org/pi/families/resources/understanding-child-abuse.aspx.

Hamm, M.P., Newton, A.S., Chisholm, A. et al. (2015). Prevalence and effect of cyberbullying on children and young people: A scoping review of social media studies. *JAMA Pediatrics, 169*(8), 770–777. doi:10.1001/jamapediatrics.2015.0944.

National Network of Hospital-Based Violence Intervention Programs. (n.d.). *Trauma-informed care.* Retrieved from http://nnhvip.org/trauma-informed-care/.

Patchin, J. W., & Hinduja, S. (2006). Bullies move beyond the schoolyard: A preliminary look at cyber-bullying. *Youth Violence and Juvenile Justice, 4*(2), 148–169.

U.S. Department of Health and Human Services. (2013). *Child welfare outcomes 2008-2011: Report to Congress.* Retrieved from https://www.childwelfare.gov/topics/systemwide/statistics/can/natl-state/.

U. S. Department of Health and Human Services. (2014). *Trauma-informed care in behavioral health services.* (HHS Publication No. (SMA) 14-4816). Retrieved from http://store.samhsa.gov/product/TIP-57-Trauma-Informed-Care-in-Behavioral-Health-Services/SMA14-4816.

U.S. Department of Justice. (2013). *Stalking victims in the United States–revised.* Report from the Office of Justice Programs. (Report NCJ 224527.) Retrieved from http://www.bjs.gov/index.cfm?ty=tp&tid=973.

U. S. Department of Justice. (2015). *Raising awareness about sexual abuse; facts and statistics.* Retrieved from https://www.nsopw.gov/en-US/Education/FactsStatistics?AspxAutoDetectCookieSupport=1#technology.

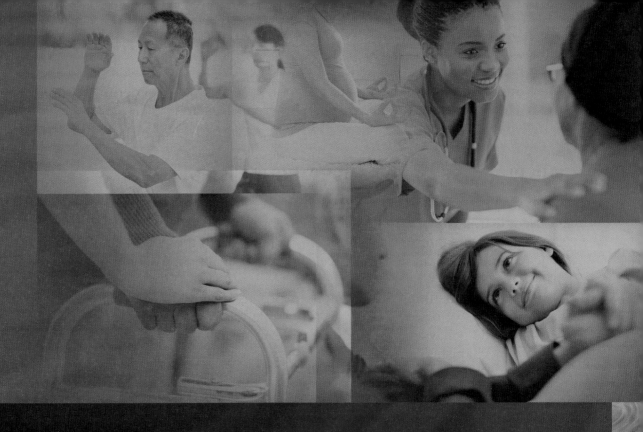

# Defense Mechanisms

## OBJECTIVES

After completing this chapter, you should be able to:

- State the purpose of defense mechanisms.
- Name common defense mechanisms.
- Define rationalization, projection, displacement, daydreaming, escape into illness, repression, and withdrawal.
- Explain how occasional use of a defense mechanism can contribute to good adjustment.
- Compare substance dependency and defense mechanisms.
- Define alcoholism, addiction, tolerance, drug dependency, and codependency.

## KEY TERMS

| | | |
|---|---|---|
| Abstinence | Fetal alcohol syndrome | Psychotherapy |
| Addiction | (FAS) | Rationalization |
| Alcoholism | Habituation | Repression |
| Codependency | Hallucinogenic | Self-deception |
| Dependency | Hypnosis | Withdrawal |
| Dysfunctional | Perception | |
| Enabler | Projection | |

There are certain mental devices that all of us use at times in order to feel more comfortable and make our behavior seem reasonable to ourselves and others. These devices are known as *defense mechanisms*.

## THE PURPOSE OF DEFENSE MECHANISMS

When we find ourselves in a situation that we cannot handle effectively, feelings of threat are aroused: fear, anxiety, hostility, frustration, or other negative feelings. Inability to handle the situation is a threat to one's self-esteem, in addition to the possibility of physical or psychological harm. When an individual feels unable to deal with a situation, a defense mechanism may be used.

Defense mechanisms are attempts to protect against loss of self-esteem. They help us handle feelings of discomfort, make it possible to "save face," provide an *apparently* logical reason for the behavior used, and enable us to maintain self-respect in spite of the outcome. Defense mechanisms can be useful—provided they do not become habitual devices for avoiding reality. Defense mechanisms can help us, or they can become crutches that substitute for more effective ways of dealing with difficult situations.

As a health care professional, being able to recognize common defense mechanisms will help you understand behavior. It is also desirable that you recognize your own use of defense mechanisms in order to develop effective ways of dealing with difficult situations. This chapter explains seven common defense mechanisms: rationalization, projection, displacement, daydreaming, escape into illness, repression, and withdrawal. The remainder of the chapter addresses substance dependency. You will encounter friends, perhaps family members, and patients who have some type of substance dependency.

## RATIONALIZATION

**Rationalization** involves offering an apparently reasonable, socially acceptable explanation for behavior, when the true reason would be too painful for the individual. Thus, rationalization helps relieve disappointment, provides a means for avoiding a situation perceived as threatening, and avoids admitting an inadequacy that would be damaging to self-esteem. Unfortunately, rationalization is a form of self-deception; frequent use of rationalization is self-defeating because it displaces efforts to improve one's competence in dealing with life situations. Consider the following example of a young girl using rationalization.

Mary has been invited to a party. The other girls know the latest dance steps. Mary does not dance. Although Mary wants to be a part of the group and have a good time, she thinks this party will place her at a disadvantage in relation to the other girls. To Mary, missing the party is preferable to being embarrassed. Mary's mother is in poor health, but she is not so sick that Mary needs to stay home with her and miss the party. Nevertheless, her mother's health provides a graceful way to avoid the party.

### For Discussion and Reflection

Have you ever used rationalization to avoid an uncomfortable situation? For example, have you ever told someone you could not participate in an event because you had to work, complete an assignment, etc., when in reality you simply preferred to avoid the event?

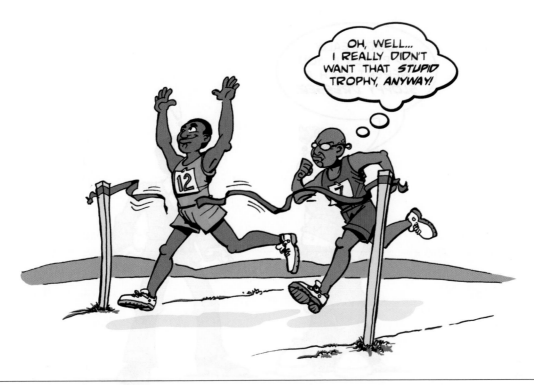

**FIGURE 11-1 Rationalization**

By rationalizing, Mary has avoided admitting to herself the degree of fear she feels at being unable to "hold her own" at the party. She has also given a socially acceptable reason for her absence. When rationalization is used habitually, it becomes an *unconscious* mechanism. Friends of the habitual rationalizer may be unaware of the fears and anxieties that are the basis for hard-to-understand behaviors. They may regard the habitual rationalizer as a person who always makes excuses.

## PROJECTION

**Projection** is a device for placing blame for one's own inadequacies on someone else or on circumstances. Projection is also used to attribute one's own unfavorable characteristics and desires to someone else; a person who is often critical of other people may be exhibiting projection. When projection is used to an extreme, the individual develops distorted **perceptions** of life situations and of people.

James is a health occupations student who is not making satisfactory grades. In discussing his academic standing with the counselor, he says that he cannot study at home because his mother wants him to help around the house. When one of the instructors corrects James on his technique in performing a procedure, he complains that the instructor does not like him. When hostility develops between James and a classmate, James explains the situation by saying that his classmate is jealous because James is dating Joanne.

Every undesirable situation in James's life is explained as the fault of something or someone other than himself. His use of projection is preventing an honest appraisal of his problems and how he himself helps create them. Other people may be saying, "Why doesn't James wise up?" But James is more comfortable projecting blame than looking at himself. He avoids having to admit to himself that he has some shortcomings.

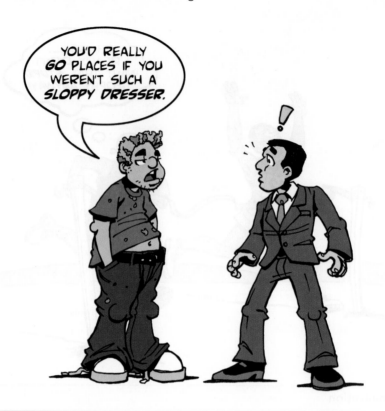

**FIGURE 11-2** Projection

Some people blunder through life using projection and other defense mechanisms instead of learning to see themselves and situations realistically. Each of us makes a mistake at times. *Being able to recognize how we contribute to an undesirable situation and being able to learn from our mistakes lead to growth as a person.* Frequent use of projection interferes with such growth. Projection is self-deception and a distortion of reality.

## DISPLACEMENT

Displacement is the redirection of strong feelings about one person to someone else. Displacement occurs when there is fear or inability to direct the feeling toward the object or person who aroused the feelings. Usually, displacement involves negative feelings, but it can also occur with positive feelings.

Bob is a health care professional with hostile feelings toward his supervisor. He is well aware that the supervisor makes out the assignments and the schedule; also, the supervisor must recommend any member of the staff for a raise. It would be unwise for Bob to be openly hostile to one who has so much control over his daily work and over progress in his career. Bob recognizes this and is always pleasant to the supervisor, even doing a little "apple polishing" at times. Whenever Bob has a conference with the supervisor, the next person he sees is likely to become the object of his hostility. Sometimes Bob carries his hostility home and is irritable and short tempered with his family or the family pet. Bob is displacing the hostility he feels for the supervisor to others who did nothing to create his negative feelings.

Obviously, displacement creates interpersonal problems. Family and friends may be tolerant for a while, especially if they recognize that the hostility has been aroused by someone else. They may even take sides with the individual and attach unflattering names to the person who aroused the anger. Usually, however, the person who habitually displaces negative feelings is perceived by others as irritable and "hard to get along with."

You have learned that the energy generated by negative feelings needs to be worked off, preferably through physical activity. Displacement is an *unhealthy* method of using negative energy. It is an undesirable pattern of behavior, both because of the self-deception involved and because of its unfavorable effects on relationships.

## ESCAPE INTO ILLNESS

Escape into illness involves periodic illnesses that serve a definite purpose, but the individual is not aware of the purpose. Illness as an escape usually has its beginnings in childhood. Parents tend to be especially attentive when a child is sick, even if the illness is a minor one. Sometimes busy parents do not give children much more attention than is necessary for the daily routine, until a problem arises involving the child. Then the child becomes the center of attention. When the problem has been taken care of, the busy routine may be resumed, with the child again receiving only necessary attention. Thus, the child learns that illness is rewarded with parental notice and concern.

If illness during childhood is rewarded by special attention, gifts, permissiveness, sweets, or other things desired by children, then illness serves a definite purpose—the reward of being "special" and of having privileges *not usually allowed when well*. If the parents permit a child to use illness to avoid a dreaded situation and/or to gain advantages available only during an illness, then these early learnings can become an unconscious mechanism that will influence behavior throughout life. Once the child has learned that a headache, a cold, or other minor physical complaint can serve a purpose, illness may be used to get special attention or to avoid certain situations. Eventually, the purpose is no longer in the conscious mind and periodic illnesses have become "real."

Many people habitually use escape into illness as a means of avoiding some of their life problems. When the stress of accumulating problems reaches a certain point, or when an anticipated event arouses fear or anxiety, a minor illness can conveniently provide temporary escape. The symptoms experienced are real; the misery the individual feels is real. There may even be great annoyance at the inconvenience caused by this illness, yet the pattern of behavior is based on the individual's inability to face certain situations. Let's look at Joe, who is enrolled in a program for surgical technicians.

Joe is 19 years old, a high school graduate. He likes sports and has high ideals about team spirit and fair play. He can hold his own with his age group, whether in sports or in standing up for his beliefs.

The surgical technician program proved very interesting to Joe—until the class went into the operating room. Suddenly Joe had some feelings he did not understand. Patients on stretchers, containers of body organs, hospital staff members with masks and floppy gowns—it was a frightening and unreal world to Joe. After several days, Joe's negative feelings about the operating room were stronger than on the first day. Increasing familiarity did not relieve his intense feelings, whereas most of his classmates had become accustomed to the sights and smells of the operating room suite.

Over the weekend, Joe could think of nothing but the operating room and its effect on him. He went bowling with the gang, but he made a poor score and could not get into the

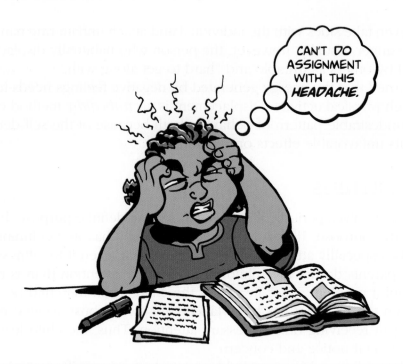

**FIGURE 11-3 Illness can provide escape from an unpleasant situation.**

upbeat mood of his friends. On Monday morning, he could not eat breakfast. When his mother anxiously inquired about his health, he said he must have hurt his back when he was bowling. Joe, with his mother's encouragement, went back to bed and slept all day.

Joe was not pretending to be sick. His doubts and fears had mounted to the point that stress was manifested as physical symptoms. Joe really did feel terrible! His retreating into illness was an unconscious escape.

At this point, Joe's early learnings will influence the behavior pattern of the next few days. If he has learned to use illness as an escape, his back pain will become worse and he will withdraw from the surgical program because of a "bad back." If Joe is able to face life realistically, he will eventually recognize that his emotional reactions to the operating room are affecting him unfavorably. An honest and realistic appraisal of himself in relation to the job requirements of a surgical technician should be made. If Joe is not temperamentally suited to the operating room, he should feel free to withdraw from the program on that basis, without the need to project blame on his "injured back."

Sometimes a person develops insight into tendencies to use escape into illness and, through determination and effort, learns to face problems rather than trying to escape them. Many people, however, have used this device for years and are unable to develop insight into the purposes of the illnesses without professional counsel.

## REPRESSION

**Repression** is the forcing of an unpleasant memory into the subconscious mind. Once a memory has been forced into the subconscious mind, it cannot be recalled at will. Although deeply buried, the memory is still a powerful influence on behavior. Repression occurs most often with painful experiences of childhood, but it can also occur with an adult experience.

Anyone who has had a traumatic experience may repress the memory because the experience is too painful to keep within conscious awareness. Family members may, at some future time, be surprised to hear that individual say, "I don't remember that," or actually deny that such an experience ever occurred. Repression is less susceptible to conscious control than the defense mechanisms discussed previously.

Repressed memories usually come to light only during **psychotherapy**. Many therapeutic sessions are necessary to bring repressed memories back into the conscious level. **Hypnosis**, possibly with age regression, is sometimes used to identify and/or help a patient "relive" a traumatic experience that has been repressed. This is usually accomplished with only a few hypnosis sessions. These methods require the skills of a psychiatrist or psychologist with specialized training.

You, as a health care professional, should be aware of the influence of repressed memories on behavior. A traumatic experience, especially during childhood, may exert a powerful influence on adult behavior, even though the adult does not recall that experience. As a health care professional in contact with pediatric patients, try to prevent the child's experience with the health care system from being psychologically traumatic.

## WITHDRAWAL

**Withdrawal** as a defense mechanism involves either shutting off communication or removing oneself physically from a situation that is perceived as threatening. Withdrawal may be the strategy of choice in a situation in which danger is likely, as in a disagreement when the other person becomes physically threatening. Extremes of withdrawal are characteristic of some psychiatric conditions. A less extreme, but quite serious, example of withdrawal is the desertion reaction of some pediatric patients if no member of the family stays with the child. Lying in the fetal position, a tendency of some chronically ill patients and many geriatric patients, is also an example of withdrawal. If your role as a health care professional will involve caring for patients who exhibit these types of withdrawals, you will study these conditions in other courses.

In every health care role and in your personal life, you will see examples of withdrawal used as a coping strategy in difficult situations:

- If a discussion becomes unpleasant and you refuse to participate further, you are using withdrawal.

- If a conference with the supervisor arouses anger and you excuse yourself from the conference, then you are withdrawing physically.

- If you do not do assignments and have made low grades on the tests, then drop the course the week before exams, you are withdrawing to avoid the threat to your self-esteem that a failing grade represents.

Suppose your first position as a health care professional requires that you work with someone you dislike. Every day you have one or more contacts with this person, and each encounter leaves you angry or unhappy. Except for this one person, you like your job very much. Should you resign? Should you keep the job in spite of these daily annoyances? This situation requires a decision between "fight" or "flight." You can stay on and try to cope

**For Discussion and Reflection**

After reading the explanation of withdrawal above, describe a time you have used this defense mechanism to avoid an uncomfortable situation. Looking back, was withdrawing a helpful choice, or could you have resolved the situation in a more productive way?

with your reactions to this person, or you can "flee" to another job.

There are times when it is a better strategy to withdraw physically from a situation than to put up with the problems it involves. There are other times when the satisfactions of a situation can balance the unpleasantness. Decisions about whether to withdraw or remain should be made on a *rational,* rather than an *emotional,* basis; but the probable long-range effects of the alternatives should enter into the decision.

## SUBSTANCE ABUSE AND DEPENDENCY

Defense mechanisms involve mental tricks—the use of the mind to deal with uncomfortable situations. Another approach to dealing with difficult experiences is the use of substances that have physical effects, thereby providing some relief from stress or diminished awareness of discomfort. Like the defense mechanisms, these substances—tobacco, alcohol, and drugs—provide an escape. With repeated use, one may develop **addiction** to one or more of these substances.

### Nicotine Addiction

It is now known that nicotine, contained in all tobacco products, is highly addictive. Evidence that tobacco is a major threat to health has been increasing for several decades. As a result, many public buildings and most hospitals have been declared smoke-free environments and smoking is prohibited on airlines. Many smokers refuse to give up their habit until they experience a major health problem, such as a heart attack. Others choose to give up smoking as part of a larger plan for a more healthful lifestyle. But for those smokers who choose to continue their habit, current societal restrictions are sources of frustration and anger.

Why do people smoke? The usual reason is that smoking provides relief from feelings of stress. For many people, the primary reason is social; this is the appeal to teenage smokers, for whom conformity to group behavior patterns is important. For an individual whose parents were smokers, the smell of a cigarette, cigar, or pipe may arouse pleasant childhood memories and feelings of comfort and security. Once a person has become addicted to nicotine, smoking is a response to subtle signals from the body that it needs a nicotine "fix."

The decision to give up tobacco may be made voluntarily or under pressure from one's physician, family, or friends. Many smokers are able to give up their habit simply by deciding to do so. When an addictive substance is no longer available to the body, physical symptoms of withdrawal occur. (This meaning of "withdrawal" is different from its meaning as a defense mechanism.) Nicotine withdrawal results in nervous agitation and intense craving for a cigarette (or whatever form of tobacco the individual uses). People who cannot tolerate withdrawal symptoms may use nicotine chewing gum or a skin patch. Psychotherapy also can provide assistance through hypnosis or relaxation with guided imagery.

As a health care professional, you will encounter people who either continue to smoke or are trying to quit. These people may be patients, coworkers, family, or friends. Learn about the dangers of tobacco and the various approaches to giving up tobacco products, so you can be a source of information for anyone who seeks your help.

## Alcohol Abuse/Alcoholism

The use of alcohol, like tobacco, may begin as a social activity and a desire for peer approval and acceptance. It is readily available, more affordable than most drugs, and present in many homes, making it accessible to children and adolescents.

Social use of alcohol can provide quick relief from stress, anxiety, guilt, insecurity, and other uncomfortable feelings. These effects may lead to occasional abuse—overindulgence to the point of becoming intoxicated. Regular use of alcohol over a period of time can result in psychological **dependency** and, eventually, physiological addiction—**alcoholism**. The distinction between occasional abuse and alcoholism is clear cut:

1. An alcoholic's drinking is compulsive (i.e., cannot stop after a reasonable number of drinks).

2. After a period of **abstinence** (hours), the alcoholic experiences withdrawal symptoms that can only be relieved by taking a drink.

Intoxication and alcoholism carry a high price tag. According to the Centers for Disease Control, in 2013, over 10,000 people were killed in alcohol-related traffic related accidents. In 2012, about 1.3 million drivers were arrested for driving under the influence of alcohol or narcotics. In industry, high rates of absenteeism, errors, low productivity, and occupational accidents are attributed to alcohol. Alcohol is involved in a large percentage of crimes, especially murders, and in domestic violence, child abuse, and sex offenses. Alcoholism is now recognized by the courts as a disease (not punishable), but the individual (alcoholic or not) can be prosecuted for any crimes committed while under the influence of alcohol.

Why do people drink? Alcohol provides *escape*. Although classed as a central nervous system depressant, alcohol is considered by many people to be a stimulant, because it lowers inhibitions and releases muscular tension. Unfortunately, these relaxing effects are accompanied by diminished judgment, thinking skills, and memory—effects that make the drinker a danger to him- or herself and others. The use of alcohol to escape the feelings of despair and hopelessness that characterize clinical depression and the depressive phase of manic depressive illness is common. If such patients have also developed alcoholism, their clinical status is "dual diagnosis."

Why do some people progress from social drinking to dependence on alcohol? Many factors have been implicated: physiological, metabolic, nutritional, genetic, emotional, and social. Regardless of causative factors, the condition is treatable, but only when the individual can admit to needing help. This may occur only after numerous arrests, hospitalizations, and various losses (job, spouse, home) have occurred. Medical treatment is required for acute phases, especially during withdrawal, and the ongoing support and encouragement of family and friends is crucial to an alcoholic's long-term recovery.

Effective treatment includes helping the individual learn to face reality and deal with life problems, instead of trying to escape them. This learning can be facilitated by counseling and participation in group therapy. Alcoholics Anonymous (AA), whose membership consists of recovering alcoholics, has proven to be effective for many people. AA emphasizes *total abstinence* from alcohol; newcomers are encouraged to avoid having a drink and to cope one day

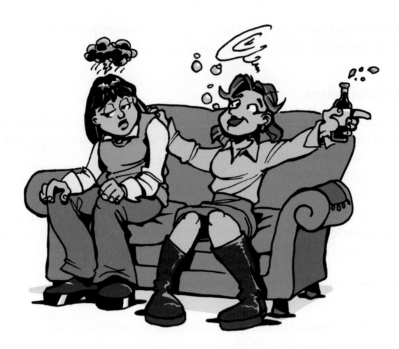

**FIGURE 11-4** Alcohol and drugs provide escape from depression, stress, and problems, but the escape is only temporary.

at a time. Making it through one day is achievable for many people, but vowing to "never take a drink again" is a promise too easily broken. Researchers have found that no one treatment approach works for everyone, and today a variety of treatment models for alcoholism are available. Treatment may include medication, behavioral therapy, support groups, and treatment of co-occurring physical or mental health conditions.

One consequence of drinking has emerged during the last two decades: **fetal alcohol syndrome (FAS)**. This disorder is the result of a woman's drinking during the prenatal period. *Even one or two glasses of wine per day during early pregnancy increases the probability that the baby will be born with FAS, since alcohol penetrates the placental barrier and enters the fetal bloodstream.* Serious damage to the brain results, so the baby is born with an *untreatable disability.* The newborn infant is small, has characteristic cranial and facial features, and may have deformities of the limbs. Growth and development will be inhibited; an intellectual disability may be diagnosed when the child is old enough for testing. This condition is so definitely related to drinking during pregnancy that the National Institute on Alcohol Abuse and Alcoholism issued a statement in 1980 that *pregnant women should totally abstain from alcohol consumption.*

## Drug Abuse

The use of drugs is so pervasive in modern society that few people are unaffected. Any drug can be abused, but those most likely to be abused are drugs that relieve pain, alter one's mood, have a stimulant effect (provide a "high"), relieve anxiety, or have a **hallucinogenic** effect. Regular use of these types of drugs leads to **habituation**, which is psychological dependence on the drug. If usage continues over a period of time, *tolerance* may develop, meaning that larger and larger doses are required to get the desired effect. *Addiction* exists when there is a physiological need for the drug at regular intervals. *Drug dependency* and *chemical dependency* are now the preferred terms, without concern about whether the patient's condition is habituation or addiction. *Withdrawal,* when used in relation to drug dependency, refers to the symptoms that occur when a drug is withheld. These symptoms range from nervous agitation and anxiety to psychotic behavior and convulsions, depending upon the specific drug being withdrawn.

The National Institute on Drug Abuse (2015) has noted the following trends in the use of illegal drugs in the United States:

- In 2013, 24.6 million Americans over the age of 12 reported using an illegal drug in the past month. This represents 9.4 percent of the population.

- Drug use is highest among 18–20-year-olds. Almost one-fourth of this age group reported using illegal drugs within the past month.

- The use of marijuana has increased since 2007, with 19.8 million Americans reporting using the drug in the past month. As of 2015, marijuana is legal for recreational use in 4 states and legal for medical use in 23 states. Therefore, not all use of marijuana can be called illegal, depending on the purpose of its use and the state in which the user lives.

Based on 2013 data, the number of Americans over age 12 who reported using drugs within the past month was as follows:

- 6.5 million Americans reported using prescription medication such as painkillers, tranquilizers, stimulants, and sedatives for non-medical purposes.

- 1.5 million Americans reported using cocaine.

- 595,000 million Americans reported using methamphetamine.

While some individuals are able to use illegal drugs recreationally without long term-effects, doing so is a risky proposition. Each year, millions of Americans struggle with addiction and drug dependency. In 2013, over 22 million Americans over age 12 needed treatment for drug or alcohol use (SAMHSA 2014, p.93). As a health care professional, you are almost certain to encounter individuals whose families, careers, finances, and health have been impacted by drug use. When appropriate, based on your job role and your employer's guidelines, you will have the opportunity to share information about treatment options and recovery support groups in your community.

## CODEPENDENCY

**Codependency** is a situation in which the **dysfunctional** behavior of an alcoholic or drug abuser meets some need of the spouse or another close family member. The role of rescuer or protector becomes such an important part of the codependent's life that the possibility of giving up that role is quite threatening. Family members may have spent years "rescuing" the addict and pleading for a change in behavior. They cling to the belief that life would be good if and when the addict takes control and gives up the addictive substance. Eventually this interaction becomes an important part of life activities; the rescuer role fulfills an important need. At that point, family members *unconsciously* encourage and support the addiction. If the addict undergoes treatment, family problems increase because family members who are codependent cannot cope with the new behavior of the former addict.

A codependent's *conscious* belief is that the family's problems will be resolved when the addiction has been treated. The reality is that a codependent *unconsciously* functions as an **enabler** by facilitating the addiction. Enabling takes many forms, such as "lending" the addict money that the enabler knows will be used for drugs, even though the addict promises to use the money for food and rent. In the case of alcoholism, the enabler may insist on going to parties where alcohol will be served or continue to keep liquor in the home for personal use, knowing that its presence is a temptation for the alcoholic. In the mental health field, codependency is itself considered a condition that requires therapy.

Where codependency exists, treatment of the addict must include treatment of the code-pendent person also. Ideally, the entire family will be involved in therapy, so that any dysfunctional family dynamics may be corrected. The addict must learn to cope with life problems effectively, without escaping into a drug-induced euphoria or relying on the codependent for solving his or her problems. The codependent must learn to encourage the addict to be self-reliant and must be willing to give up the role of rescuer, protector, and caregiver. *Effective treatment of an addict must involve family members.* Otherwise, the "cured" addict will return to a dysfunctional family situation that does not support being drug-free. A difficult adjustment for the recovering addict is giving up old friends and associates who continue to use drugs. New relationships must be developed that include a drug-free lifestyle and ongoing support and encouragement as the recovering addict struggles against the temptation to resume the use of drugs. The desire to experience that drug-induced state of euphoria may remain, even after years of being drug-free.

## DEFENSE MECHANISMS AND ADJUSTMENT

All of us need to use adjustment mechanisms at times, including defense mechanisms. At one time or another we all have unhappy experiences, problem situations to face, and obstacles to overcome. We all experience disappointment and failure at intervals. We all need to feel good about ourselves, but our self-esteem is always at risk—vulnerable to negative experiences. When circumstances threaten self-esteem, we tend to become defensive.

A situation that you perceive as threatening may not bother your best friend. Conversely, you may be puzzled about your friend's defensive reaction to a situation you consider to be ordinary. Some of us become defensive whenever we are criticized. Some of us become apprehensive when we are expected to show achievement. Some of us become uncomfortable in the presence of an authority figure. Some of us distrust others, always expecting a put-down or criticism. Threat, then, is quite personal. It is based on our own specific areas of sensitivity, the psychological scars that are the result of hurtful experiences in our past.

### The Patient

As a health care professional, keep in mind that illness and hospitalization represent a threat to most people. Therefore, you are likely to see many examples of defense mechanisms as you work with patients. If you work with psychiatric patients, you will need to learn about other mechanisms and about behavior deviations that psychiatric patients manifest. In the meantime, observe behavior and learn to recognize defense mechanisms.

When you become aware that someone is using a defense mechanism, realize that the person feels threatened by a situation. It is *not your role to point out the defense mechanism.* Your role is to *reduce the degree of threat the individual feels.* Through reassurance, acceptance, and sincere interest in the patient's well-being, you can usually reduce a patient's need for defensive behavior.

## The Health Care Professional

How can you use knowledge about defense mechanisms to improve your own adjustment? First, keep in mind that defense mechanisms can be useful in relieving discomfort or negative feelings. Suppose a friend drops in just as you are about to leave home for a movie. At first, you feel quite irritated, but then you tell yourself, "I didn't really want to see that movie anyway." Having thus rationalized, you disposed of the angry feelings toward your friend and are free to enjoy the unexpected visit.

*The key to healthful use of a defense mechanism is awareness.* If you are aware of using a defense mechanism and of your reason for using it, then you are probably using it healthfully.

Suppose, on the other hand, your supervisor criticizes your performance frequently, but each time you place the blame on someone else or on circumstances. For example, the supervisor comments that you should have explained a procedure to your patient before carrying it out, but your reaction is, "I didn't have time." For every criticism you have an excuse. Then your use of projection is an obstacle to improving your performance as a health care professional. *Self-deception and distorted perception of situations are incompatible with learning and improved performance.*

In striving to improve your own adjustment, be aware of the frequency and purposes of the defense mechanisms you use. As you learn to recognize your use of each defense mechanism, you will be able to identify the types of situations that are threatening to you. Then you can seek ways of effectively dealing with such situations. If you have a habit of projecting blame, you may have to force yourself to admit a shortcoming now and then. Eventually, you will find it easier to admit being wrong or having made an error. By discarding the defense mechanism, you open the way to learn from experience.

As you become more aware of your tendencies to use defense mechanisms, you will begin to recognize those you have previously been using unconsciously. With increased understanding of yourself and your use of defense mechanisms, you will be ready to eliminate **self-deception**, learn to face reality, and use appropriate behavior in a variety of situations. Through practice in dealing with problems rather than "fleeing" from them, you will improve your skill in solving problems—even those that involve some unpleasantness. At that point, you will have less need for defense mechanisms.

## ACTIVITIES

1. Reflect on your own behavior, and rate each of the following defense mechanisms as follows:

    0 = I never or almost never do this

    1 = I sometimes do this

    2 = I often do this.

    a.  I tend to use rationalization when I must choose between responsibility and fun.

    *Example:* This is often true for me. When I want to watch television, I convince myself that I have studied enough and understand the material. The next day, I wish I had studied. I will rate this item 2.

    b. I do not like to be criticized, even when I know the criticism is true.

    c. I am easily hurt by other people's remarks. It seems to me that people are too ready to be critical or to say unkind things.

    d. I have a lot of trouble with teachers (parents, supervisors, etc.) because of things other people did. I also have a lot of bad luck.

    e. Other people often make me angry (or unhappy), but I usually do not let them know it. I wait until I am home and then "let off steam."

    f. Sometimes my daydreams are more pleasant than what is going on around me. Then I have trouble keeping my mind on my work.

    g. It seems as though my colds always come when we have a big test scheduled (substitute some other type of threat if it is more applicable to you).

    h. I don't believe in getting upset. When the going gets rough, I leave.

    i. Some people irritate me, so I don't talk to them unless I have to.

2. Select one item above that you gave a rating of 2. State how you could modify your use of this defense mechanism.

3. Select a defense mechanism you have used in the past week.

    a. Explain the defense mechanism in your own words.

    b. Describe the situation in which you used this defense mechanism.

    c. Explain why that situation elicited defensive behavior.

    d. Consider the situation from your own viewpoint and, as best you can, from the viewpoint of other people who were present.

    e. List two or more ways you could have dealt with the situation without using a defense mechanism.

4. Participate in a class discussion on the topic: "Watching television/social media/the Internet serves as an escape for many people."

5. Your Uncle Bob was an alcoholic. The family often expressed sympathy for "poor Mary Lou," who put up with his drinking for many years. When Uncle Bob died unexpectedly, the family believed Mary Lou could now enjoy a life free of the problems Uncle Bob had created. Several months later the family was amazed to learn that Mary Lou had married Joe, who was known to be an alcoholic. Explain Mary Lou's behavior.

6. You work at Community Hospital. A family friend, Joe (who married your Aunt Mary Lou in the previous activity), often seeks your company at family gatherings. Today he says to you, "I really want to stop drinking. I've tried several times, but sooner or later I fall off the wagon. Can you help me?" Consider the following:

    a. What will be your first step in helping Uncle Joe?

    b. What role could you play over the next year as Uncle Joe works on controlling his drinking? List specific actions you could take and indicate whom you could involve.

7. Search online to find the following sources of help in your community. Note the phone number and types of services available for each:

   a. Alcoholics Anonymous

   b. Alcohol abuse 24-hour helpline

   c. Drug abuse 24-hour helpline

   d. Your local community agency for alcohol and drug abuse

## REFERENCES AND SUGGESTED READINGS

Centers for Disease Control and Prevention. (2015). *Injury prevention and control: motor vehicle safety.* Retrieved from http://www.cdc.gov/motorvehiclesafety/impaired_driving/impaired-drv_factsheet.html.

Huebner, Robert, and Kantor, Lori. (2011). Advances in alcoholism treatment. *Alcohol Research & Health, 33*(4), 295–299. Retrieved from http://pubs.niaaa.nih.gov/publications/arh334/295-299.htm.

National Institute on Drug Abuse. (2015). DrugFacts: nationwide trends. Retrieved from http://www.drugabuse.gov/publications/drugfacts/nationwide-trends.

Substance Abuse and Mental Health Services Administration. (2014). Results from the 2013 national survey on drug use and health: Summary of national findings. NSDUH Series H-48, HHS Publication No. (SMA) 14-4863. Rockville, MD: Substance Abuse and Mental Health Services Administration.

## SOURCES OF ADDITIONAL INFORMATION

**Alcoholics Anonymous,** http://www.aa.org
For over 50 years, AA has offered community support for alcoholic individuals.
**Narcotics Anonymous,** http://www.na.org
Narcotics Anonymous offers community support for individuals recovering from drug addiction.

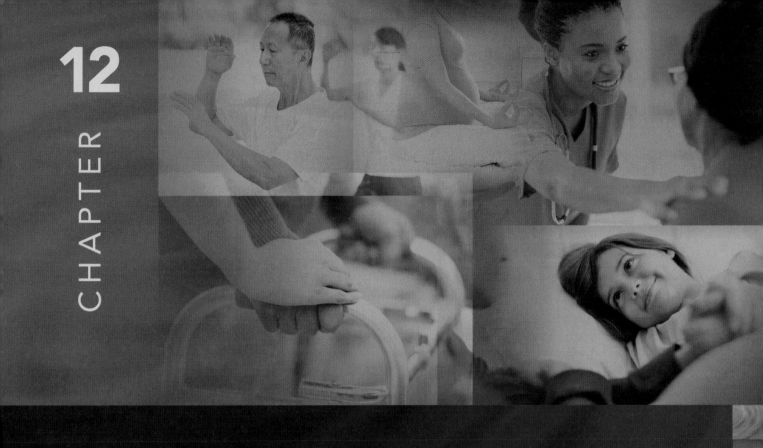

# Frustration and Inner Conflict

## OBJECTIVES

After completing this chapter, you should be able to:

- Name internal and environmental factors that could be sources of frustration.
- Explain prejudice as a source of frustration for members of certain groups.
- Discuss emotional reactions to frustration.
- Describe a general approach to dealing with frustration and preventing unnecessary frustration in one's life.
- Define inner conflict and explain how it differs from interpersonal conflict.
- List steps for resolving inner conflict.

## KEY TERMS

| | | |
|---|---|---|
| Alternative | Digital | Proficient |
| Analgesic | Frustration | Prognosis |
| Aspirations | Incompatible | Prosthesis |
| Attitude | Manipulative | Subtle |
| Capabilities | Narcotic | |
| Debilitating | Perfectionism | |

You are now aware that everyone experiences threats to adjustment at intervals and reacts to such threats according to learned patterns of behavior. **Frustration** is a threat that tends to arouse negative emotions and evoke aggressive or defensive behavior. The effects of frustration can seriously interfere with interpersonal relationships and adjustment.

Frustration exists when progress toward a desired goal is blocked. Everyone feels frustrated at times, but how we react to frustration determines to a large extent whether or not we reach the desired goal.

## DEGREES OF FRUSTRATION

Frustration may evoke irritation or a major emotional reaction. Minor frustrations occur almost daily: The car won't start when we are in a hurry; a pencil point breaks just as we begin a test; we miss the bus; someone keeps us waiting; a button pops off when we do not have time to sew it back on. Such experiences arouse feelings that range from annoyance to intense anger—these feelings are due to frustration.

Major frustrations involve larger aspects of living. A person whose job is not satisfying—who has many job-related problems or has been passed by repeatedly for promotion—has frustrations in the workplace. A mother who wants a career but feels "trapped" by home responsibilities experiences frustration involving her life situation.

Minor frustrations cause annoyance for a relatively short period of time, though a frustration encountered in the morning often sets the pattern of the day. On such days we might comment, "I should have stayed in bed today." Major frustrations, however, may affect the individual's total personality—behavior patterns, values, beliefs, moods, attitudes, and general outlook on life. Major long-term frustrations can negatively impact an individual's adjustment.

## CUMULATIVE EFFECTS OF FRUSTRATION

Minor frustrations are significant if they lead to a buildup of negative feelings, with sudden release over a seemingly minor incident. A series of frustrations during the day may be the underlying cause of Dad's explosion when Johnny asks for twenty dollars. Or Dad may show his annoyance on Friday after giving Johnny three dollars every morning. Unknown to Johnny, his requests for money are frustrating Dad's efforts to make his money hold out until payday. Knowing that Johnny has to have lunch money does not help Dad with his own frustration.

People differ in their tolerance for frustration. Some react emotionally whenever their goals are blocked, and others show the effects of frustration only when it is major. Most people react to minor or moderate frustration with some type of action to resolve the problem; but when frustration is overwhelming, performance deteriorates.

Occasionally the news media report an incident of bizarre or violent behavior. A tobacco farmer who believed his livelihood was being taken away from him by government intervention in the tobacco industry drove his tractor to Washington, DC, and threatened to set off explosives. Workers who went to their workplace and shot colleagues, supervisors, or innocent bystanders have given rise to new terminology; "going postal" refers to this type of behavior because it has occurred several times in the postal system. Although each case of such behavior would require detailed study for a full understanding of the individual's behavior, it is likely that cumulative frustration and a sense of powerlessness for dealing with the sources of frustration were major factors.

# SOURCES OF FRUSTRATION

Blocking of progress toward a goal can arise from many sources: personal characteristics, the environment, other people, illness, or prejudice.

## Self

Each of us is influenced by many different factors in setting our goals. Whether or not these goals are in accord with our own **capabilities** and the opportunities available to us has a bearing on the amount of frustration likely to occur.

As high school seniors, Jack and Paul shared an interest in the health field. Both boys discussed their futures with the school counselor, taking into consideration many types of information, including high school records, achievement and aptitude test scores, vocational interest surveys, personal interests, family finances, and other factors.

Paul's record indicated that he could probably be successful in college. Family finances were strained, and Paul did not like to think of four or more years of school. He liked the idea of becoming a laboratory assistant, so he enrolled in the nearby technical institute. After completing his course with honors, Paul accepted a position in the local hospital. Soon he asked the laboratory supervisor to teach him some of the complex procedures, but he was told that only the registered medical technologists were allowed to do these tests. Paul felt resentful and became increasingly hostile toward his coworkers. He felt he was quite capable of doing more than he was allowed to do. Paul had settled for objectives too low for his potential. As a result, he was frustrated in his job because he was not allowed to function like the more highly trained technologists. Yet, because of the expense and long-term preparation required to become a medical technologist, Paul did not set his goal in accordance with his abilities.

On the other hand, Jack applied to a college, even though he had difficulty with high school subjects. The school counselor had encouraged Jack to plan vocational goals rather than academic ones. Jack's mother always said she wanted her son to be a doctor, so Jack had grown up with the idea of attending medical school. He refused to recognize evidence that he probably would not be able to succeed in college courses. After failing three out of four courses at the university, Jack came home confused and upset about his failure. He had set his objectives too high, in spite of guidance that could have helped him plan more realistically.

Frustration, then, can result either from trying to reach what is unreachable or from achieving unchallenging goals. A career goal should be carefully selected on the basis of all information available about the individual and occupations in which the person is interested. Career goals are important to achievement, development of one's potential, job satisfaction, and, ultimately, to adjustment and happiness.

Goals are also involved in short-term aspects of living. To some youngsters, failure to make the Little League team is a shattering experience. Athletic ability is, to a great extent, based on physical characteristics and motor skills. If one's goal is to make the football team in spite of small physical build and limited stamina, then frustration is almost certain to occur. If one enjoys singing, the short-term goal of being accepted into the school chorus is probably realistic. On the other hand, the goal of becoming a pop star is realistic only for those few who have rare talent, resources to develop the talent, and the determination and perseverance to strive many years for that goal.

Goals are more realistic when related to what we enjoy and learn readily. Satisfaction is greater if goals continue to offer challenge. In measuring goal progress, it is better to compare yourself today with yourself in the past, rather than with other people. Aspiring to be "the best" in anything is more likely to lead to frustration than aspiring to "continue to improve."

## The Environment

Environment—either physical or social—can be a source of frustration. The environment is less subject to control than one's goals and **aspirations**. As adults, we learn to accept some frustrations, such as rain on the day of a picnic or lack of snow for skiing.

The opportunities an environment offers should be considered in making long-range plans. If you decide to follow a career for which there is no locally available opportunity, frustration will occur unless resources can be made available or a move to another community can be arranged.

Sometimes the customs and practices of a community are the source of frustration. The health care professional who wants to improve health habits in a community must give careful consideration to the established beliefs, values, and customs of that community. Cultural aspects of the social environment may block efforts to change established practices.

## Other People

Many obstacles can be overcome through persistence, problem-solving techniques, or an approach that removes the obstacle or allows one to get around it. When the obstacle is a person, however, overcoming the obstacle is more difficult.

Paul's laboratory supervisor was an obstacle to his learning advanced techniques, even though the supervisor was basing the decision on hospital policy, role differentiation, and Paul's lack of educational foundation for the judgments required by advanced procedures. Suppose Jack had been refused admission to college. Then the admissions committee would constitute an obstacle to his attending college.

In some cases, people are obstacles because of their beliefs, prejudices, attitudes, superior ability, dependency, and many other factors. When achieving a goal requires changing an **attitude** or belief of the person who is an obstacle, then the frustration is not likely to be overcome easily; people do not readily change their values and beliefs. In competition, the abilities of other people determine whether or not an individual makes the team, wins a gold medal, or gets a promotion. When the obstacle is a competitor's superior ability, then personal effort to surpass such ability is necessary to reach the goal.

## Illness

Illness may cause either minor or major frustration, depending upon the duration of illness and the patient's life situation. A minor illness that lasts a few days may simply be an inconvenience, or possibly a welcome relief from the daily routine—a chance to stay home and take it easy. But even a minor illness can create intense frustration if it interferes with some important event.

If the illness is serious or life-threatening, the patient experiences numerous frustrations. The individual may feel that he or she is losing control of his or her life. Suddenly

### For Discussion and Reflection

Consider a situation within the last month that frustrated you. Was the frustration major or minor? What frustrated you about the situation?

someone else (i.e., a doctor) is telling the patient what he or she must do. Often these mandates include major life changes: stop smoking; change jobs to minimize stress (or physical exertion or exposure to hazardous situations); stop playing tennis; eat fresh vegetables; do not eat red meat; stop drinking alcoholic beverages; stop drinking sodas; exercise at least 20 minutes every day; stay in bed a minimum of 10 hours a day; have at least two rest periods; stay out of the sun between 11 a.m. and 3 p.m.; agree to a course of chemotherapy (or radiation); go to a medical center for special tests or treatment. Whatever the mandate includes, it will impact the patient's lifestyle. The significance of each thing that must be given up determines the degree of frustration. The specific treatment may also be a source of frustration, especially if there are side effects.

Frustration is usually experienced as anger. When you, as a health care professional, realize that a patient's behavior seems to be an expression of anger, consider what impact the illness is having on the patient's life. Show interest in the patient's life situation with an expression of caring and concern, such as, "I imagine this illness is really changing your life." If the patient is willing to talk about the effects, it will help defuse the anger. As you carry out your responsibilities for health care, be aware that the recipient of your services is a person who may be angry and/or sad about the losses involved as his or her life is disrupted by illness.

## Prejudice

Federal legislation has attempted to remove prejudice as an obstacle to educational and job opportunities. Unfortunately, the passage of a law does not change deeply rooted beliefs or the behavior patterns of a lifetime. Yet this legislation has increased awareness of the extent to which prejudice creates obstacles based on income level, race, age, gender identity, sexual orientation, or handicap. Such prejudices of employers and school officials continue to create obstacles for many people, but in more **subtle** ways than in the past. At this time, a person who has been discriminated against because of one of the conditions covered by equal rights legislation may petition the courts to remove the obstacle. Some professional groups and consumer advocate organizations provide legal assistance to people whose rights to equal opportunity have been violated.

## EFFECTS OF FRUSTRATION

Each of us reacts to frustration according to patterns we have learned throughout life. These reactions, therefore, vary from one person to another, but they often involve either hostile behavior or withdrawal. Frustration arouses negative emotions: fear, anger, disappointment, anxiety, resentment, or a combination of these. Both behavior and emotional reactions to frustration are influenced by the importance attached to the goal as well as the individual's adjustment. A person who is insecure and inclined to perceive frustration as a threat is likely to feel a mixture of fear and anger. A person who is self-confident is likely to feel some degree of anger, with little fear. The person who is easily discouraged is likely to give up when there is an obstacle to success. Quitting, remember, is a form of withdrawal. The person who is stimulated to try harder in the face of difficulty is likely to react to an obstacle by increased effort or a change in strategy.

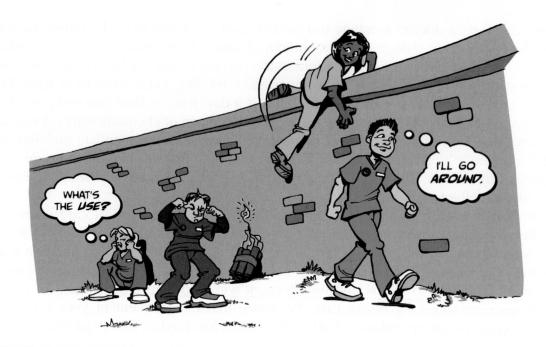

**FIGURE 12-1 Each person reacts to frustration in his or her own way.**

## FRUSTRATION AND BEHAVIOR PATTERNS

Everyone who has cared for a baby or young child has seen examples of behavioral responses to frustration. The pattern of response is learned behavior, largely based on how others react to the child's frustration. Ideally, an adult would recognize that the child is frustrated and take action to assist the child or remove the source of frustration. Frequently, however, the child's need is not recognized and the frustration is viewed as misbehavior. Thus, patterns become established based on whether or not the child's behavior led to satisfaction of a need.

### Early Learning

Experience with frustration may begin almost with birth. The infant who is fed according to a rigid schedule, rather than when hungry, experiences frustration as well as the physical discomfort of hunger. Each developmental task (such as turning over, sitting, and standing) requires many efforts before success is realized. Early efforts to perform such activities are frustrating, but the infant persists until bodily control has been mastered. Many infants show distress when these early efforts result in failure.

Toddlers know what they want long before they can state their needs verbally. When a toddler is unable to make wants known, the reaction may involve falling to the floor, kicking, or crying. The child's frustration is due to inability to communicate verbally—a lack of competence for the task attempted. The parent who does not understand frustration may punish the child. Then the child feels anger as the result of frustration and fear as the result of punishment. Such experiences affect the child's learning about frustration and also about the "right" to express feelings. The parent, without realizing it, is teaching the child that it is "wrong" to express negative feelings. This can be the beginning of ineffective patterns for dealing with frustration. It can also be the beginning of a pattern that you have already learned is undesirable—suppression of emotions.

## Childhood

During childhood, many frustrations result from the child's lack of competence for tasks being attempted, parental restraints, and rules at school, in clubs, and other organizations. Adults should make a conscious effort to help children understand the necessity for placing limits on behavior, especially where there are groups of children. Yet, even when the need for rules is understood, the child is frustrated when these limits interfere with a desired activity. If the frustration is great, the child may feel resentment toward the source of the rule—a parent, teacher, club sponsor, or whatever authority figure seems to be preventing a desired activity. If punishment is also involved, fear and distrust of authority figures may develop. Rebelliousness or hostility toward authority, beginning with such childhood experiences, may later interfere in relationships with authority figures, such as supervisors in the job setting.

## Adulthood

Adults experience frustration in many forms and in every aspect of living. For the majority of people, probably the most common frustration is lack of enough money to have the material possessions desired. The major adaptations required by marriage, parenthood, and a job all involve numerous frustrations. Even after one has learned to function within the various roles of adulthood, frustrations periodically occur in each role.

As a health care professional, you are likely to have patients who are experiencing frustration. Illness and injury interfere with one's life. Loss of income due to inability to work and difficulty in performing self-care tasks, such as buttoning a shirt, are common problems for patients. Some patients, however, have long-term frustrations. The amputee who must learn to use a **prosthesis**, the stroke patient who has lost the use of one side of the body, and the laryngectomee who cannot speak are examples of patients who live with frustration. Be aware that some of your patients are experiencing intense frustration; try to anticipate their needs and be sensitive to the feelings they are experiencing.

## PERFECTIONISM AND FRUSTRATION

A personal trait that leads to frequent frustration is **perfectionism**. This trait probably has its roots in childhood, with the child seeking parental approval through performance of assigned tasks, school work, or athletics. Parents' efforts to motivate a child to improve performance may result in the child learning that no performance is ever good enough ("Well, it's good that you passed the audition for chorus. Now, I expect you to be a soloist by the end of the year."). In this situation, one child may give up hope of winning unqualified approval; another may become determined to please, to turn in the perfect performance that is sure to win approval.

The perfectionist may expect perfection from him- or herself or from others, especially a spouse, one's children, or coworkers. When perfectionism is focused inward, the individual views any less-than-perfect performance as unacceptable, even humiliating ("You may make mistakes, but not me!"). This person may agonize over a mistake or social blunder that others hardly notice. Self-forgiveness is not even considered.

The person whose perfectionism is directed outward is repeatedly disappointed in the performance of other people. Being intolerant of mistakes or poor performance by others, the perfectionist tends to be critical and irritable, leading to poor relationships within the family and on the job. These high expectations of self and others inevitably result in frustration for a perfectionist.

## COPING WITH FRUSTRATION

You will experience frustration at intervals throughout life. This is a good time to evaluate your behavior patterns and decide whether you need to find new ways of dealing with frustration. By learning to handle frustration effectively, you can spare yourself much unhappiness and increase the proportion of satisfying experiences in your living.

There are numerous ways of dealing with frustration. The most desirable method of handling one particular frustration may be inappropriate for handling another. The general approach requires three steps:

1. Expect a certain amount of frustration in living and avoid overreacting emotionally or using defense mechanisms to avoid dealing with the problem.

2. Recognize frustration when it occurs.

3. When experiencing frustration, evaluate the situation and use the systematic procedure described next to select an approach for dealing with the obstacle.

### Overcoming the Obstacle

There is no guaranteed way to overcome any and all obstacles. Recognize that the negative feelings of the moment are due to frustration, and then use a rational approach to solve the problem at hand. If dealing with the frustrating situation can be delayed, it is helpful to put it out of your mind for a while; take time to "sleep on it." You may then be able to return to the problem with a fresh viewpoint and with less emotional influence on your thinking. The following questions can help in planning to overcome the obstacle:

- Exactly what goal am I trying to reach?
- What is preventing my reaching that goal? (Identify the obstacle.)
- How can I overcome or get around this obstacle? List *all* possible ways to deal with the obstacle.
- How is each possible solution likely to affect my achieving the goal?
- How is each possible solution likely to affect the way I feel about myself?
- How is each possible solution likely to affect other people?
- Is this *my* goal, or did someone else set this goal for me?
- Which solution is most likely to help me reach my goal?
- Is the goal important enough to me to justify the expenditures (time, effort, energy, money) required for reaching the goal?
- What other benefits (such as new competencies, widened experience, and future opportunities) am I likely to gain from continued efforts to achieve the goal?

- Shall I persist in striving for this goal? Or shall I substitute another goal?
- Make a decision.
  a. If you decide to continue to strive for that goal, select a means for dealing with the obstacle and follow through with it.
  b. If your first effort does not remove the obstacle, try another approach.
  c. If you decide not to continue to strive for that goal, modify the goal or substitute a different goal.

> **For Discussion and Reflection**
>
> What is one of your career or personal goals? When you honestly assess your abilities and resources, is this a realistic goal? If yes, what are some short-term goals or steps that can help you move toward your long-term goal? If your original goal is not realistic, what are other options you could explore?

## Preventing Frustration

It is also desirable to use a preventive approach to frustration. As illustrated by the cases of Jack and Paul, unrealistic goals can be the source of much frustration. Long-term goals, such as preparing for a career, usually include numerous short-term goals. There may be many frustrating experiences before the long-term goal is reached. If the short-term goals provide stepping-stones to be reached one by one, then frustration is offset by achievement of these intermediate goals.

## INNER CONFLICT

Another common cause of poor adjustment is inner conflict. Perhaps you are accustomed to thinking of conflict as a fight or argument. Such conflicts involve two or more people and are *interpersonal* conflicts. Inner conflict, on the other hand, exists *within one person*. Other people may contribute to a person's inner conflict and others may be affected by the behavior resulting from inner conflict, but it is the individual with the conflict who is most affected.

Inner conflict exists when an individual has two **incompatible** needs or goals, or when the individual must choose between two or more **alternative** means for meeting a need or achieving a goal. The conflict arises because of the incompatibility of these needs, goals, or means, but other behavior influences may also be involved. One's value system, standards of behavior, beliefs, interests, personality traits, character traits, and self-concept may all contribute to inner conflict.

The person who has an inner conflict is usually aware of the need to choose between two goals or two courses of action. However, the individual may be unaware of the basic needs, values, interests, beliefs, and other factors that contribute to the conflict.

## Conflict between Needs

Adolescents are often faced with a conflict between the need for acceptance by the peer group and the need for maintaining their beliefs about "right" and "wrong" behavior. Suppose someone in Bill's crowd proposes a risky adventure involving behavior Bill believes to be wrong. Bill must choose between participating in the adventure or refusing to participate.

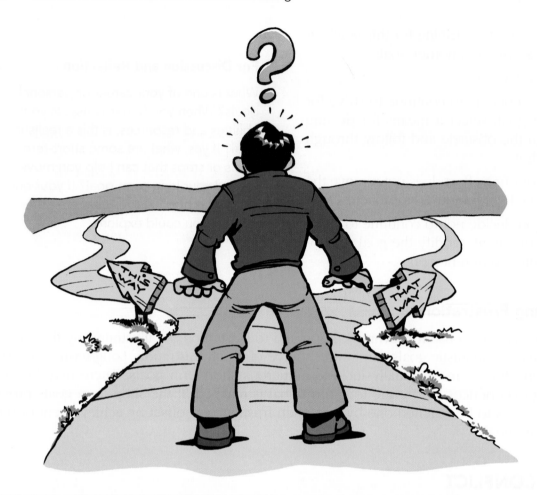

**FIGURE 12-2 Inner conflict exists when a person must choose between different ways to meet their needs.**

His need to belong, feel accepted, and be approved by members of his peer group is in conflict with his need for maintaining his standard of behavior, beliefs, and self-concept— "I am a person who does not do things that are wrong." Going along with the adventure requires lowering his standards of behavior, which is a threat to his beliefs, values, and self-concept. Opposing the proposed adventure involves risking his status with the group, which is a threat to his need to belong. Through no fault of his own, Bill is in a situation that requires a decision between two alternative actions, both of which threaten something he values.

## Conflict between Means

Conflict also exists when a goal can be reached in two or more ways. Mrs. P. has a chronic condition that causes her much discomfort. She usually relies on **analgesic** drugs, but more and more often she must have a **narcotic** to obtain full relief from pain. Her physician now warns her that continued use of drugs will have undesirable effects. He recommends surgery to correct her problem.

Mrs. P.'s goal of restored health requires choosing between habitual use of drugs and surgery. To be free of pain, she must use one means or the other. When Mrs. P. was a child, her oldest brother died during an operation. Since then, she has heard numerous stories about

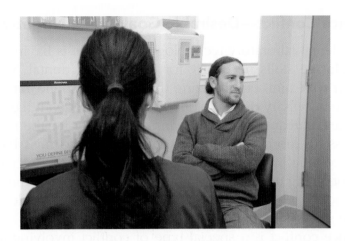

**FIGURE 12-3** Patients may experience frustration or inner conflict when receiving a diagnosis or making decisions about their treatment.

unsatisfactory surgical results, each one adding to her fear of surgery. Now, the thought of going to the operating room terrifies her, yet she desperately wants to be free of pain. To Mrs. P., with her deep-seated fear of the operating room, this conflict between two remedies for her health problem may be far more distressing than the physical discomfort associated with surgery.

## TYPES OF INNER CONFLICT

Regardless of whether a conflict is between needs, goals, or the means for achieving them, the individual must choose between alternatives. These alternatives may be positive (desirable) or negative (undesirable). Even in a choice between two positives, unhappiness may result from giving up one alternative. The degree of difficulty in making a decision is often influenced by whether the alternatives are both positive, both negative, or positive accompanied by a negative outcome.

### Approach-Approach Conflict—Two Desirable Goals

Approach-approach conflict involves two needs or goals that are incompatible. Al is working in the local hospital as a nursing assistant. He enjoys his work and is especially good with elderly patients. His supervisor calls him into the office and states that he has been recommended to the director of the practical nursing program. The supervisor points out the advantages of being a licensed nurse and indicates belief in Al's potential for succeeding in the program. Al is proud that the supervisor has so much faith in him. He is suddenly fired with ambition to improve himself through educational preparation for a career.

When Al tells his girlfriend about his exciting opportunity, she says, "But how can we get married if you are not going to have any income for a year?" Al is eager to get married and has been saving for the costs of setting up a home. Any delay in these plans will be just as disappointing to him as to his girlfriend.

Al has two goals, each of which he would like to reach as soon as possible. He is eager to get married, but he is also aware of the advantages of educational preparation for his job. He cannot get married immediately and at the same time enroll in the practical nursing course. Al has a conflict between two strong but incompatible needs—they cannot be met at the same time.

## Approach-Avoidance Conflict—Desirable Goal with a Negative Effect

Ryan is enrolled in a dental laboratory technology course. He is having difficulty developing some of the **manipulative** skills necessary for constructing dental prostheses. His teacher discusses the problem with him, emphasizing that he must spend more time on laboratory practice to develop the necessary **digital** skills. The only time Ryan has for this extra practice is the period the basketball team practices. Ryan is top scorer for the team.

Ryan wants to pass his lab course, but to do so he has to miss basketball practice. To achieve his goal of becoming **proficient** as a dental laboratory technician, Ryan has to accept the negative aspects of giving up his prized position on the team: feeling disloyal to the team and relinquishing an activity that gives him much satisfaction. Regardless of which choice he makes, Ryan will lose something that he values.

Approach-avoidance conflict is a special type of conflict involving a desirable goal with undesirable effects. The individual alternates between trying to reach a certain goal and abandoning the goal. The decision to abandon a goal usually occurs as the individual approaches achievement of the goal or when the time for a desired event approaches.

Emily is a dental assistant who is engaged to Jake. Emily gets along well with her parents. She especially likes her room, which she decorated and furnished during her first year as a "career woman." When she comes home from her job, her mother has dinner ready. Emily's only home responsibility is cleaning her own room. She is able to save a large portion of her paycheck. Getting married and moving into an apartment requires that Emily give up these benefits of living with her parents. On the other hand, she loves her fiancé, wants her own home, and wants to have a family.

Emily has set the wedding date several times. Repeatedly, when ordering the wedding announcements could not be delayed any longer, she has broken the engagement. Jake is persistent and has accepted each delay with good humor. But each time the date approaches for achieving her goal (getting married, having her own home, starting a family), Emily develops intense feelings (anxiety? panic?) that she relieves by breaking off the engagement. Thus, she avoids achieving the goal that would involve giving up the advantages of living with her parents.

## Avoidance-Avoidance Conflict—Two Negative Alternatives

Avoidance-avoidance conflict exists when an individual must choose between two alternatives, both of which will have a negative outcome. Carolyn is a student in a medical assistant program. Last week her best friend in the class broke an expensive piece of equipment and returned it to its storage case without reporting the breakage. Carolyn was present at the time, and her friend insisted that Carolyn promise not to tell anyone. Today, Carolyn learns that another student in the class has been blamed for the broken equipment and told to pay for it.

Carolyn has strong feelings about loyalty to friends. She also has strong feelings about keeping promises, honesty, truthfulness, and fair play. Carolyn knows who actually broke the equipment, but the guilty person refuses to report herself. Carolyn can break her promise to this friend and report the incident, or she can keep silent and permit an innocent person to take the blame. Carolyn's values are involved, yet either course of action will violate personal traits on which she places a high value. Carolyn's self-concept is also involved: she does not want to be a person who breaks promises, nor does she want to be a person who permits an injustice when she could prevent it. She has to choose between loyalty to her friend and her sense of fairness. She has to choose between telling the truth and breaking a promise.

How Carolyn handles this situation will probably be determined by her values. She must place a higher value on one set of traits than the other in order to select an alternative. If she reports the breakage, then honesty and fair play assume a higher place in her value system than loyalty to friends and keeping promises.

Carolyn's behavior patterns will affect how she works through this conflict. She may put off a decision and, by her inaction, allow the wrong person to be blamed. She may project blame by saying to herself that it is her friend's responsibility to tell the truth. She may rationalize by telling herself it is not really her business. Which choice she makes and how she justifies that choice to herself will result from many years of forming behavior patterns to deal with unpleasant situations.

> **For Discussion and Reflection**
>
> Consider a time when you felt torn between two possible courses of action. After reading about types of inner conflict, would you describe your experience as approach-approach conflict, approach-avoidance conflict, or avoidance-avoidance conflict?

## HOW TO DEAL WITH INNER CONFLICT

Inner conflict may be handled effectively *only by making a decision between alternatives*. Obviously, the choice will be better if the individual recognizes that a conflict exists and identifies the competing needs or goals. Insofar as possible, the feelings and values related to the conflict should also be examined.

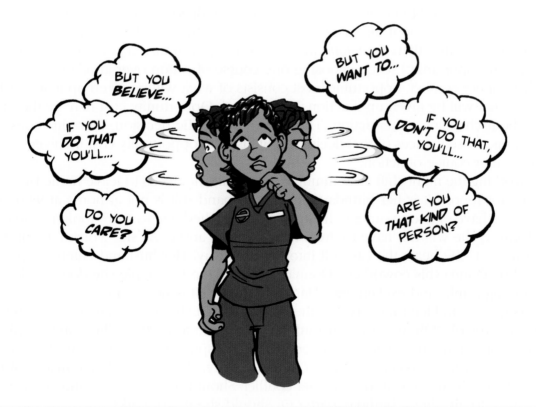

**FIGURE 12-4 Inner conflict can only be resolved by making a choice.**

## Thinking through a Conflict Situation

The following steps provide a rational approach to resolving a conflict:

1. Recognize that there is a conflict.

2. Identify the two incompatible needs (or goals).

3. Examine the situation in terms of interests, values, immediate needs, long-term needs, and other relevant factors.

4. Decide how each need could be met (or each goal achieved).

5. Think through the probable effects of each possible action: what will be gained, what will be lost, and whether or not the action would be in accord with your beliefs, value system, interests, goals, and needs.

6. After thorough consideration of the probable effects of each possible choice, make a decision.

7. *Fully accept your decision.* One alternative has been selected; the other has been discarded. Do not flounder in doubt about whether the right choice was made. Set out to prove that you made a good decision. Do not develop feelings of guilt or failure about the alternative that was discarded. Remember: *A choice had to be made.*

## Identifying Opportunity Cost

In business, a concept known as "opportunity cost" may be used to assist in making decisions. This concept, when applied to inner conflict, can help the individual focus on presumed facts; by so doing, vague fears about alternative actions can be translated into information—the basis for a *rational*, rather than an *emotional*, decision. Opportunity cost refers to what one must give up (an opportunity) when choosing one course of action over another.

In resolving inner conflict, opportunity cost consists of what will be given up if action 1 is pursued, and what will be given up if action 2 is pursued. Opportunity cost may be the basis for anxiety about choosing either action. The cost of a specific decision, then, includes not only the obvious consequences of that decision, but also the opportunity cost involved in not following the other course of action.

Anna is working the night shift at Community Hospital; she needs to leave home by 10:15 to be on time for report. It is her birthday, but her husband still is not at home at 9:00. She and her husband have only one car, and he knows she is scheduled to work tonight. She puts on her uniform so she will not have to dress after he does arrive. As she worries about why he is not home yet, she hears the car pull into the driveway. Her husband enters, laughing, accompanied by Donna (his coworker), Donna's husband, and a couple she does not know. They are carrying drinks and exclaiming, "Happy birthday!" It is now 9:45.

Anna gets glasses and ice for everyone, then explains that she must leave for work. She is greeted by a chorus of, "Oh, no! It's your birthday. We came to party." When Anna explains that she cannot stay and party, that she is needed at the hospital, her guests suggest, "Just call in sick. They'll never know you are having a birthday party." Leaving aside the matter of her husband's behavior, let us look at Anna's inner conflict. Should she stay home and enjoy these guests who want to give her a birthday party? Or should she go to work?

The *reward* of choosing to call in sick and stay home would be that Anna has a birthday party, enjoys socializing with friends, and becomes acquainted with the new couple. The *cost* of staying home would be that Anna uses a sick day she might need later. The *opportunity cost* of this choice could be a sense of guilt for lying to the supervisor and leaving her coworkers short-handed. Anna is conscientious; her self-esteem would be affected negatively if she fails in her duty. Possibly, her supervisor would learn that she is not sick but stayed home to party.

The *reward* for choosing to go on duty as scheduled would be that Anna retains her self-respect, her self-esteem is not threatened; she does not harbor guilt about her behavior. Also, Anna still has that sick day in reserve in case she needs it. The *cost* of not staying home to party was missing her own birthday party and the annoyance of her husband and the guests about her leaving. The *opportunity cost* was not having a chance to become acquainted with the new couple.

Note that identifying the rewards, costs, and opportunity costs of each alternative paves the way for a *rational,* rather than *emotional,* decision. So adding the concept of opportunity cost to your problem-solving method can facilitate the resolution of an inner conflict.

## INNER CONFLICT AND ADJUSTMENT

The approach just described illustrates the familiar saying, "You can't have your cake and eat it too." Even minor conflicts cause a certain amount of inner discomfort until they are resolved. If you put off doing an assignment in favor of more pleasant activities, you eventually reach the point of having to resolve the conflict. You must either decide to do the assignment instead of some preferred activity, or decide not to do the assignment and accept the consequences. You are probably a little uncomfortable as long as you continue to put off the decision.

Many people react to conflict with indecision, either procrastinating as long as possible or making one choice and then changing to another. Only a firm decision truly resolves a conflict. Sometimes the decision is necessarily accompanied by an unfavorable effect, either on oneself or on others. *The ideal result in handling conflict is to gain the desired goal with the least possible undesirable effect. In many situations, a new solution to the conflict can be discovered by talking the situation over with a trusted friend, relative, or coworker.*

## INNER CONFLICT AND THE HEALTH CARE PROFESSIONAL

As a health care professional, you can make good use of your understanding of conflict and its effects on behavior and emotional states. Health care professionals frequently have inner conflict. The responsibilities of being a health care professional are great. Health care professionals often possess confidential information. People tend to put health care professionals into conflict situations by asking about patients or seeking health advice. The necessity for providing many health services on a 24-hour basis requires that some health care professionals have a schedule different from that of their families. Staffing problems give rise to occasional changes in time off, sometimes on short notice. Urgent situations require working overtime, being "on call," or returning to work unexpectedly after putting in a full day's work.

The health care professional who is dedicated to serving others and has a strong sense of duty is likely to experience conflict between loyalty to the job and loyalty to the family. There may be occasions when there is a conflict between responsibilities and "rights" as a person.

Medical ethics and the policies of your place of employment can help you with some of these conflicts. For example, when a close friend asks about a patient, your *ethical responsibility* to hold in confidence what you learn about patients in the course of your job helps you resolve the conflict between responsibility and desire to have your friend's approval. At times, you may have to justify your *sense of duty* when job requirements interfere with plans involving family or friends. Thinking about such possible conflicts in advance can help you resolve them if they actually occur.

## INNER CONFLICT AND THE PATIENT

Many patients have inner conflict related to their illness. Mr. B. has orders for strict bedrest, yet he feels capable of returning to work. He has a conflict between his need for self-interest (perhaps self-preservation) and his need to fulfill his job responsibilities. Ms. J., who is having diagnostic studies, may have a conflict between the need for relief from distressing symptoms and the fear of learning something unfavorable as a result of the studies.

Family members, too, have inner conflict when decisions must be made. It is difficult to agree to painful procedures on someone you love, yet refusing permission for the procedure may contribute to continued illness or the loved one's death. The decision on whether or not to consent to surgery involves many emotions, including the possibility of guilty feelings if the outcome is unfavorable. An emotionally wrenching conflict for family members is a decision to discontinue life support. Even if the patient's status fits the conditions specified in an advance directive, an inner conflict exists for each person involved in the decision. Some physicians try to protect families from decisions that may lead to guilty feelings. However, it is desirable that the family be involved in decisions about painful or **debilitating** treatments and the use of life-support systems for persons whose illness involves a hopeless **prognosis**.

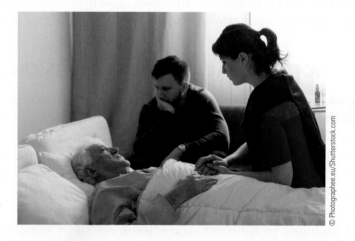

© Photographee.eu/Shutterstock.com

**FIGURE 12-5** Family members often experience inner conflict when making difficult treatment decisions for a loved one.

# USING KNOWLEDGE ABOUT INNER CONFLICT

As a health care professional, be aware that some of the distress you see in patients and their families is due to inner conflict. With such understanding, you are better able to accept behavior that appears unreasonable and accept emotional reactions that seem out of proportion to the seriousness of the illness. Be aware, too, that sometimes the physician has given the family or patient information that you do not have, such as an unfavorable prognosis.

Applying knowledge about inner conflict to your personal life can help you resolve conflict situations rationally to achieve the best possible outcome for you and your family. Applying your knowledge of inner conflict to relations with patients can help you be more understanding and more accepting of your patients and their families.

## ACTIVITIES

1. Your goal for a particular course is a B grade. The examination is two weeks away. In the meantime, you have three laboratory reports and a term paper due. Develop a plan that will increase the probability of your feeling prepared for the exam and also completing the other assignments. Explain how your plan would minimize the frustration likely to occur.

2. You have a 2-year-old male patient who is to be hospitalized for about a month. During the first days in the hospital, the child tries to talk to those caring for him, but no one can understand him. He frequently throws himself down in bed and kicks violently; sometimes he bangs his head on the crib.

   a. Explain the child's behavior.

   b. How should you as a health care professional react to this behavior?

   c. How could those in frequent contact with this child best help him?

   d. Describe this child's primary need.

   e. List some possible long-term effects on the child if health care professionals:

      (1) Label the child "spoiled" and avoid the child whenever possible.

      (2) Make a sincere effort to understand what the child is trying to say.

3. You have accepted a well-paid position in a large health agency. Job descriptions have been written for each position. The job description for your position lists the procedures you will be permitted to do, omitting several that you learned in your health occupations course. You resent not being allowed to perform these procedures. What are some possible approaches to dealing with this situation? Describe each approach fully in terms of your goals, possible actions, possible effects of each action, and the solution you believe is most likely to help you reach your goal.

4. Consider one conflict you have had during the past month.

   a. Describe how you handled the conflict.

   b. Describe the effects of your handling of this conflict.

c. State two possible alternatives for resolving the conflict.

d. In the light of your knowledge about inner conflict, how do you now think you should have handled this particular conflict? Justify your answer in terms of basic needs, value system, emotional effects, and short-term or long-term goals.

## REFERENCES AND SUGGESTED READINGS

Fogler, H.S., LeBlanc, S.E., Rizzo, B. (2013). *Strategies for creative problem solving. 3rd edition.* Upper Saddle River, NJ: Prentice Hall.

Heath, Chip & Heath, Dan. (2013). *Decisive: How to make better choices in life and work.* New York: Random House.

Krogerus, Mikael & Tschappeler, Roman. (2012). *The decision book: 50 models for strategic thinking.* New York: Norton.

# Effective Human Relations and Communication

The technological advances of the health field tempt the health care professional to become absorbed in complex equipment and the details of technique. To the patient, however, the *social climate* that health care professionals create has great importance. Each contact with a member of the health team affects the patient's peace of mind, emotional state, and outlook. *Scientific breakthroughs and sophisticated procedures cannot replace the human element in patient care.*

Section IV is designed to help you learn ways to promote a favorable outlook for the patient. Remember to relate to each patient as a human being and develop your own personal technique for identifying patient needs. As you learn to select the behaviors that promote favorable reactions in others, you will also enrich your personal life. Thus, you can grow not only as a health care professional, but also as a thoughtful, self-directing person, gaining increased satisfaction in living and at the same time enriching the lives of others.

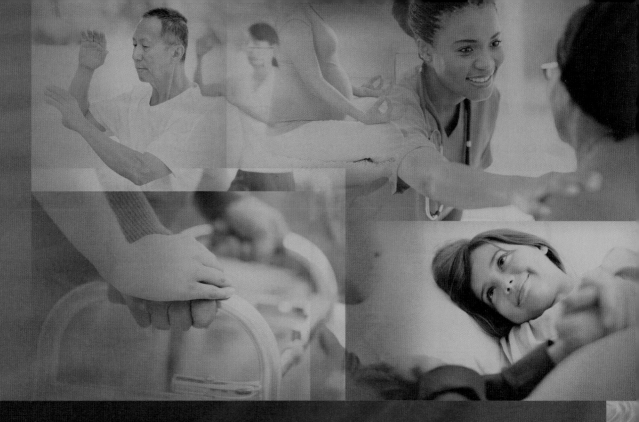

**CHAPTER**

**13**

# Effects of Illness on Behavior

## OBJECTIVES

After completing this chapter, you should be able to:

- Describe physical and emotional effects of illness.
- Discuss how to assess a patient's emotional reaction to illness.
- State guidelines for providing effective care for a hospitalized child.

## KEY TERMS

Desertion reaction
Disguised behavior
Incapacitated

Lethargy
Mindset

Separation anxiety
Verbalize

Illness is always a threat to one's sense of security. Even a minor illness or injury poses a challenge to an individual's physical and emotional well-being. Illness disrupts everyday routines, causing discomfort and inconvenience and often arousing feelings of fear, anger, or grief. These feelings are often manifested through the patient's behavior, but are not verbalized.

In other courses you are learning about specific illnesses: symptoms, diagnostic procedures, therapeutic techniques. Such knowledge is essential to safe and efficient performance as you provide patient care. Your *effectiveness* as a health care professional, however, is dependent upon your skill in applying knowledge about human behavior to relationships with patients. An effective health care professional/patient relationship promotes the patient's well-being. For one patient, reassurance in large amounts is needed to counteract fear and anxiety. For another patient, you may need to build confidence in the health team in order to gain the patient's cooperation in following the therapeutic plan.

Trying to provide a therapeutic atmosphere that is favorable for each patient is an ongoing challenge. Human variability is so great that no one method will work for all patients. By applying your knowledge about human behavior and the effects of illness, you can become sensitive to patient behaviors and their possible significance in terms of mental and emotional needs.

## PHYSICAL EFFECTS OF ILLNESS

Patients not only experience the signs and symptoms of a specific illness, but also various physical effects related to emotional reactions, change in daily routine, drugs, and numerous other factors. Examples of such general physical effects are fever, pain, nausea, lack of appetite, urinary problems, and difficulty with elimination. The overall effect may range from extreme **lethargy** to extreme restlessness. These general effects may be just as distressing to the patient as the symptoms of a specific illness. *The patient's complaints about general or vague effects should be noted.* These general symptoms may indicate either physical or emotional needs. Since interpretation may be beyond the scope of your role, report such complaints to your team leader or supervisor.

## EMOTIONAL EFFECTS OF ILLNESS

Most people react to illness with negative emotions that vary in type and intensity.

- Some patients are mildly annoyed at being sick; others are quite angry.
- Some patients are apprehensive; others are almost in a state of panic.
- Some feel sorry for themselves, while others react with pronounced self-pity.
- Some people feel bitter about their misfortune; bitterness is a combination of anger and self-pity.
- Some patients readily **verbalize** their feelings. The patient who says, "Why me?" is probably expressing anger.

Obviously, the words alone do not carry the full message. Be alert for additional evidence about the patient's emotional reaction to illness: facial expression, tone of voice, body posture, choice of words, and emphasis given to certain words.

Negative feelings may also be expressed through **disguised behavior**. The patient who is very talkative may be covering up fear. The patient who is eager to please may be covering up fear, hostility, or other negative feelings. Such patients are just as much in need of understanding and interest from health care professionals as those who verbalize their feelings. Do not make the mistake of thinking that the patient who is pleasant does not have fears and anxieties; for these patients, too, illness is a threat. *Each patient reacts to threat in a very individual way.*

## GENERAL EFFECTS OF SERIOUS ILLNESS

During serious illness there is some depression of mental and emotional functioning. The individual's energy resources are being utilized to cope with the physical stress of illness. There is likely to be decreased awareness of surroundings and lessened concern about life problems. A calm, interested, and caring manner on the part of health care professionals is essential to provide these patients with emotional support, reassurance, and, hopefully, some relief from fear.

Sometimes a patient who has been very cooperative during the serious stage of illness shows a marked change in behavior as convalescence begins. Energy resources are no longer fully required for coping with physical demands. The patient is now more aware of discomfort. There is energy for emotional reactions and for conscious attention to symptoms and life problems. You may find it difficult to cope with this change in behavior, because you probably believe the patient should now exhibit a positive emotional state. Accept a patient's behavior as indicative of needs and problems, rather than condemning behavior because it is different from what you think it should be.

## INFLUENCES ON PATIENTS' REACTIONS TO ILLNESS

As a health care professional, you will see situations involving pain, discomfort, disability, and even death. The atmosphere of the health agency is your work environment, but to a patient, it may seem unfamiliar and uncomfortable. The equipment you use daily and the clinical

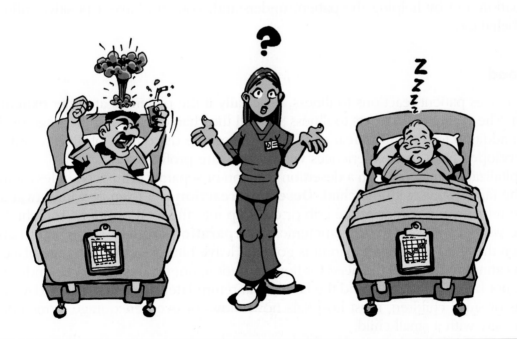

**FIGURE 13-1 People have various reactions to illness.**

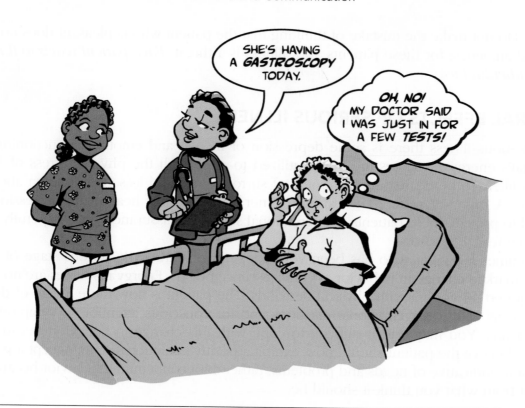

**FIGURE 13-2** Help your patient understand the situation by using appropriate vocabulary.

sights, smells, and sounds that are so familiar to you may be frightening to other people. Most patients will benefit from your taking time to explain a procedure and to answer questions, no matter how routine that procedure has become for you. By dealing with the strangeness of a situation and by helping the patient understand, you can have a positive influence on patient behavior.

## Childhood

Age influences patient reactions to illness, especially if the patient is at either extreme of the life span. The young child reacts to illness with all the characteristics of the stage of development, in addition to the child's fear of strange places, the discomfort of illness, and expectations developed from past experiences with health care professionals.

Hospitalization may result in a desertion reaction or separation anxiety, unless some member of the family stays with the child. **Desertion reaction** is a form of withdrawal in which the child retreats to a corner of the crib or curls up into the fetal position. The child is unresponsive when caregivers try to communicate. **Separation anxiety** is a type of panic reaction when the child realizes the parent is going to leave him or her in a strange place. Young children cannot understand the need for hospitalization; nor do small children understand that they are not being abandoned and the family will return later. Because of these two common reactions of small children, most hospitals now allow, or even encourage, a member of the family to stay with a small child.

How to work effectively with sick children of various ages is a full course of study. By observing some general rules, however, you will improve your effectiveness with young patients.

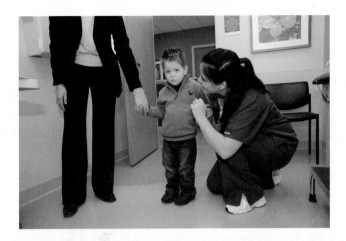

**FIGURE 13-3** As a healthcare professional, it is your task to win the child's confidence.

- Accept each child according to his or her current stage of development.

- Allow the young patient to express feelings—do not suggest that a 3-year-old "be brave" and not cry when something hurts.

- Do not expect cooperation from those who are too young to understand. Be aware that the child does not understand what is happening.

- Accept that the child is afraid.

- Remember that children often sense the feelings of adults. If you have negative feelings, the child is likely to sense your true feelings. Some child behavior is actually a reaction to the feelings of an adult.

As a health care professional, it is your task to win the child's confidence. *When a treatment or diagnostic procedure must be done, indicate that you accept the child's feelings and are sorry that the child is having pain.* Be aware that any traumatic experience will influence the child's behavior throughout this illness, create negative feelings toward health care professionals in general, and influence behavior in future illnesses.

## Senescence

Most elderly people fear becoming bedridden or otherwise losing their independence. For the senescent patient, any illness is especially threatening. This may be the illness that will render the patient helpless. An elderly patient may have greater anxiety than you think is justified by the particular illness. Such patients need your sincere interest and concern as they cope with the threat their illness represents.

In caring for an elderly patient, encourage independence insofar as it is reasonable. The need for help with buttoning a shirt may be due to arthritic hands—very different from a child who needs help with buttons! Consider the following guidelines:

- Do not assume that the elderly patient's need for help with some aspects of daily living also means that the patient is to be treated like a child.

- Allow the patient to make decisions whenever appropriate, rather than insisting that the patient conform to every routine of the facility.

- Keep in mind that some routines are for the convenience of the staff and may not be in the best interest of every patient.

Above all, remember that this elderly person, now somewhat dependent on you, was at one time independent and self-reliant. The loss of one's independence is a difficult loss to accept.

## Life Role

One's life role assumes great importance during illness. The mother with small children has anxiety about their care while she is **incapacitated**. Possibly, there is also anxiety about her ability to fulfill her responsibilities as a wife and mother. Her reaction to illness may be quite different from that of a woman with the same illness whose family is less dependent on her.

Occupational role also influences the degree of threat. Illness can seriously threaten job security; even if one's job is secure, there may be loss of income. Sick leave, salary continuation plans, whether or not one works on commission, whether or not insurance will help with the costs of illness—all influence the amount of anxiety the patient feels. If there is permanent disability, a change of occupation may be necessary. For most of your patients, you will not know the details of their life situation; hence, you cannot know what their worries are. You can, however, be sensitive to manifestations of anxiety, and you can listen when a patient indicates a need to talk.

## Adjustment

The usual adjustment of a patient has much influence on reactions to illness. The patient who has a sense of security and usually copes with life problems effectively is very likely to cope with illness effectively also, even though adjustment will not be as good as usual. *Even for the well-adjusted person, illness is accompanied by inconvenience and discomfort, which alters the degree of adjustment.*

Those same personality traits and patterns of behavior that influence adjustment also influence how one reacts to illness. A person who is inclined to use defense mechanisms will continue this pattern during illness. The person who is inclined to find escape from unpleasantness will try to avoid facing the reality of illness. Sometimes the defense mechanisms fail the individual during illness; then the patient may be unable to cope with the situation. When the usual patterns of coping fail, the individual may become fearful and may even panic. Patients who seem overly anxious may not know how to cope with illness.

## Dependency

Some people are quite independent, in the sense of being self-reliant. Others are inclined to lean on someone else whenever possible. This trait is known as dependency. People who are extremely dependent may react to illness in a way that reflects this characteristic. It is expected that the sick be dependent on others; therefore, illness justifies dependency. During illness, *dependent persons* escape the self-reliance normally expected of adults. Therefore, *unconsciously* wishing to prolong an illness, they find it difficult to admit they are improving. New complaints may be offered as evidence that they are still sick.

It is easy to be critical of such patients. Yet if you had that patient's life problems, background, and patterns of behavior, then you would probably be using the same behavior pattern the patient is using. Instead of being critical, the health team should plan ways for such a patient to resume self-care progressively during convalescence.

## Cultural Background and Language Barriers

Another influence on patient reactions to illness is cultural background. The United States has experienced an influx of people from all over the world. They come from Central and South America, Asia, the Middle East, Africa, and Eastern Europe. Each culture has certain beliefs about sickness, death, and dying. In some cultures, members of the family and the community care for the sick. Hospitals and doctors may be viewed with suspicion and are consulted only if the situation becomes desperate. When a person moves from that type of culture to one where medical care is a common occurrence, admission to the hospital may be perceived as meaning the patient's illness is hopeless.

The patient with a limited understanding of English presents a special challenge to health care professionals. The patient may have difficulty describing symptoms or conveying needs—frustrating for both patient and health care professional. Such patients should be given careful explanations of procedures and routines to alleviate fear and prevent misunderstandings. Many hospitals now have a roster of translators for patients who do not understand English. These patients present an opportunity for the health care professional to learn about the patient's culture, perceptions of illness, and lifestyle.

Cultural differences also include religion and membership in one of the American subcultures. The patient whose religious beliefs influence diet and other practices needs assurance that the practices will be respected. Patients from a minority group may expect prejudice from caregivers. Efforts to show that they are accepted may even arouse suspicion. There is no room for prejudice in providing health care, however. Your philosophy of individual worth should guide you in providing quality care for each patient, regardless of cultural background.

## Past Experience

Experience creates in each of us a mindset toward certain types of experience. **Mindset** influences how we perceive a situation. How we perceive the situation influences how we react. The patient who has had unfavorable experiences with sickness, health care professionals, or health agencies is likely to perceive greater threat than a person who has not had such unfavorable experiences. The patient who has a mindset that health care professionals are cold and impersonal may perceive coldness even in a friendly care professional. If the patient expects inefficient care, then examples of inefficiency will be found. Evidence of defensiveness, distrust, hostility, or fear toward health care professionals may indicate traumatic past experiences.

You cannot undo past damage quickly. Mindset is a fixed expectation that is not easily modified; it creates readiness to behave according to the *expectation*, rather than according to the specific situation. When you encounter a patient who seems to have had unfavorable experiences with health care professionals, do not expect to establish rapport immediately.

However, your efforts may be more effective than you realize and pave the way for new and more favorable attitudes in the future.

## THE CHALLENGE FOR HEALTH CARE PROFESSIONALS

As a health care professional, you will sometimes be extremely busy performing all the procedures required to complete your assignment. Both time pressure and workload can be quite stressful. At such times you may tend to focus on task completion, rather than identifying patients' needs, being aware of patients' emotional reactions to their illnesses, and understanding that certain behaviors are reactions to illness. Actually, *giving your attention to human relations as you perform various procedures* will help you manage your own stress. You will be able to enjoy interacting with each patient and be less aware of job pressures.

### Relating to the Patient

Practicing effective human relations is not time-consuming; it is a matter of *where you focus your attention*. Familiar procedures do not require a lot of concentration, so you can focus on relating to the patient while you carry out a procedure. If you do need to concentrate on the task, you can simply state to the patient, "I really need to focus on what I'm doing; we'll talk some more when I have finished."

Relating to your patients effectively requires certain attitudes: genuine concern for others, the belief that other people are important, and willingness to see a situation from the patient's point of view. In fact, these three attitudes are essential to feel empathy for another person. The caregiver who truly feels empathy for a patient is likely to be perceived by the patient as warm and caring.

Certain personal traits also contribute to effective relationships, especially sincerity, truthfulness, and honesty. In addition, behavior patterns affect relationships. Attentiveness, giving one's full attention to the patient, is absolutely necessary to convey caring and concern. Two health care professionals who carry on a conversation with each other while performing a procedure on a patient are sending the message: "We are not really interested in you as a human being. We are just here to do this task." Making eye contact at frequent intervals also

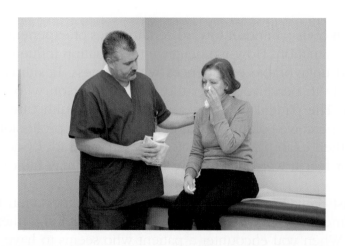

**FIGURE 13-4 It is important to convey caring and concern for the patient.**

conveys attentiveness. Have you ever tried to have a conversation with someone who looked over your shoulder or kept glancing around the room while you were talking? If so, you probably felt that the other person was not really interested in you or what you had to say. Probably the most important of all caring behaviors involves just "being there" when someone needs comfort and emotional support. Being there may or may not include conversation. It may involve simply taking the patient's hand in yours for a moment, or simply asking, "Do you need anything?"

## Communicating with the Patient

Your purpose in communicating with a patient affects your communication style. Interviewing a patient to obtain information, instructing the patient in self-care, explaining a procedure or the patient's care plan, or conveying empathy are examples of different purposes that would require somewhat different approaches. Regardless of purpose, however, it is important to convey caring and concern for the patient. Communication includes both verbal and nonverbal messages, so you should become aware of your own communication style, especially your use of body language as you communicate verbally. Chapter 15 discusses verbal and nonverbal communication in greater detail.

## ACTIVITIES

1. Consider some past illness you have experienced. Describe your reactions to this illness in terms of the following:

   a. Perception of threat

   b. Emotional effects

   c. Physical discomfort

   d. Your behavior when you were uncomfortable

   e. Inconvenience of the illness

   f. Effects on your daily habits

   g. Effects on your state of adjustment

   h. Patterns of behavior you used to cope with the illness

   i. Influence of one or more personality traits on how you reacted to illness

   j. Expectations or mindset that affected your relationship with those caring for you

> **NOTE**
>
> Reactions to illness occur even if the illness is a minor one. If you have never had any illness that could provide a basis for this activity, interview a friend or member of your family who has had a recent illness.

2. You have been having annoying symptoms for several months. Then a new symptom appears—one that you know is a warning sign of cancer. When you consult your

physician, she recommends hospitalization for diagnostic studies. Picture yourself on admission to the hospital. Using parts a through j in Activity 1, think through the reactions you might have under these circumstances.

3. As a health care professional, you probably would react somewhat differently than a layperson when you have a potentially serious illness. How is being a health care professional an advantage? How is being a health care professional a disadvantage?

4. It has been said that doctors and nurses make "poor" patients. Why?

5. Your neighbor comes to you to talk about her recent experiences with diagnostic studies. She states, "The doctor says there is nothing physically wrong. He says I should stop being so nervous. I don't know what he means." How could you help this neighbor understand what the doctor means, without exceeding your role as a health care professional?

6. A member of your family has a disorder that can only be treated by extensive lifestyle changes. List specific suggestions for helping this relative make the necessary changes.

7. A friend informs you that her husband has a malignancy and describes some changes in his behavior. How could you help her understand her husband's behavior?

8. You are assigned to a patient whose treatment includes bedrest. As you prepare to give a bed bath, you put on gloves. The patient says angrily, "Am I so dirty that you can't touch me with your bare hands?" How will you respond?

## REFERENCES AND SUGGESTED READINGS

Di Benedetto, M., Lindner, H., Aucote, H., Churcher, J., McKenzie, S., Croning, N., & Jenkins, E. (2014). Co-morbid depression and chronic illness related to coping and physical and mental health status. *Psychology, Health & Medicine, 19*(3), 253–262. doi:10.1080/13548506.2013.803135.

Hartley, Carolyn, & Wong, Peter. (2015). *The caregiver's toolbox: Checklists, forms, resources, mobile apps, and straight talk to help you provide compassionate care.* Lanham, MD: Taylor Trade.

Horn, Danea. (2013.) *Chronic resilience: 10 sanity-saving strategies for women coping with the stress of illness.* San Francisco, CA: Red Wheel/Weiser.

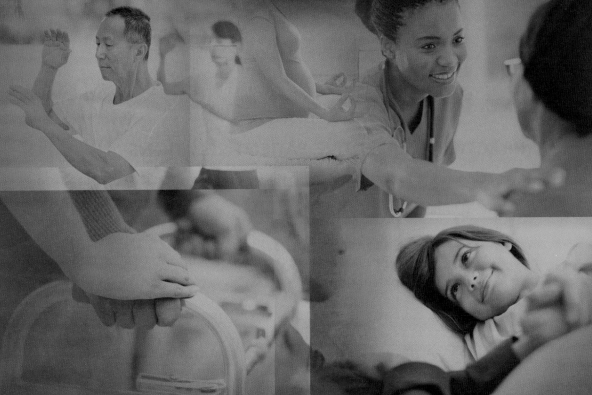

# Human Relations and Coping with Patient Behavior

## OBJECTIVES

After completing this chapter, you should be able to:

- Describe strategies for positive interactions with patients.
- Explain common patterns of patient behavior and appropriate ways health care professionals can respond.
- Discuss common emotional reactions patients may have to illness.
- Communicate effectively with patients.

## KEY TERMS

Covert
Egocentric

I-statements
Overt

Passive aggression
Regression

Behavior is highly individualized. Each person has typical patterns of behavior for various situations, including reacting to the stress of illness. Do not expect to know exactly why each person behaves in a certain way. You can, however, be aware of *possible* reasons for behavior and thus be more accepting of whatever behavior the patient does exhibit. If you demonstrate an accepting attitude rather than a judgmental attitude, you will be able to develop more effective relationships with patients and coworkers.

## PRACTICING EFFECTIVE PATIENT RELATIONS

To become an effective health care professional, you will be expected to:

- Know your job.
- Perform well all tasks within the scope of your responsibilities.
- Understand and apply the concepts and facts relevant to each task.
- Observe safety precautions.

Most of the courses you are now studying prepare you to fulfill these requirements. But to be truly effective, you must also focus on developing human relations skills. As you improve your skills in interacting with coworkers and patients, you will find your work more satisfying, and you will gain confidence in handling a variety of challenging situations.

## HELPING PATIENTS ADJUST TO ILLNESS

Your patients come to the health agency with the effects of illness added to their usual problems. There are some—perhaps many—stressors in their life situations; illness is an additional stressor. To some people, the health care facility is a strange place. For some, it is so threatening that the patient enters only as a desperate effort to get help. Patients may also be worried about how they will cope with the high costs of health care. In a stressful situation such as the hospital, the patient uses patterns of behavior that have proven useful in past threatening situations.

### Identifying a Patient's Needs

You are learning about influences on patient behavior. Use this knowledge to understand and accept each patient as a person. You do not serve Mrs. Jones's needs when you tell your coworkers "she just acts like that because she has a conflict." You may or may not be right about the cause of her behavior. Your role is to be aware of *possible* meanings of behavior in terms of patient needs. Recognizing some of the possible influences on behavior is the key to identifying patient needs, not the source of conversational topics.

If you think a patient's behavior indicates unmet needs, discuss the patient's behavior with your supervisor. Sometimes, the health team needs to study a patient situation in an effort to identify needs. The need driving a particular behavior may not be obvious at first. For example, children may cry because they are tired, hungry, afraid, or missing a parent. Similarly, an adult may display aggressive, hostile, or uncooperative behavior for a variety of reasons—they are worried about finances, in pain, angry with family members for "not being there for them," and so on.

Striving to understand the behavior of your patients should be approached in a *thoroughly ethical and responsible way.*

Each person's behavior is highly individual. We each have typical patterns of behavior for various situations:

- Reacting to stress
- Feeling out of control

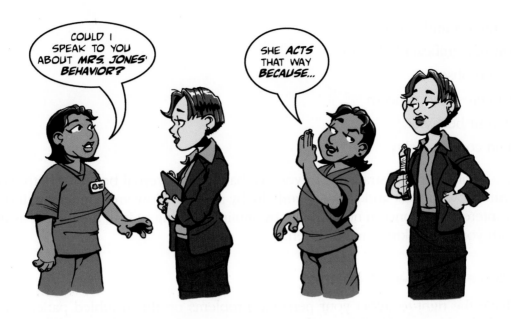

**FIGURE 14-1 There are ethical and unethical ways to discuss patient behavior.**

- Feeling afraid or anxious
- Expressing anger
- Expressing worry

You may never know exactly why each person behaves in a certain way. However, you can be more accepting of patients' behavior by considering *possible* reasons for the behavior. By choosing to have a non-judgmental attitude toward your patients rather than a judgmental one, you will be better able to form effective relationships. *Keep in mind that skill in interpersonal relations comes through applying your knowledge and understanding to every relationship with another person—at work, at home, and in all activities involving other people.*

## Being Sensitive to Feelings

Unpleasant behavior is usually due to a negative emotional state, ignorance, or an unfavorable attitude. When patients behave in undesirable ways, it is almost always the result of inner feelings; these feelings affect the patient's well-being. *When you encourage a patient to adopt a positive, realistic outlook, you contribute to that patient's well-being.* Negative feelings indicate a need; try to identify the need and respond appropriately.

## GENERAL GUIDELINES

Practicing the strategies that follow will improve your ability to interact effectively with patients. As you read the description of each strategy, consider how you could use each approach not only with patients but also with friends, family, or coworkers.

- Set aside your own personal problems.
- Accept the patient.

- Show interest and concern.
- Recognize significant behavior.
- Listen and observe.
- Show interest and concern.
- Adapt your behavior.
- Maintain confidentiality.

Practice applying these strategies to your verbal and nonverbal behavior both. For example, you can show interest and concern verbally by asking, "How are you feeling today?" You can show interest and concern nonverbally by smiling, turning to face the patient as he or she speaks with you, and taking time to listen.

### Rising above Your Own Problems

Do you have the right to inflict your personal problems on this troubled patient? Your role is to provide health care. To do so effectively, you must handle your own problems of living well enough to give your full attention to your patients. When you report for work each day, the problems of your personal life must be set aside until you have completed that day's work. *You cannot deal with job problems and home problems at the same time.* Put personal matters aside while you are on the job, so you can give your full attention to your patients. With practice over time, the ability to rise above your own problems will increase your effectiveness as a health care professional.

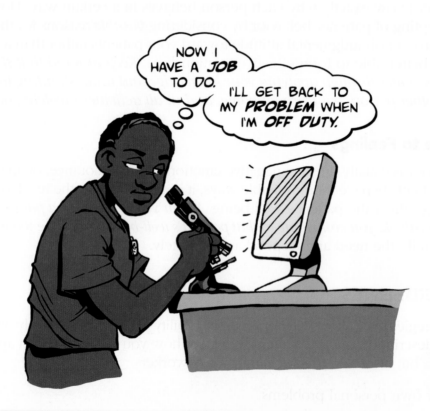

FIGURE 14-2 **Do not carry your personal problems to work with you.**

## Accepting the Patient

Each patient needs to feel accepted by health care professionals. Many patients are sensitive to any evidence of irritation, impatience, indifference, or hostility on the part of a health care professional. Accepting every patient may require effort, because each of us has some prejudice or lack of understanding toward those who are different from ourselves. Through increased experience with a variety of people, you can grow in understanding of others—provided you avoid a critical or judgmental attitude. This is the key to learning to accept others—*recognize that other people are like you in many ways, even though different in other ways.*

Accepting someone includes accepting that person's behavior—even if it is not pleasant. There may be good reason for a patient's irritability or criticism. It is not realistic to expect everyone to be pleasant all of the time; such an expectation is especially unrealistic in regard to people who are sick.

Occasionally, a patient's behavior *is* unacceptable. Then, without showing anger or fear, the health care professional can use an **I-statement** to indicate that such behavior is unacceptable. An I-statement is a sentence which states how you think or feel about a behavior or situation. Rather than an accusatory you-statement, which can put the other person on the defensive, an I-statement communicates your feelings or needs without expressing blame or criticism of the other person. The following are examples of how you could begin an I-statement:

* I need . . .
* I would appreciate . . .
* I feel uncomfortable when . . .

In contrast, you-statements can sound as though you are blaming:

* You need to . . .
* You made me uncomfortable when . . .

With practice, using I-statements can help you communicate concerns clearly and directly without blaming the other person.

## Showing Interest and Concern

While you are caring for a patient, give that patient your full attention. Address the patient by name, listen, respond appropriately, and show willingness to act on any requests. In many situations, hospital routine requires that things be done at a certain time; usually, an explanation will gain the patient's cooperation. In other situations, health care professionals unnecessarily force patients into a routine. If a patient customarily bathes at bedtime, why insist upon a morning bath while in the hospital? Some patients deeply resent unnecessary interruptions or changes in their daily routine. Before insisting that such patients conform to the usual hospital routine, be sure that such conformity is really necessary.

> **For Discussion and Reflection**
>
> Consider a time when a friend, family member, or coworker behaved in a way that you found unacceptable. How did you respond? If this situation were to occur again, how might you use an I-statement to respond to the other person?

## Listening and Observing

The patient who has fears and anxieties can benefit from talking out these feelings. Most patients, however, do not readily "open up." Be sensitive to subtle indications that something is bothering the patient. Linger in the patient's unit to chat casually and respond to any hint of anxiety by showing interest in how the patient feels. Be available as an interested listener. A patient's readiness to express feelings to you is, in a sense, a test of the effectiveness of your relationship with that patient. Usually acceptance, demonstrated interest, and concern pave the way for a patient to express fears, anxieties, and uncertainties.

## Recognizing Significant Behavior

Nonverbal behavior often provides a clue to the patient's feelings. Consider the following examples of patient behavior:

- Nervous movements, restlessness
- Unwillingness to participate in conversation
- Not making eye contact when speaking
- Sleeping excessively
- Watching television when you are speaking to them

The patient who states, "My doctor says I should have surgery," is probably signaling a need to talk about it. You can shut off conversation, or you can encourage it by your response. Saying, "I know that. I took your preoperative orders from the doctor," may be interpreted by the patient to mean, "This health care professional doesn't care how scared I am." On the other hand, if you respond, "How do you feel about having surgery?" the patient is more likely to verbalize feelings about the impending surgery.

When you encourage patients to express feelings, you are providing a valuable service. A patient may gain more from verbalizing anxieties than from taking a tranquilizer. Asking open-ended questions can encourage patients to open up about their concerns. Several ways to ask open-ended questions and to respond to patient feelings are discussed below.

## Using Appropriate Responses

When patients make "loaded statements," it is usually effective to repeat what the patient has said, using essentially the same words but with a questioning inflection. This type of response, known as *echoing*, is a safe response; it does not give information, and it does not show your reaction to what the patient said. It merely says to the patient that you heard; the rising inflection in your voice implies, "Please continue. I am listening." Some patients will not understand the meaning of the rising inflection and simply be annoyed by your use of echoing.

It is good to have a range of communication techniques so you can use the most appropriate one for a particular situation. Some other useful techniques are: reflecting, clarifying, validating, questioning, and confronting. *Reflecting* is similar to echoing, but requires that you restate what the patient said, indicating that you have heard the message and are aware of the patient's feelings. Your response may begin with a phrase such as, "It sounds like. . ." or "It seems like you. . ."; this type of response is also called *mirroring*. When you use reflecting, you are essentially providing a mirror for the patient to view what he or she just said. The patient then has an opportunity to confirm, deny, or modify the meaning of the comment.

*Clarifying* is a technique used to test your interpretation of what has been said. After stating something like, "Let me see if I understand what you mean," you state the message, as you understand it, in your own words. The speaker can then confirm or deny that you understand the intended meaning. This may require several repetitions before the speaker will agree that you understand the message.

*Validating* is a technique used to check the meaning of certain nonverbal behaviors of the speaker. Often, the spoken message conveys one meaning, but certain nonverbal clues indicate a different meaning or indicate that the speaker's emotional state is different from what the verbal message implies. The technique for validating involves such statements as, "I sense that. . ." followed by a description of a feeling or "I notice that. . ." followed by an observation of some behavior, posture, or facial expression. This technique invites the patient to express feelings, doubts, anxieties, worries, annoyances, and frustrations.

*Questioning* is often required in the performance of patient care, usually to obtain specific information. Questioning can also be used as a therapeutic tool and as a means of avoiding a misunderstanding. Questioning should be done with a caring attitude. It is better to ask only one question, allow time for the patient to answer, then converse briefly before asking another question. It is especially important that you listen while the patient responds and allow the patient to finish before you speak again.

## Adapting Your Behavior

Accept each patient as a worthy person. Remember that the patient's behavior is an effort to deal with the present situation. If it becomes apparent that you are having an adverse effect on the patient, change your behavior. Some patients enjoy a cheerful, talkative health care professional; others find cheerfulness annoying. As you become more sensitive to the feelings of others, you will be able to adapt your behavior to each patient.

## Maintaining Confidentiality

Legally and ethically, health care professionals are required to protect patients' privacy and to hold patients' health information in confidence. In 2003, the Health Insurance and Portability and Accountability Act (HIPAA) Privacy Rule took effect. This federal legislation protects the privacy of individuals' medical information. Clients are generally given information about their privacy rights on their first visit to a particular health care office or facility. HIPAA stipulates that consumers have the right to request copies of their medical records, and to correct any errors they may contain. Consumers also have the right to decide who can receive their medical information and for what purposes. Violations of the HIPAA Privacy Rule may be reported to the Department of Health and Human Services Office of Civil Rights.

An exception to confidentiality is information *relevant to the patient's well-being*. For this reason, it is unwise to commit yourself to promises. If a patient offers to tell you something that requires a promise "not to tell," do not be flattered that the patient wants to share a secret. Even more important, do not make such a promise. Simply state, "Whatever I learn about a patient is kept in confidence, unless the patient's well-being requires that I share the information with the health care team." Then indicate that you are listening if the patient wishes to talk.

Suppose you made such a promise to Mr. Z, a very personable young man who has been admitted to the hospital with a possible bleeding ulcer. After extracting a promise of secrecy from you, he confides that his brother is bringing clothes tonight, and they are going to slip out of the hospital and "hit the bars." What should you do, once you know that his "secret" involves a plan that would be harmful to Mr. Z? Should you break your word and report his plan to your supervisor? Should you keep your word and not tell his secret? Suppose he really does slip out of the hospital? Suppose you report his plan; when your supervisor confronts him, he denies everything. Avoiding any promise of secrecy can prevent getting caught in such a trap.

## COMMON BEHAVIOR PATTERNS OF PATIENTS

### Egocentrism

Most people become **egocentric** during illness. This means that the patient becomes self-centered—the primary concern is with self. Much of the demanding behavior that health care professionals (and families) resent in patients is actually a manifestation of the egocentric reaction to illness. This behavior can test your acceptance of the patient, yet egocentrism is just as much a reaction to illness as physical symptoms. If you accept egocentrism as a reaction to illness, you will find it easier to tolerate a patient's self-centered behavior.

### Regression

**Regression** involves reverting to behaviors that are appropriate to an earlier level of development. The most extreme form of regression is lying in the fetal position and not responding to one's surroundings. This is often seen in elderly patients who have been bedfast for a long period of time.

In the home, a young child may regress when a new baby arrives. For example, a toddler who has mastered drinking from a cup may ask for a bottle. Regression can be seen with patients of all ages. Dependence on others for personal care, when one is capable of self-care, is an example of regression.

### Unfriendly Behavior

Place yourself in the following situation. Today you are assigned to Mr. A., who is totally indifferent to all your efforts to be pleasant. You feel annoyed and wonder why you are wasting good cheer on this cold, unfriendly person.

Then you tell yourself that there may be reasons for Mr. A.'s behavior. Your thoughts run through some of the possible reasons. "Maybe Mr. A. fears his illness, but he does not want me to know he is frightened. Perhaps he does not admit to himself that he is frightened. He may have had unfavorable experiences with health care professionals and is transferring hostility from his previous experiences to me."

There is no one way to cope with an unfriendly patient. Every person reacts as an individual and may or may not be aware of the reaction or its effects on other people. Do not take unfriendliness personally. Accept it for what it is: a manifestation of how the patient feels at the moment. Maintain your own pleasant manner. Continue to show interest and concern. Visit the patient's room at intervals, but not so frequently that you are an annoyance. Sometimes your efforts will pay off without your knowing; your sincerity and interest lead to trust and the patient begins to respond to you.

## Aggressive Behavior

Aggression may be physical or verbal. Physical aggression is most likely to occur if the patient is a child, is emotionally or mentally disturbed, is inebriated, or is in an irresponsible state. A simple aggressive act such as pushing your hand away may indicate fear, anger, or other negative emotional reactions to you or to what you are planning to do. It may be an effort at self-defense. If the aggression is more serious—an actual attack on you, for example—you must handle the situation as best you can to avoid being hurt and then summon help from a professional worker. Because there are legal and ethical implications in handling aggression, avoid any action that could result in your being accused of assault on the patient. Protect yourself from injury, but secure the assistance of your supervisor as quickly as possible.

A child is likely to use physical aggression defensively, due to the expectation of pain. The child's age, condition, and other factors determine the best way to handle aggressive behavior. If you are in doubt about how to work with a particular child, discuss the problem with the pediatric supervisor and obtain specific instructions. Your general approach, however, must include an accepting attitude. Never say to a child, "You are bad." Instead, tell the child you cannot accept kicking, biting, or whatever form the aggression is taking. Set limits to the behaviors you will accept. Even if the child does not respect these limits (e.g., no kicking), he or she will understand why you are using restraints during a procedure. When you have finished working with the child, demonstrate acceptance with friendly behavior. Keep in mind that the child who fights you is manifesting an intense emotional state.

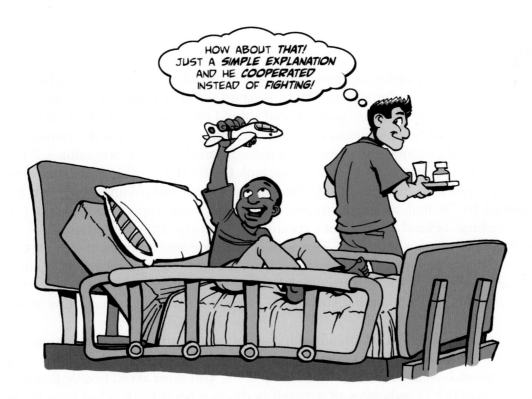

**FIGURE 14-3 A patient who understands a procedure is more likely to cooperate.**

With adults, aggressive behavior is usually in the form of verbal attack or resistance. Verbal aggression may involve criticism, loud talking, profanity, or arguing. If the patient is critical, listen to the complaint and how it is described. If there is a valid complaint, corrective steps should be taken immediately. If the complaint does not seem to be valid, consider the complaint to be an expression of feelings. Arguing may be a disguised request for an explanation: the patient is challenging you to justify some aspect of the therapeutic plan, some policy of the health agency, or some procedure.

**Passive aggression**, on the other hand, is likely to consist of overt or covert noncooperation. In **overt** noncooperation, the patient balks—refuses to take medicine, accept a treatment, undergo a diagnostic procedure, or carry out some self-help routine. **Covert** noncooperation involves deceit. The patient wants the health team to think he or she is cooperating, but actually is not. Patients who ask that their medication be left on the bedside table ("I'll take it later") may intend to flush it down the toilet. If you discover that a patient has been covertly noncooperative, you will probably feel anger. It is hard to accept that someone has deceived you. But consider for a moment: why would a patient not cooperate with the therapeutic plan?

Perhaps the patient fears drug reactions and believes that quietly disposing of the drug is easier than trying to explain to health care professionals "who do not understand how I feel about drugs." Perhaps the patient's religion discourages the use of drugs. Perhaps the patient knows (or thinks) that this is a terminal illness and does not want to prolong life, if the cost is pain and helplessness or depleting the family's financial resources. Whatever the reason for this noncooperation, you may be sure it makes sense to the patient. It is your responsibility to (1) refer this problem to the professional staff, (2) remain nonjudgmental toward this patient, (3) accept that you may never understand the reasons for the patient's behavior, and (4) remember that noncooperation serves a purpose for the patient.

## Hostility

Dealing with verbal or passive aggression is largely a problem of dealing with hostility. Team planning is more likely to be effective than isolated efforts by one or two members of the team. In general, each health care professional should give undivided attention to the hostile patient, listen without defensiveness or argument, indicate respect for the patient's feelings, show concern, and encourage expression of thoughts and feelings. Sometimes, it is effective to reflect what the patient has just said: "You think the food is terrible." At other times it may be more appropriate to question, using the patient's ideas but adding your own interpretation followed by "Is that what you mean?" It may be more appropriate to test your guess about the feelings behind the patient's comments: "Are you unhappy about this?" Or, "You seem to be quite angry about this." Use a pleasant tone and phrases that help the patient feel free to express feelings. Your responses should convey acceptance, caring, and willingness to listen. Sometimes such an approach has unexpectedly good results. The patient, after airing feelings, may say something such as, "I guess that's a pretty small thing to be fussing about."

The worst thing you can do with a hostile patient is to return hostility. This simply confirms the patient's belief that you do not care or understand—your hostility has justified the patient's hostility. To avoid hostile behavior toward the patient, you *must* avoid hostile feelings. Accept the patient's hostility as indicative of a need, perhaps a need to develop trust in the health care team. If you develop negative feelings toward a patient, avoid defensiveness, criticism, arguing, short answers, or otherwise showing your negative feelings. If the patient detects your negative feelings, someone else should be assigned to care for that patient.

## Crying

Crying can result from any degree of anger, fear, or grief. Some people cry whenever they experience sentimental feelings. Crying is an emotional release and should not be stifled.

When you find a patient crying, avoid such comments as, "Let's stop crying now," or "You are much better, so there is nothing to cry about." These remarks may make you feel better, but they indicate to the patient that you are not trying to understand the patient's feelings.

Sometimes it is appropriate to ask the reason for the crying. At other times, it is better just to show acceptance, encourage freedom to express feelings through crying, and wait for the patient to volunteer information. It is not difficult to find out if the patient is crying because of pain and discomfort, fear, or sadness. If the crying seems to be due to personal problems, avoid prying questions, which could be an invasion of the patient's privacy.

With the crying patient, always indicate that you approve of crying as a means of relieving feelings. Sometimes holding the patient's hand or placing your hand over the patient's hand provides reassurance and conveys your interest and concern. Offer to stay, but if the patient shows a preference for being left alone, then say you are available if anything is needed, and leave. But return after 15 to 20 minutes and use appropriate behavior to respond to the patient's status at that time.

Each situation with a crying patient must be handled according to your best judgment and knowledge about the patient. Exactly what to say and do is dependent on the patient's situation. In every case, however:

- Do not offer false hope.
- Do not make promises you cannot keep.
- Do not minimize the patient's cause for crying.
- Do not express disapproval of crying.

## Noncooperation

When an adult patient is uncooperative, there is usually a reason. Most adults recognize that cooperation with the health team is in their interest. Some possible reasons for noncooperation are lack of understanding, misinformation, suspicion or distrust, preference for one's own way of doing things, or negative feelings.

To understand a patient's failure to cooperate, inquire in an interested but uncritical manner about the reason for the patient's behavior. You may find that an explanation is needed, the patient needs to be taught a health principle, a false belief needs to be corrected, a misunderstanding needs to be cleared up, or feelings of fear or distrust need to be relieved.

Patients cannot be forced to cooperate. Cooperation must be gained by eliminating the cause of noncooperation. If you are unable to learn why the patient is not cooperating, discuss the situation with your supervisor. Sometimes the problem must be referred to the patient's physician. If cooperation is essential to recovery, then it must be secured in some way. If the patient is objecting to a procedure that is not essential to recovery or well-being, then the physician may discontinue it rather than antagonize the patient.

## The Overly Friendly Patient

Occasionally, you may have a patient who is overly friendly. Such behavior may consist of personal questions or physical contact. The person who begins to ask personal questions may be trying innocently to make conversation or may be attempting to establish an overly familiar relationship. It is better to avoid discussing your personal life and your own experiences with patients. Instead, direct the conversation to the patient or to impersonal topics. One health care supervisor tells staff, "We are *friendly* to our patients, but it is not our role to be their *friends*."

Situations involving familiarity should be discussed with your supervisor. Be sure to report facts—what actually happened. Do not color your report with what you would have liked the situation to be, with judgmental statements, or with opinions. The supervisor can best assess the situation if you give an accurate account of what the patient said or did and what you said or did. The supervisor's professional judgment can provide guidelines for members of the health team who are caring for the patient.

## Inappropriate Sexual Behavior

Occasionally a patient may display inappropriate sexual behavior. The behavior may include sexual remarks, inappropriate touching, or self-exposure. In inappropriate sexual behavior occurs, you can use the techniques described below to let the patient know that the behavior is unacceptable and to set limits. However, if the behavior persists or if you feel unsafe, you should seek assistance from other staff immediately and notify your supervisor. You should also be familiar with your employer's policies and procedures regarding sexual harassment.

## Responding to Inappropriate Behavior

The following techniques can be used to set limits in response to inappropriate patient behavior: "I think, I feel, I want" and the positive/negative warning (Cambier and Gordon, 2013).

The "I think, I feel, I want" technique involves a series of I-statements:

- The first sentence describes or assesses the situation.
- The second sentence includes a statement of how the inappropriate behavior makes you feel.
- The third sentence states the appropriate behavior you expect from the patient.

For example, if a patient has made a sexually suggestive remark to you, you might reply as follows: "I think you meant that as a joke. However, I feel uncomfortable with your remark. I want our conversation to remain professional if I am going to continue your treatment."

The *positive/negative warning technique* sets limits by stating the positive outcome if the patient behaves appropriately as well as the negative outcome if the patient persists in inappropriate behavior. To use this technique, follow these steps:

- State the appropriate behavior you would like the patient to exhibit.
- State the positive outcome if the patient behaves appropriately.
- State the negative outcome that will occur if the inappropriate behavior continues.

- Follow through with either the positive or negative outcome based on the patient's continued behavior.

If a patient intentionally exposes himself or herself during treatment, you might reply as follows: "If you stop lifting your gown, I will stay with you and help you get stronger. However, if you continue to show me your genitals, I will leave and cancel the rest of this treatment" (Cambier and Gordon, 2013).

**For Discussion and Reflection**

Think of a time someone's behavior has made you feel uncomfortable, whether in a health care setting or another setting. How did you respond? Was your response effective in stopping the behavior?

Following an incident of inappropriate behavior, follow your employer's policies and procedures regarding documentation of the behavior. If you are unsure about your employer's policies and procedures, ask your supervisor.

## CONCLUSION

In this section, you have studied several topics that will help you be sensitive to the needs of a patient and understand common behaviors of patients:

- Physical and emotional effects of illness
- General effects of serious illness
- Influences on a patient's reaction to illness (age, life role, usual state of adjustment, dependency, cultural background, past experience)
- Common behavior patterns
- Strategies for coping with certain problem behaviors

You have also studied several topics that are relevant to you as a health care professional—*the beliefs and attitudes that you personally bring to the role*—and are important aspects of your personal effectiveness:

- Acceptance of each patient as a worthwhile human being (including tolerance for those who are different from you)
- Interest in and concern for each patient
- Willingness to listen
- Accuracy in observing
- Ability to recognize significant behaviors
- Respect for confidentiality
- Being sensitive to a patient's feelings and providing emotional support as needed
- Willingness to try to identify needs and serve each patient in accordance with those needs
- Ability to put your personal problems aside while caring for patients
- Willingness to adapt your behavior as needed to interact effectively with a variety of patients exhibiting many different behavior patterns

These topics deal with how you relate to your patients. Another major aspect of good human relations is how you communicate, verbally and nonverbally. In Chapter 15, you will practice interpreting verbal and nonverbal behavior. In each of these units, you will have the opportunity to participate in role-play situations as a means of polishing your communication skills and increasing your sensitivity to the real messages sent to you by another person.

## ACTIVITIES

1. Write a brief description of a situation in which a patient exhibited a pattern of behavior discussed in this unit. Describe how a health care professional could respond using one of the techniques discussed.

2. Develop a brief role play with a classmate in which one of you plays the role of the patient and the other plays the role of the health care professional. Briefly describe the type of setting or health agency you will depict, as well as the patient's reason for seeking health care. As the "patient," select one of the following behaviors to demonstrate (the classmate playing the role of health care professional should select an appropriate response to the behavior demonstrated):

   Option 1: Demonstrate the role play to the class or a small group of classmates. The observers can identify the patient behavior that was demonstrated and discuss additional options for responding appropriately.

   Option 2: Practice this activity in groups of three, with the third classmate taking the role of observer. Rotate roles until all three have practiced each role. The observer can identify the patient behavior demonstrated and provide feedback about the response of the health care professional.

   List of patient behaviors to demonstrate:

   Egocentrism

   Regression

   Hostility

   Crying

   Aggression

   Asking staff to "keep a secret"

3. Conduct an informal interview with a friend, relative, or acquaintance currently working in health care. What types of patient behavior have they encountered? What responses have they found to be most helpful?

## REFERENCES AND SUGGESTED READINGS

Cambier, Z., & Gordon, S.P. (2013). Preparing new clinicians to identify, understand, and address inappropriate patient sexual behavior in the clinical environment. *Journal of Physical Therapy Education, 27*(2), 7–15.

Greene, J., & Hibbard, J. H. (2012). Why does patient activation matter? An examination of the relationships between patient activation and health-related outcomes. *Journal of General Internal Medicine, 27*(5), 520–526.

Lubetkin, E. I., Zabor, E. C., Brennessel, D., Kemeny, M. M., & Hay, J. L. (2014). Beyond demographics: Differences in patient activation across new immigrant, diverse language subgroups. *Journal of Community Health, 39*(1), 40–49. doi:http://dx.doi.org/10.1007/s10900-013-9738-1.

Nilsen, M. L., Sereika, S. M., Hoffman, L. A., Barnato, A., Donovan, H., & Happ, M. B. (2014). Nurse and patient interaction behaviors' effects on nursing care quality for mechanically ventilated older adults in the ICU. *Research in Gerontological Nursing, 7*(3), 113–125. doi:http://dx.doi.org/10.3928/19404921-20140127-02.

Raja, S., Hasnain, M., Vadakumchery, T., Hamad, J., Shah, R., & Hoersch, M. (2015). Identifying elements of patient-centered care in underserved populations: A qualitative study of patient perspectives. *PLoS One, 10*(5), doi:http://dx.doi.org/10.1371/journal.pone.0126708.

Sirri, L., Fava, G. A., & Sonino, N. (2013). The unifying concept of illness behavior. *Psychotherapy and Psychosomatics, 82*(2), 74–81. doi:10.1159/000343508.

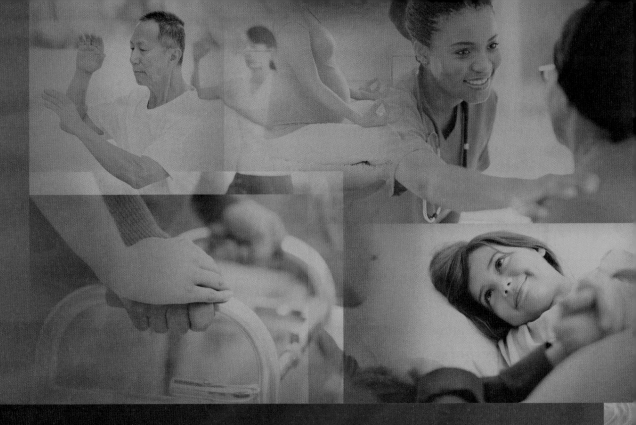

# Practicing Effective Communication

## OBJECTIVES

After completing this chapter, you should be able to:

- Explain the meaning of "skill in interpersonal relations."
- Describe selective observing.
- List examples of nonverbal behavior that may convey a message.
- Interpret the message of nonverbal behavior.
- Discuss reasons for communication breakdown.
- List ways to minimize ambiguity in verbal communication.
- Practice strategies for sending a clear message.

## KEY TERMS

| | | |
|---|---|---|
| Ambiguity | Expectation | Selective observing |
| Assumptions | Inconsistency | Stance |
| Clarification | Paraphrase | |
| Enunciation | Paraverbal | |

You have heard much about "good human relations" since you began your preparation for a career in the health field. Skill in interpersonal relationships may be thought of as *controlled* interaction with others. It means control over what happens by *consciously deciding* what to say or do to bring about the response you desire from another person.

When your behavior arouses positive feelings in others, then it is likely that the behavior of the other person toward you will be favorable. On the other hand, your behavior can arouse negative feelings in others: anxiety, anger, a sense of threat, self-pity, feelings of being "put down," or just plain irritation. When your behavior arouses negative feelings, then the behavior of the other person toward you may be unpleasant: noncooperation, complaints, withdrawal, or disagreement with whatever you say.

Any interaction with another person involves three types of communication: verbal, para-verbal, and nonverbal.

- *Verbal* communication uses words and language to convey a message.
- ***Paraverbal*** communication refers to *how* a verbal message is spoken—the tone of voice, volume, and rate of speech.
- *Nonverbal* communication refers to body language and facial expressions.

Many experts have stated that nonverbal communication accounts for half or more of the messages we send to other people. By learning to observe others' nonverbal behavior more closely, you can make a more informed decision about how you will communicate with them. By becoming more conscious of your own nonverbal behavior, you can increase the chances that the other person will receive your message in the way you intend.

## OBSERVING AND INTERPRETING NONVERBAL BEHAVIOR

Most of us think we are observant and that our observations are reasonably accurate. **Selective observing** means that we notice some details of a situation, while completely missing many other details. Left to chance, observations are likely to be made according to one's interests or curiosity. To become skillful in observing nonverbal behavior, make it a habit to consciously observe others' nonverbal behavior.

Most people communicate feelings through nonverbal behavior, often unconsciously. But regardless of whether or not the nonverbal behavior is conscious, it signals that the person is responding to something—perhaps to you as a person, something you said or did, your tone of voice, the expression on your face, and the other person's interpretation of what it means. It is also possible that the behavior indicates the individual's response to the total situation: the stress of a job interview, anger at being ill, fear of surgery, or the expectation of an unfavorable diagnosis. Nonverbal communication, then, provides a clue to a person's inner feelings. In some cases, it is also a signal that more specific behavior, such as an angry outburst, is about to occur.

The message of nonverbal behavior is lost unless you note it and interpret the meaning correctly. To improve your use of nonverbal communication, consciously practice observing the nonverbal behavior of others. Next, practice interpreting that behavior and check your interpretation against further evidence. When you interact with another person, note any changes in facial expression, slight movements of facial muscles, position of the lips, direction of gaze, position of the eyelids, body movements, **stance** (how a person stands), general posture, and the hands—position and movements. Experts use the ability to read people to help them select members for a jury or screen job applicants.

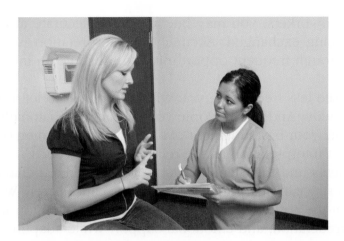

**FIGURE 15-1** **Effective communication includes understanding spoken communication and body language.**

After noting the nonverbal clues, try to interpret that behavior. Does a twitching facial muscle indicate stress? Or repressed anger? If stress, why does the individual feel stressed in this situation? Do the restless movements of the hands indicate nervousness? If so, why does the person feel nervous in this situation? What is the person's emotional state? What expectations does the person have? Are you sending nonverbal messages to which that individual is responding? By associating the nonverbal behavior of a specific person with additional evidence as it becomes available, you can learn to "read" that person with a reasonable degree of accuracy.

Interpretation of nonverbal behavior carries the risk of misinterpretation. This is a serious risk, for *misinterpretation can lead to more misunderstanding than simply ignoring the nonverbal communication.* The risk of misinterpretation can be decreased by following six steps:

1. Note the nonverbal behavior.

2. Make a *tentative* interpretation.

3. Continue to observe for more evidence, especially evidence that is easily interpreted—a display of anger, statements of disapproval, objections, or complaints.

4. Revise your interpretation if there is evidence that the first interpretation was not accurate.

5. Watch for *consistency,* that is, occurrence of a specific nonverbal behavior every time that individual is in a particular situation, such as making a decision, doing something new, speaking before a group, or coping with conflict.

6. Use verbal communication to clarify the meaning of the nonverbal behavior. For example, if it is appropriate in a given situation, you could say, "Pat, you seem upset. What's going on?"

Once you have detected the pattern and determined that certain nonverbal behaviors consistently indicate a specific feeling state of that person, you have learned to "read" that person's nonverbal behavior.

**For Discussion and Reflection**

Think about someone you know well, such as a close friend or family member. What nonverbal behaviors provide a clue to this person's mood? How do you know, even without speaking, what kind of day this person has had?

With friends and coworkers, you may become quite accurate at reading their feelings without any words being exchanged. Accuracy in interpretation is achieved only over a period of time and through frequent opportunities to observe an individual in a variety of situations.

With people you see less frequently, you will not be able to learn the meaning of their nonverbal clues as readily. And, with people you see only occasionally or for brief periods of time, you must make your best judgment of the probable meaning of nonverbal behavior and try to confirm that interpretation as the relationship proceeds.

In relating to patients and their families, look for nonverbal behavior that may mean a buildup of feelings, especially fear, anxiety, confusion, and anger. When you detect such signals, it is likely that the patient would benefit from extra attention in the form of sincere interest, concern, consideration, and emotional support while adapting to strange surroundings and illness.

The special attention you provide may encourage the patient to talk. You might invite questions with, "Is there something you would like me to explain? I will try to answer any questions you have." You may be able to answer some questions but find it necessary to refer others to appropriate persons—the patient's physician, the supervisor, or another department of the health facility. You will be safe in giving information about routines and the facility itself. Questions about the patient's condition should be handled by others, usually the physician. Your role is to provide emotional support for the patient when you listen to questions, show sincere concern, and state that you will pass any questions you cannot answer on to the person who can provide answers.

A *full exploration of feelings* is best left to professionals with counseling skills. However, you can encourage *expression of feelings* and still remain within your role as a health care professional. Be aware that your patient is a human being going through a stressful experience, indicate your willingness to listen, and give your full attention to the patient. But, in order to recognize those who need an understanding listener, you must receive the message. A *message of need is most likely to be sent nonverbally*.

The following exercises are designed to help you practice recognizing and interpreting nonverbal communication.

## EXERCISE 15–1: OBSERVING NONVERBAL BEHAVIOR

### Purpose

In this exercise, you will discuss the messages conveyed by a series of nonverbal behaviors.

### Instructions

1. Work in groups of two. One partner will be the actor and the other the observer. In round 2, you will reverse roles.

2. Without speaking, the actor will demonstrate each of the nonverbal behaviors listed. After each behavior, the observer will comment briefly on the message he believes the behavior is sending. (There are a number of possible explanations for each behavior.)

### Nonverbal Behaviors: Round 1

1. Cross your arms.
2. Roll your eyes.
3. Look at the floor.
4. Jiggle your leg for several seconds.
5. Fiddle with your pencil or pen.
6. Sit up very straight in your chair.

### Nonverbal Behaviors: Round 2

1. Clench your fists.
2. Sigh loudly.
3. Smile.
4. Tap your fingers on the table repeatedly.
5. Look at your watch.
6. Make direct eye contact with your partner.

## EXERCISE 15–2: OBSERVING AND INTERPRETING NONVERBAL BEHAVIOR

### Purpose

In this exercise you will observe and interpret nonverbal communication and test your interpretation against the person's explanation of the thoughts and feelings that accompanied the nonverbal behavior.

### Instructions

1. Divide into groups of four. Two people will be actors and two will be observers. In round 2, you will reverse roles.
2. Select one of the situations below to role-play. The actors may take a few minutes to plan their performance.
3. Actors role-play the situation for three minutes. During this time, observers list the nonverbal behaviors they see and note what was happening in the role-play when the behavior occurred. One of the observers should call time after three minutes.
4. Observers describe the nonverbal behaviors they witnessed and offer a possible interpretation for each behavior. Actors confirm whether each interpretation matches what they were thinking or feeling at the time.
5. Reverse roles so that the actors are now observers and the observers are now actors. Repeat the exercise using a different situation.

### Role-Plays for Exercise 15–2

1. Janelle often arrives late to work and asks to leave early. Her supervisor decides to discuss the matter with her.

2. Rob, an experienced lab technician, notices a new technician using sloppy procedures and taking shortcuts. Concerned about accuracy and a reprimand from the supervisor, he confronts his coworker.

3. Arturo has recently immigrated to the United States and must get a physical for his new job. He has never been examined by a doctor before, and his English is limited. A nurse sits down to help him fill out paperwork and to get a medical history.

4. Mrs. Jones, an elderly patient, is hard of hearing. She takes several prescription medications. She asks a staff person to explain how much of each medication she should take and when.

5. Fifteen-year-old Lisa has come to the clinic for a pregnancy test, which is positive. A clinic worker gives her the test results and discusses her options with her.

## VERBAL COMMUNICATION

Workers in the health field spend much time communicating with others: patients and their families, visitors to the health agency, other members of the health team, and supervisors. As a health care professional, you need a high level of communication skill. Whenever and wherever people talk to one another, communication problems may occur.

We often assume that whatever we say to another person is understood—that the listener gets the meaning we intend to convey. In reality, there are numerous sources of communication breakdown:

- Our language permits different meanings for many words.
- Speech and hearing factors may distort what is heard.
- Nonverbal messages may differ from the spoken message.

Many examples of misunderstanding, noncooperation, criticism, and other forms of conflict between people can be traced to a communication problem. Your preparation for working in the health field includes practice in improving your communication skills so you will have a minimum of communication problems.

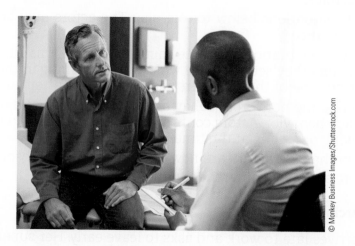

**FIGURE 15-2 Workers in the health field spend much time communicating with others.**

## AMBIGUITY

**Ambiguity** is the state of being *ambiguous*, or vague and unclear. The opposite of ambiguity is clarity. The word *unambiguous* is sometimes used to mean completely clear or free of ambiguity.

It is difficult to avoid ambiguity in verbal communication for a number of reasons:

- A word may have several different meanings.
- The word used by the speaker may not be the best word for expressing the desired meaning.
- A pronoun may not clearly indicate whom or what it represents.

For example, the word *smart* is used by some people to mean very intelligent; another person uses *smart* to mean sassy or disrespectful. Can you think of other meanings for this one word?

Some words or phrases have double meanings. They can be interpreted literally, or they may be used to mean something entirely different. The following joke illustrates this type of ambiguity:

A: *"This cat is really good for mice."*

B: *"How can you say that? He is afraid of mice. He even runs from them."*

C: *"That's just what I mean. He is very good for the mice."*

A pronoun that may refer to more than one noun is another source of ambiguity. Suppose a patient tells the nurse, "Dr. Brown and Dr. White (both males) both came by to see me last night. They think I'm doing fine. He even said I may go home today." Does "he" refer to Dr. Brown or to Dr. White?

In attempting to avoid ambiguous statements, you should:

- Use words that have a single, precise meaning whenever possible.
- Use the best word for what you want to say.
- Use a noun to indicate who or what; if you use a pronoun (he, she, it, they), it should clearly refer to *one specific noun* used in the same sentence.

## DISCREPANCIES IN A MESSAGE

Most of us are careless about verbal communication, especially when we are trying to attend to many things at once. In haste, we say *approximately* what we mean, then *assume* that the message received by the listener is the same as the message we intended to send. Also, we sometimes send one message nonverbally and state a different message verbally. Which message is the listener to believe?

Message discrepancy means that the message sent and the message received differ in meaning. The difficulty may be with

> **For Discussion and Reflection**
>
> Consider a situation in which you experienced a communication breakdown with another person. Were you the sender or the receiver of the message? What might have caused the breakdown? How was the situation resolved?

the sender of the message or the receiver. When the problem is with the sender, it may be caused by:

- Ambiguity in the message.
- **Inconsistency** in the verbal and nonverbal messages.
- Poor **enunciation**, causing some words to sound like other words with a different meaning.
- Use of language the listener does not understand. (This is likely to occur if the listener is a child, a person from a different culture, or an elderly person who may not be familiar with newer meanings of a word.)

If the problem of message discrepancy lies with the receiver, it may be caused by:

- Poor hearing.
- Selective listening (the individual listens only to certain parts of a statement).
- Inability to understand the words used by the speaker, such as medical terminology.
- Acceptance of the wrong message when there is inconsistency in the sender's verbal and nonverbal communication.

An example of inconsistency in verbal and nonverbal messages is the crying patient who says, "I'm all right. I feel fine." Sometimes the health care professional who is alert to nonverbal messages can pick up the true situation, as when a patient says, "There is nothing really wrong with me. The doctor says these are just routine tests." At the same time, the patient's countenance reflects a high level of anxiety. Whenever there is inconsistency in verbal and nonverbal messages, the listener must decide which message to believe.

In your endeavors to convey messages that are received (interpreted) as you intend:

- Avoid ambiguous statements.
- Select words and phrases the listener will understand.
- Speak clearly.
- Control your nonverbal signals to avoid sending a message that is different from your verbal message.
- Face the person to whom you are speaking.

## PARAVERBAL COMMUNICATION

Tone of voice is a key aspect of paraverbal communication, or *how* you say a message apart from the actual words used. You have probably heard a parent or teacher scold a child, "Don't take that tone with me!" Tone of voice can be as important as the choice of words in conveying a message to a listener. Responding to someone who is angry in a calm tone of voice often helps defuse the person's anger. On the other hand, an impatient or harsh tone of voice may hurt or anger the listener. Becoming conscious of your tone of voice helps your listener take your words in the spirit you intend them. Tone is particularly important when talking on the telephone because the listener does not have the benefit of seeing your facial expressions and other nonverbal behavior.

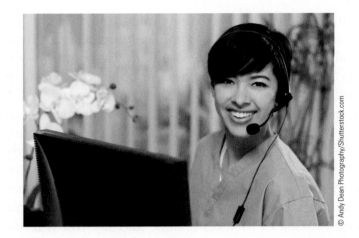

**FIGURE 15-3** Tone is particularly important when talking on the telephone because the listener does not have the benefit of seeing your facial expressions and other nonverbal behavior.

Two other components of paraverbal communication are volume and rate of speech. You have likely experienced listening to someone who spoke so quietly that you strained to hear each word. Very quiet speech may send a message that the speaker is shy, anxious, or afraid. Likely, you have also heard someone speaking too loudly, which can give the impression that the person is angry or upset. When someone speaks at a very slow rate, the listener may become impatient, question the intelligence of the speaker, or feel that the speaker is being condescending. On the other hand, a very fast rate of speech may send the message that the speaker is in a hurry, and the listener may have difficulty catching all the information in the message.

As you communicate with others, notice both their use of paraverbal communication and your own. You may have heard the phrase, "It's not what you say, it's how you say it." By consciously choosing a tone of voice, volume level, and rate of speech which fits the message you want to send, you can increase the chance that your message will be received accurately.

## EFFECTIVE LISTENING

In addition to expressing ideas clearly, a good communicator takes care to "hear" others accurately. The following techniques will help you become an effective listener:

- Give your full attention to anyone who is speaking to you.
- Listen to the words and observe nonverbal behavior in an effort to get the "real message."
- **Paraphrase** or restate what the person says to make sure you have understood correctly.
- Use questions to clarify the speaker's intended meaning, especially (1) if the speaker uses ambiguous or unfamiliar words and (2) if the verbal and nonverbal messages are inconsistent.

## ASSUMPTIONS AND EXPECTATIONS

Underlying many communication problems are **assumptions** and expectations held by the speaker or by the listener. An assumption is *acceptance of something as fact without any evidence or proof.* Sometimes we assume that another person "knows" how we feel or what we are thinking, even though we did not verbally express our thoughts or feelings. In fact, the person to whom we are speaking may be completely unaware of how we feel or what we are thinking. Or the other person may make assumptions about how we think or feel and the assumptions are completely wrong! Making assumptions is certain to create misunderstandings and communication breakdowns.

Another frequent cause of communication problems is the expectation of a person, either the sender or receiver of the message. An **expectation** means thinking that something will occur. An expectation can cause the receiver to "read into" a message something that the sender did not intend. For example, suppose your supervisor walks in while you are taking a shortcut on a task, then later the supervisor sends for you. Having been "caught" taking an unauthorized shortcut, your expectation is that the supervisor is going to correct you. You are probably set to defend yourself or to accept blame and say you will not do it again. But perhaps, instead of reprimanding you, the supervisor says, "I noticed you were not following procedure. Let's take a close look at the method you were using. It may be more efficient than our present procedure." Let us hope you did not misinterpret the supervisor's opening statement before you found out that your expectation was wrong! Sometimes an expectation can even lead the listener to "hear" a message that is quite different from the words spoken. This takes the speaker by surprise because the speaker is unaware of the other person's expectations.

## IMPROVING COMMUNICATION SKILLS

Improving your communication skills requires that you test your habits as both a sender and a receiver of messages. Fortunately, the same practice that helps you become more precise in your sending can also contribute to your skill in listening. As you become sensitive to ambiguities, inconsistencies, assumptions, and expectations, you will ask for **clarification** rather than risk a misunderstanding.

The following exercises are structured to provide practice in speaking, listening, and interpreting messages. In Exercise 15-3, you will increase your awareness of how the tone of a message can alter the meaning you convey to your listener. In Exercise 15-4, you will practice expressing your ideas clearly and listening effectively to the ideas of others.

When you have made progress on each of these skills, the probability of your having a communication breakdown is less. As an effective communicator, you will also be more effective in establishing good relationships.

---

**EXERCISE 15–3: USING TONE TO ALTER THE MEANING OF A STATEMENT**

### Purpose
In this exercise, you will practice using and listening to different tones of voice.

### Instructions
1. Work in groups of two. One partner will be the speaker and the other the listener. In round 2, you will reverse roles. Note that although the statements are the same in both rounds, the tones of voice used are not.
2. Role-play the following situations, using the tone of voice indicated. After the speaker has made the statement, the listener comments on how the tone affects the message he or she "hears."

## Role-Plays: Round 1

In this exercise, you will practice making statements that convey your intended meaning to another person, with minimal chance of misinterpretation by the listener.

1. A nurse says to a patient, "Are you ready for your treatment, Mr. Jones?"

   Tone: impatient

2. A supervisor says to an employee, "I expected you at work an hour ago. What happened?"

   Tone: concerned

3. A patient says to a health care professional, "There was a mistake on the last bill I received from your office."

   Tone: hesitant

4. A lab supervisor asks a lab technician, "Are those test results ready yet?"

   Tone: curious

5. A health care professional comments to a coworker, "Here we are, working the late shift again."

   Tone: resentful

## Role-Plays: Round 2

1. A nurse says to a patient, "Are you ready for your treatment, Mr. Jones?"

   Tone: kind

2. A supervisor says to an employee, "I expected you at work an hour ago. What happened?"

   Tone: irritated

3. A patient says to a health care professional, "There was a mistake on the last bill I received from your office."

   Tone: demanding

4. A lab supervisor asks a lab technician, "Are those test results ready yet?"

   Tone: hurried

5. A health care professional comments to a coworker, "Here we are, working the late shift again."

   Tone: joking

## EXERCISE 15–4: EXPRESSING IDEAS AND LISTENING EFFECTIVELY

### Purpose

In this exercise, you will express your opinion on a topic as clearly as possible. You will also use the listening techniques described earlier to check your understanding and to gain more information about another person's opinion.

## Instructions

1. Organize into groups of three. Each person should get a turn to play the role of the speaker, the observer, and the listener. The roles are described below.

2. The opinion statements that follow will serve as the basis for your discussion. Select a different opinion statement for each of the three rounds.

3. The speaker will discuss an opinion (agree or disagree) about one of the statements. The listener will use the listening skills described in this unit to check for understanding and to gain more information. After three minutes, the observer will call time and will provide feedback about the communication skills and listening skills observed.

**Speaker** Your objective is to communicate your opinion clearly to the listener. Select for discussion one of the opinion statements listed following this exercise. Explain why you agree or disagree with the statement. Feel free to use your personal knowledge and experiences to support your opinion.

**Listener** Your objective is to use effective listening techniques to gain a full understanding of the speaker's opinion. You are not to express your own opinion while playing the role of listener.

**Observer** Your objective is to provide feedback for the speaker and listener according to these guidelines:

- How clear was the speaker's first statement of opinion?
- How did the listener show that he or she was listening?
- Which listening skills did you observe?
- What additional information did the speaker share as a result of the listener's responses?

## Opinion Statements to Serve As a Basis for Discussion

1. Health care professionals should be allowed to go to classes during duty hours if they want to work on a higher certification.
2. Most people entering a health career want to help the sick.
3. Women make better health care professionals than men.
4. Every health care professional wants to stay up to date.
5. Patients should not expect health care professionals to listen to their personal problems.
6. The government should take over the costs of health care.
7. A woman who is pregnant has the right to decide whether or not she will continue the pregnancy.
8. Sex education should not be allowed in the public schools.
9. Managed care is the best system for providing health services.
10. Select a health-care related topic of your own based on current events or information you are studying in your health occupations program.

# COMMUNICATION AND THE HEALTH CARE PROFESSIONAL

So far we have explored three types of communication: nonverbal, verbal, and paraverbal. In everyday situations, all three types of communication occur simultaneously, working together to create an overall message. As you practice your communication skills in the workplace and elsewhere, the following guidelines can help:

- When someone is upset, angry, or afraid, often the most helpful approach is to listen to their concerns. Most individuals will calm down once they feel that their concerns are being heard.

- An anxious or upset individual is unlikely to "process" information from you at that time, so keep your own statements as clear and brief as possible.

- Pay attention to both verbal and nonverbal messages.

- If you are unsure what another person means, follow up with clarifying questions or by restating the message to check for understanding.

- If you can remain calm and professional in your communication, others are more likely to do the same. By remaining calm, you can avoid escalating a negative situation.

## ACTIVITIES

1. The next time you watch a sitcom on TV, concentrate your attention on one of the lead actors and note examples of nonverbal communication. Did any specific example lead to a misunderstanding or conflict between two of the characters?

2. The next time you watch a comedian who does imitations, note the various mannerisms and facial expressions the comedian portrays. Comedians are keen observers of human behavior, and imitators are especially observant of small bits of behavior that characterize an individual. Note the specific mannerisms portrayed in the actor's imitation of a certain person.

3. Use your next movie or TV evening to study the communication styles of the actors. Especially note examples of the following:

    a. An actor who has a frozen countenance (facial expression does not change) most of the time. What nonverbal behaviors does this actor use to communicate?

    b. An actor who uses subtle changes in facial expression. What "body language" does this actor use to supplement facial expression?

    c. An actor who conveys feelings primarily through facial expression. Does this actor also make use of body language to communicate feelings and/or reactions to the action occurring?

    d. Turn down the volume for at least five minutes during a television show and observe the characters' facial expressions and body language without sound. Can you follow the plot, based on the actors' nonverbal communication?

4. As you watch television or a movie, note examples of:

    a. Communication breakdown.

    b. Poor listening skills on the part of one or more characters.

c. Message discrepancy.

d. Nonverbal communication unnoticed by other characters.

## REFERENCES AND SUGGESTED READINGS

Body language in health care: a contribution to nursing communication. (2015). *Revista Brasileira de Enfermagem, 68*(3), 430–436. doi:10.1590/0034-7167.2015680316i.

Cuddy, Amy. (2015). *Presence: bringing your boldest self to your biggest challenges.* New York: Little, Brown, and Company.

Fleming, Carol. (2013). *It's the way you say it: becoming articulate, well-spoken, and clear.* San Francisco, CA: Berrett-Koehler.

Schiavo, R. (2015). Addressing health disparities in clinical settings: Population health, quality of care, and communication. *Journal of Communication in Healthcare, 8*(3), 163–166. doi:10.1080/17538068.2015.1107352.

# SECTION V

# Death and Loss

You have now learned about human behavior, ways people react to threat, and how to communicate effectively. This knowledge will be especially valuable as you work with people who are struggling to cope with loss. The ultimate losses are death (loss of one's own life) and bereavement (loss of a loved one).

In order to provide effective care to a terminally ill patient or to help those who are facing the loss of a loved one, the health care provider must have arrived at full acceptance of his or her own mortality and must have resolved any "unfinished business" related to past losses.

The purpose of Section V is to help you acknowledge your own mortality, clarify your beliefs about death, and become sensitive to the needs of terminally ill patients and their families.

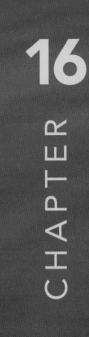

# CHAPTER 16

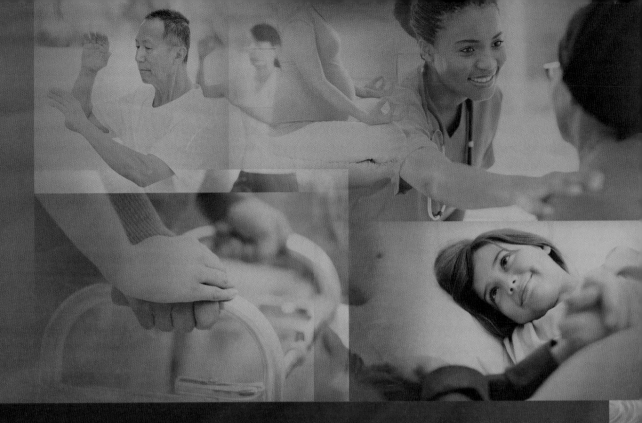

# Grief and Loss Throughout Life

## OBJECTIVES

After completing this chapter, you should be able to:

- Explain why loss is a part of everyone's life.
- Discuss strategies for coping with loss, sadness, and depression.
- Explain possible causes of suicide.
- Describe how a suicide can affect surviving friends and family.
- List emotional and physical effects of grief.
- Describe how grief can affect behavior.
- Name the five stages of the grief process as described by Dr. Elisabeth Kübler-Ross.
- List indications of unresolved grief.
- Discuss strategies for assisting the family of a dying patient.

## KEY TERMS

| | | |
|---|---|---|
| Anticipatory grief | Displacement | Survivor guilt |
| Bereavement | Grief work | Transference |
| Condolences | Mortality | |

Life involves a continuous series of changes that require us to adjust and readjust. Some of these changes represent a gain of some type—new home, new member of the family, graduation, new job, or a promotion. Some changes represent a loss—being fired, losing an important object, losing a spouse through divorce, losing a loved one through death.

Many events involve both gains and losses. Moving to a new home is exciting, but it involves losing the familiarity of the old home and relationships in the old neighborhood. Graduation is usually a happy event—it symbolizes moving on to bigger and better things. But graduation also means giving up a favorite teacher, no longer spending much of the school day with your classmates, and giving up a familiar role for a new role and new responsibilities. You expect the big events of life to have a happy effect, so it is confusing to find that, instead of being happy, you are sad or even depressed. These negative feelings are due to awareness (perhaps at the unconscious level) of losses that will result from an otherwise happy event.

Most people do not need to learn how to be happy about a gain, but many people do not know how to cope with loss. Loss definitely is one of life's most important lessons because unexpressed grief is a powerful influence on behavior and on emotional/mental health.

## LEARNING TO COPE WITH CHANGE AND LOSS

If we learn early in life to deal effectively with the small losses that are part of living, then we are better prepared to deal with those losses that cause a radical change in our life situation. If we do not learn to "let go" of whatever was lost and to grieve appropriately for each loss, then there is an accumulation of suppressed emotions—grief, anger, guilt, and fear. Suppressed emotions are eventually expressed in some form, such as uncontrolled outbursts, depression, or inability to cope with daily life problems. Failure to express such feelings is characteristic of people who develop phobias, commit suicide, or develop alcohol/drug dependency.

Actually, we have a choice. We can learn to accept the inevitable losses of life and express our grief appropriately, thereby maintaining control and emotional well-being. Or we can go through life without learning how to deal with loss—reacting with anger about the "unfairness" of life or suppressing our grief, thereby risking loss of control when these feelings eventually erupt.

Dr. Elisabeth Kübler-Ross (1926–2004) was a psychiatrist who worked with dying patients for many years. According to Dr. Kübler-Ross, the dying process extends throughout life, and each of us goes through the stages of this process repeatedly as we experience specific life changes, especially those that involve some type of loss. The best preparation for dealing with death, according to Dr. Kübler-Ross, is to learn to grieve appropriately for the small losses that accompany any major life change. Once we have learned to grieve, we are able to cope better with the big losses that will, inevitably, occur in each of our lives. Learning to cope with loss involves several specific steps:

1. Recognize the losses involved in a life event.

2. Grant yourself the right to grieve for each loss—no matter how small.

3. Recognize and accept the various emotions involved in your reaction to a specific loss.

4. Allow yourself time to grieve.

5. Accept that grief is a *process* that extends over a period of time.

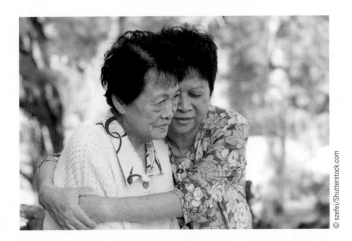

**FIGURE 16-1 The significance of a loss is very personal.**

## SIGNIFICANCE OF LOSS

Losses are of many types: objects, people, relationships, jobs, money, body image (e.g., amputation, radical mastectomy), or intangibles such as beliefs, faith, one's sense of security, self-esteem. The significance of a loss is very personal. A person's reaction to a loss *reflects its meaning to that person*, rather than its value as perceived by others.

Some types of loss may be experienced at any time throughout life: moving, personal relationships, death of a loved one, personal property, health. Reactions to such losses are influenced by the period of life in which they occur. Children often do not understand the reasons for a loss, and adults may fail to note or accept the child's emotional reaction. Adults have the advantage of being involved in some decisions that result in a loss, such as moving, so their emotional reaction is tempered by an understanding of the reasons for the decision. For elderly people, a great loss is losing control over decisions that affect the remainder of their lives. Moving into a child's home or into a nursing home results in partial loss of control over one's daily activities. The reaction to such a change often includes hopelessness and resignation. The most devastating loss is the loss of life—one's own or that of a loved one.

## LOSSES DUE TO DEATH

The impact of a death on each survivor is influenced by numerous factors, including age of the survivor, relationship to the deceased, the survivor's past experience in coping with significant losses, age of the deceased, and circumstances surrounding the death. For example:

- Was the death expected? Did it follow a lengthy terminal illness?
- Does the death represent a release from pain and suffering?
- Was the death sudden and unexpected? In this situation, the survivors must cope with shock initially, then with loss.
- What was the age of the deceased? If the deceased was elderly and the survivors believe that he or she had "lived a good life," the loss is easier to accept. If the deceased was young, grief is likely to be accompanied by anger and a sense of injustice.

**For Discussion and Reflection**

Think back to your childhood. At what age did you first experience death, whether the death of a pet, a friend, or a relative? What was your family's attitude toward death?

Certain circumstances surrounding a death have an especially powerful impact on survivors:

- **The death was accidental**. Was the accident due to someone's negligence or carelessness? If so, anger and blaming may delay the beginning of a healthful grieving process. If a survivor was involved in the accident, that person may feel that he or she was responsible for the death. Or, that person may experience **survivor guilt**, wondering "What right did I have to survive?" or believing "I should have been the one who died." Anyone who is experiencing survivor guilt needs professional counseling.

- **The death was related to violence or criminal activity (mugging, burglary, or drive-by shooting).** Survivors of this type of death must deal with anger and perhaps a desire for revenge, as well as grief.

- **The death was a murder or homicide.** Survivors must deal with shock initially, then questions of "Why?" and "Who?" If the killer was a member of the family, survivors may divide into two groups. Some will refuse to believe the perpetrator's guilt and will loyally support his or her defense. Others will direct anger at the accused and seek "justice" for the deceased. In both cases, these emotions interfere with the grief process.

- **The deceased was on life support.** Who made the decision to discontinue it? Even when a living will and advance directives exist, the decision to discontinue life support is difficult for family members. If some family members disagree with the decision, then the decision maker has to cope with their criticism in addition to personal feelings about making that fateful decision.

- **The death was due to self-inflicted injury—suicide.** This type of death is especially difficult for survivors. Because suicide is widely misunderstood, it is important that health care providers understand this type of death.

## SUICIDE

Any suicide attempt is a medical emergency. Although suicide is viewed as a mental health problem, it can be understood only within the context of the person's life situation: social isolation, abuse, pain, disfigurement, disability, loss of a body part, severe mood swings, the "voices" heard by a schizophrenic, or any life circumstance that has become intolerable. For a desperate individual, death may seem to be the only way to escape. Members of certain groups are at high risk for suicide: teenagers, the elderly (especially divorced or widowed men), and anyone who is seriously depressed.

Any death by suicide places family members and associates of the deceased in a soul-searching position:

*Why did I not recognize the signs that he or she was in such distress?*

*Why was I not more sensitive to his or her unhappiness?*

*What did I do that caused this terrible act?*

*Why did I not express my love?*

*Why was I so critical?*

*Why did I not insist that he or she seek help?*

*What could I have done to prevent this act?*

For parents there may be many questions, most pertaining to "how could I have been a better parent?" For siblings, the entire range of emotions is possible, depending upon the relationship with the deceased. For surviving spouses, the emotional impact may range from relief to a devastating sense of loss, depending upon the quality of the marital relationship. Friends and associates may be affected differently by suicide than by a death due to accident or illness. Some of the questions just listed may haunt those who associated with the deceased on a daily basis, especially the question, "What could I have done to help?"

Following a suicide, survivors have to deal not only with their loss, but also with psychological trauma: guilt, anger, remorse, confusion, helplessness, or feelings of failure for not having been a better parent, sibling, or friend. Suicide by a child or teenager may affect an entire school, setting off an epidemic of suicides or suicide attempts within the school population.

Suicide is considered an honorable death in some cultures. In certain Asian societies, someone who has lost honor, for whatever reason, is *expected* to commit suicide. Today there is a resurgence of belief in *honorable suicide* among fundamentalist groups throughout the world. The role of suicide bomber is willingly assumed, usually by an adolescent or young adult, in order to destroy members of a group perceived as the enemy. This activity occurs with disturbing frequency in the Middle East. The mother of a young male suicide bomber was quoted in the news media as declaring proudly that her son had died an honorable death. If the suicide bomber acted on instructions of a terrorist organization, that organization may pay the surviving family a large sum of money for this sacrifice of a family member. But in the United States, suicide is regarded by many people as a dishonorable act. Some insurance companies do not pay if a death is due to suicide or may exclude suicide for a specific period of time.

One who completes a suicide is found dead, and therefore will not come under your care. Most people who complete a suicide have a history of suicide attempts. Who is to know when a person who survived one suicide attempt will make another attempt that becomes a completed suicide? As a health care provider, avoid thinking that any suicide attempt is "just trying to get attention." The attempt may be a call for help, but "attention" is not the motive.

Why would anyone ingest a poison or take a lethal dose of a drug? Why do some people cut themselves? Why put a bullet through one's head? The only logical answer is that the individual is desperately trying to escape an intolerable life situation, a painful or debilitating physical condition, or the hopelessness that accompanies deep depression.

*The greatest danger of suicide is when the person is coming out of a depressed state.* Many depressed persons do not have the energy to carry out a suicide. As they recover from depression, they not only have the energy, but also know that sooner or later they will again experience the hopelessness of depression. One journalist spoke of her depressed periods as a "bottomless hole" or a "black abyss" of hopelessness and despair. After two attempts, she completed a suicide just when her physician and family believed she was recovering from her latest bout of depression. The suicide of a person who is depressed is a desperate effort to escape the effects of depression.

It is likely that you will encounter a hospitalized patient who has attempted suicide. It is especially important for caregivers to keep in mind that they do not know the circumstances of that patient's life situation. Any one of us may at some time in our lives experience emotionally overwhelming circumstances. Without having experienced such conditions, we do not know how we would react. Only those who have experienced hopelessness, depression, or mood swings over a period of time can understand the distress of a person who attempts suicide.

The implications for you as a health care provider are clear. Do not judge the patient who has attempted suicide. Know that this person needs emotional support and respect. Keep in mind your philosophy of individual worth, be a compassionate caregiver, demonstrate caring, and *listen*. Anyone who has attempted suicide should be evaluated by a psychiatrist and, according to the diagnosis, given appropriate treatment. Long-term counseling is needed by most survivors of a suicide attempt, to learn effective ways of coping with depression, mood swings, and life problems.

## DEATH OF A PARENT

The death of one's parent is a unique type of loss, regardless of one's age and the age of the parent. For each of us, parents provide a link to our ancestry, our own life history, and most of what we learned as children. For a child, the immediate reaction may be anger: "How could Mommy (or Daddy) leave me?" There may also be feelings of guilt:

> *When she (he) sent me to my room I wished she (he) was dead. It's all my fault.*
>
> *If I had been a better daughter (son), Mommy (Daddy) would not have died.*
>
> *If only I had said, 'I love you' more often.*

A young child is likely to perceive the parent's death as abandonment. Loss of a parent during childhood also means the loss of parental guidance through current and future developmental tasks. The deceased parent will be missing from important life events: graduations, recitals, athletic performances, the wedding, the birth of one's own children.

The death of a same-gender parent means the loss of a parental role model. This loss is especially significant during adolescence, a time of struggling to establish one's own identity.

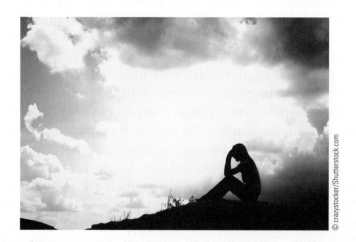

**FIGURE 16-2 Following the death of a loved one, survivors may feel sadness, depression, or guilt.**

Although adolescence is characterized by some degree of rebellion, this period of life involves developmental tasks that are best accomplished under parental guidance. Sometimes the death of a parent forces a child into an adult role. The oldest girl may assume maternal responsibilities for care of younger siblings and for managing the household. An adolescent boy may become "the man of the house" and seek work to help support the family.

After a parent dies, surviving children may be profoundly affected psychologically, especially if they do not grieve appropriately for their loss. **Displacement** may occur if feelings were not fully expressed during the mourning period; they may emerge, greatly magnified, later in life when some other loss occurs. **Transference** is manifested by seeking fulfillment from others, placing them in the position of parental substitute.

## LOSSES IN SPECIFIC PERIODS OF THE LIFE SPAN

Preparation for coping with a significant loss comes from experiencing a variety of losses throughout life. The individual who learns during childhood to grieve for small losses is better prepared to cope with a major loss than someone who has not learned to recognize and grieve for a loss. Learning to cope with loss begins in infancy; the types of loss and their significance vary according to the period of life.

### Losses of Infancy and Early Childhood

The prenatal period is a very special time for both mother and fetus. If there are no complications or difficult circumstances, the pregnant woman experiences positive feelings during most of the pregnancy. For the fetus, life in the womb is the ultimate in security and safety. At the time of delivery, the family gains a new member—one of life's happiest events. But birth is the end of pregnancy—the loss of a once-only relationship between mother and infant. If the baby is breast-fed, the mother and infant establish another very special relationship. Weaning is a small loss because it requires both mother and infant to "let go" of this special relationship.

During infancy and early childhood, any separation from the parents (or other caregivers) is perceived as loss. The child, not knowing that the parents will return, feels deserted. Sadness is a natural reaction to separation; but separation from those who represent security can also arouse fear, anger, and even guilt. When a young child is hospitalized and no member of the family remains with the child, the child's emotional reaction may be manifested as withdrawal. Early separation experiences may be the source of fears and anxieties in later life about the loss of a relationship.

The importance of parental attachments, especially during infancy and childhood, should be understood by parents who must leave their children at frequent intervals. Special efforts should be made to establish a loving relationship and minimize the child's distress at being left in day care or with a babysitter. A good day care center offers a loving and supportive atmosphere for the child, in recognition of the distress felt by an infant/child as a normal reaction to separation from parents.

Health care providers need to understand separation anxiety, spend as much time as possible with a child whose parents have left, and provide emotional support as needed. Honest, age-appropriate explanations will help the child understand what has happened. Above all, do not subscribe to the value judgment that a crying child is "just spoiled." Be aware that the crying child may believe that he has been abandoned.

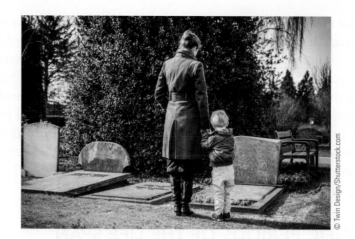

**FIGURE 16-3** When a death occurs, a child needs honest explanations, but only enough detail to help the child understand the situation.

Many changes in relationships occur during early childhood. The child achieves more independence (and less dependence) as growth and development occur. Dependency is another type of special relationship, so the child's achievements also involve changes in relationships. Entering kindergarten or school is an exciting, sometimes frightening, experience. The child loses the comfort, safety, and security of home, but gains new experiences, a peer group, and new adult contacts. The mother loses her dependent "baby" and gains a school-child who is increasingly independent.

## Losses of Middle Childhood

Throughout the school-age years a child repeatedly experiences losses and gains. Each promotion means leaving a familiar teacher and gaining a new one. There may be a loss of some classmates, although new children may come into the class at intervals. Friendships may break up, with any grief over the loss obscured by anger or guilt about the cause of the break-up. A change of school during this period includes numerous losses, which may or may not be offset by gains available in the new school. Completion of the elementary grades includes the loss of some relationships and also the loss of a familiar role. Promotion to middle school or high school usually means giving up childhood activities and entering the world of adolescence.

## Losses during Adolescence

Gains and losses related to growth and development, dependence versus independence, and promotion from one grade to another continue through adolescence. For the most part, the emotional effects of these types of losses or gains are manageable. A person with adequate adjustment copes with these changes reasonably well. But some events of adolescence have the potential for arousing very strong emotional reactions: establishing a romantic relationship, becoming sexually active, experiencing peer pressure (to smoke, to use drugs, to consume alcoholic beverages), getting a job, and graduating. During this period romantic relationships are established. When such a relationship ends, one or both parties may experience intense emotional reactions to the loss.

Adolescence is also the time when many young people obtain their first job, which requires learning a new role and includes a significant gain—one's own income. If the job is terminated, both role and income are lost; the circumstances may include loss of self-esteem.

Graduation from high school is perceived by students and their families as a happy event. The losses involved are seldom talked about. A high school graduation results in the end of many friendships. It also represents the beginning of passage into adulthood and many new responsibilities. Although some students maintain their dependence on parents through additional years of education, for many the relatively carefree life of childhood and adolescence ends forever with graduation from high school.

## Losses of the Young Adult Years

The adult period of life is characterized by vocational choices, the struggle for financial independence, establishing adult coping strategies, affirming one's sexuality through marriage or a relationship, starting a family, setting up a home, and developing a satisfying lifestyle. Each of these activities may provide much satisfaction and happiness. Each also includes the possibility of loss: getting fired from a job; ending a marriage through divorce; losing property through theft, fire, or natural disaster; losing friends or family members through death; moving, which often includes loss of a support network of friends and family.

The adult period of life involves a continuous sequence of gains and losses, both large and small. Accepting the joy that life may bring and also learning to cope with the pain of loss leads to continued growth and a full life. Trying to escape pain by avoiding life experiences that include the risk of loss, such as marriage or a loving relationship, does not lead to growth and precludes living a full life. *Part of the adult life experience is accepting the risk of losing some of what we have gained.*

## Losses of Middle Age

Ideally, middle adulthood is a period for enjoying the rewards of one's labors during the early adult years. For many, however, this is a period of continued struggle for financial survival. The expenses of a family peak as children reach high school and college. If the family's income has increased through the years, these expenses are manageable. Otherwise, adolescent members of the family may have to become wage earners.

The struggle for financial security involves relatively frequent gains and losses. For example, a promotion may mean additional salary and prestige, but result in the loss of free time if new responsibilities require longer hours or taking work home at night. Any unexpected expense may result in loss. For example, a long-awaited vacation at the beach may be lost because the car needs a new transmission.

Parents usually welcome the growing independence of their children. There may also be some sadness at the loss of the child/parent dependent relationship. As children leave home to attend school, set up their own apartments, or marry, parents experience a sense of loss. Departure of the youngest child is especially difficult. "Empty nest syndrome" is a well-known depressive reaction to this event.

During the middle adult years, many people begin to realize that they will not be able to achieve some of their career or financial goals. As this realization reaches full consciousness, the individual may experience a profound sense of loss. Attitudes toward the job may change, the quality of work may be lower, and there may be expressions of hopelessness.

Recognition of a significant loss—namely, the loss of one's youth—occurs sometime during the middle years. This may occur on a 40th or 50th birthday, or it may develop gradually as physical stamina diminishes, physical proportions change, baldness develops, wrinkles appear, or once-firm tissues become flabby. Many people accept the effects of time and adapt their lifestyles to accommodate physical changes. Some people, however, experience a "midlife crisis" and set out to prove to the world (and to themselves) that they are still young. A long-term marriage may break up during this period, as one partner seeks younger companions to bolster the belief, "I am still young and attractive." Loss of youth is very painful to those who subscribe to the current emphasis on youth and sex appeal in the mass media. Menopause represents a very significant change for a woman—namely, loss of the ability to reproduce. For a man, occasional periods of impotence threaten self-esteem.

Middle age is also the time of life when potentially serious health problems may develop. As life span has increased during the past 50 years, the incidence of chronic diseases has risen markedly. Loss of health is so unacceptable that many people, upon being told that they have a particular disease, react with, "I don't believe it."

Denying a newly diagnosed disorder is not limited to serious illness. An adult who is told that recurrent sore throats are due to allergy may refuse to have allergy studies performed. This person's self-concept may not include "I am a person with an intolerance for certain foods and other substances in my life situation." A person who is diagnosed as having early arthritis may think immediately of people with deformed hands or those who complain constantly of their joint pain. The initial reaction is, "I will not become deformed, and I will not accept continuous pain in my life." Denial eventually gives way to acceptance of the diagnosis, after the individual has had time to adjust to symptoms and changes in body function.

## Losses during Senescence

The fastest-growing population segment in the United States is 65 and older group. Because of this increased life span, we are seeing a relatively new phenomenon—elderly persons caring for their even more elderly parents. For these caregivers, death of a parent is a loss that is experienced during old age.

The senescent period of life includes more losses than gains. Physical losses eventually include diminished vision, hearing, taste, mobility, and memory. These losses usually develop gradually, but may be accelerated by any serious illness. Any chronic condition, such as arthritis, increases awareness of losses. When buttoning a shirt or tying a shoe becomes difficult, the individual is reminded daily of lost mobility and dexterity.

Psychological losses are also numerous during senescence. Retirement is a serious threat to mental health. For people who have not developed interests and activities outside of their work, there is no longer a daily routine of meaningful activity. One's work-related identity is lost. Daily interaction with coworkers is lost. Because retirement benefits seldom equal work-related income, financial loss may be significant. All of these losses are a serious threat to self-esteem, so serious that a period of depression following retirement is relatively common. This emphasizes the importance of having a purpose in life and being actively involved in meaningful activities other than work.

Social losses affect the elderly more than other age groups. Friends and close family members move or die. The loss of a specific friend may also mean the loss of a social activity shared with that person. The loss of a spouse may mean being left out of social activities in which the couple has participated for years. A son or daughter moving to another town means the loss of daily contact with immediate family, especially grandchildren. For many elderly persons, social life gradually diminishes. Loneliness and aloneness may characterize the daily life of an elderly person.

The loss that is feared by most elderly people is loss of independence. When an elderly person is deemed unable to live alone, the result is loss of one's home, loss of a familiar bed, loss of choices in what to eat and when. This loss of independence is accompanied by a loss of self-esteem. Moving to a retirement home or confinement in a nursing home involves so many losses for the individual that there is often an immediate decline in health. All too often the emotional reactions of elderly people to these radical changes in lifestyle are not recognized or acknowledged by caregivers or by family members.

## GUIDELINES FOR USING LOSS AND GRIEF AS A GROWTH EXPERIENCE

Loss involves pain. The intensity of the pain depends upon the degree of commitment to what was lost. *Coping with the pain of loss is a life skill that is essential to mental and emotional health.* There are many opportunities in health care agencies for a sensitive caregiver to recognize someone's need for emotional support when dealing with significant loss.

The following guidelines may appear simple. They are relatively easy to accept—intellectually. Accepting them at the *emotional level*, however, requires dealing honestly with one's feelings and beliefs. The result should be an increase in readiness to cope with the reality of loss and to help others who have experienced a significant loss.

1. Learn to recognize the small losses that occur in your life.
2. Accept anger, fear, and guilt feelings as part of many grief reactions.
3. Allow time for grieving.
4. Acknowledge your own vulnerability to losses and pain.
5. Acknowledge your lack of total control. You may control some aspects of your life, but some events are beyond your control.
6. Acknowledge your own **mortality**—the fact that your life will end at some time.
7. Accept that life involves change, including losses. Some changes require that we modify our belief systems to fit the new reality.
8. Following a loss, work through the feelings. When you are ready, "let go" of the past (which includes the loss).
9. Believe that you can cope with whatever loss you may experience.
10. Be supportive of those who have suffered a loss.

### For Discussion and Reflection

Identify a loss, large or small, that you have experienced in the past three years. Which of the steps above do you feel that you have accomplished in regard to "letting go" of the loss? Are there ways in which you have not finished the grief process?

## UNDERSTANDING GRIEF

Grief is a normal and natural reaction to loss that ranges from mild disappointment through various degrees of sadness, up to the intense and painful state that we call grief. **Anticipatory grief** occurs prior to the actual loss, usually during a terminal illness. **Bereavement** is separation from or loss of someone who is significant in one's life. Grief is the predominant emotional response to bereavement, although anger and fear may also be experienced. **Grief work** is a process of working through the emotional reaction to loss, reorganizing one's life patterns, and achieving some degree of adjustment. Grief work is important to future emotional and mental health. Uncompleted grief work will eventually manifest as physical illness, poor adjustment, or tendencies to avoid or overreact to situations involving loss, dying, or bereavement.

Some grief reactions include not only sadness, but also some degree of anger, hate, guilt, anxiety, or even panic.

- *Anger* is usually a major component in grief when the age of the deceased is "inappropriate" for dying, such as infancy and childhood, adolescence, young adulthood, or "the prime of life." A survivor may actually feel anger toward the deceased for "going away and leaving me." This reaction is especially likely in a child whose parent has died.

- *Anxiety* is related to the future: "How can I live without . . . (that which was lost)?" or "How can I make certain this never happens to me again?"

- *Panic* is related to the recognition that one does not have the power to control the loss of a loved one.

- *Guilt* may be concerned with control: "Could I have prevented this from happening?" or blame: "If I had been more loving, this wouldn't have happened." Children who are not old enough to understand terminal illness or death are especially prone to guilt, because a child's anger toward a family member or playmate is sometimes expressed as an explosive "I hate you!" or possibly, "I wish you were dead!" A child may recall past actions, words, or thoughts and perceive that behavior and the death or illness as having a cause/effect relationship.

Grief is painful. Grief related to loss of a loved one through death usually results in a profound grief reaction. The remainder of this unit limits discussion of grief to this type of loss.

## EFFECTS OF GRIEF

The death of a loved one has both physical and psychological effects on the survivor. Shock is the immediate reaction. Profound shock is likely if a death is sudden or unexpected, the result of an accident or act of violence, or a suicide. In contrast to sudden bereavement, a lengthy illness provides time for anticipatory grieving prior to the actual death. Intensity of the immediate grief reaction, then, is determined by whether the death was expected or unexpected, a sudden or slow process, violent or nonviolent. If shock is severe, the survivor cannot begin grief work until the physical effects of shock have subsided.

In the absence of severe shock, a grief reaction can range from little or no visible reaction to uncontrolled, destructive behavior. The immediate physical effects include tightness in the throat, a choking sensation, shortness of breath, weakness, a feeling of emptiness or a knot in the stomach, and nausea. These effects may subside within a few hours, to be replaced by loss of appetite and/or digestive problems, disturbed sleep patterns, restlessness, frequent sighing, and crying that may continue intermittently for days, weeks, or months.

The mental/emotional effects of bereavement include preoccupation with thoughts of the deceased, lack of interest in other people, irritability, difficulty in organizing thoughts or making decisions, difficulty in concentrating or remembering, feelings of hopelessness, feelings of guilt, and possibly a tendency toward blaming self or others for the loss. Some behavioral effects of grief are lack of interest in grooming, refusal to participate in previous activities or hobbies, poor performance at home or on the job, reminiscing about the deceased, idealizing the deceased (forgetting negative aspects of the deceased), and clinging to personal reminders.

These effects of grief vary in intensity and duration according to a survivor's relationship to the deceased, personal ways of dealing with strong emotion, and patterns of behavior learned in previous life crises. *How a survivor deals with grief influences future adjustment.*

## IMPORTANCE OF THE GRIEF PROCESS

Grief is a period of pain from which one recovers over time. It may also be a growth experience in which one learns to accept certain realities:

- We are vulnerable to certain life experiences, including losses.
- We are not all-powerful. We only have control over *some* aspects of our lives.
- We are mortal, not immortal.
- There will be a time for each of us when life comes to an end.
- Loss requires saying "good-bye" to some aspect of life, but loss can also mean a new beginning.
- "Letting go" does not diminish the importance of what was lost, but it does free the survivor to make the necessary adjustments for living without the deceased.

## INFLUENCES ON THE GRIEF PROCESS

Any person who has experienced a significant loss has the right to grieve. A person's grieving tends to be consistent with the personality and usual coping styles. The intensity and duration of grieving are influenced by the relationship to the deceased and past experiences with loss. Friends and family should grant each survivor the right to grieve in his or her own way.

Working through the stages of denial, anger, and bargaining prior to the actual death seems to facilitate grief work during the bereavement period. Spending quality time with the dying person—sharing memories, expressing feelings, touching and holding—facilitates anticipatory grieving and also eases the dying process. Grieving is facilitated if family members share their feelings and if relatives and friends are supportive throughout the process.

### Acceptance of Loss

Grief work begins with acceptance of the loss—the finality of death. Sometimes there is intellectual acceptance without emotional acceptance. Only when the finality of the loss is accepted at the emotional level can grief work begin. The survivor needs encouragement to "be with" his or her feelings by expressing the sadness and pain, rather than denying the feelings or hiding them from others.

## Making Final Arrangements

Participating in the tasks related to death seems to facilitate acceptance. Before or immediately after the death, someone must notify relatives, friends, coworkers, the minister, and the family lawyer; prepare an obituary; care for and remove the body; plan for the disposal of the body (burial, cremation); plan a service (funeral, memorial); purchase a cemetery lot (or decide how to dispose of the ashes if cremation is chosen); complete paperwork (death certificate, notices to insurance and annuity companies, government agencies, banks). Insofar as possible, the tasks that involve decision making should be completed prior to the actual death, because one who is experiencing powerful emotions may not be able to make important decisions.

Some people want to be involved in the final stages of the dying process, and some want to assist with final care of the body. Being present at the final moments of life is beneficial to survivors and also to the patient. Many dying patients state that dying alone is their greatest fear. For survivors, being with the patient in those last moments is preparation for emotional release. Bathing, dressing, and grooming the body provides an opportunity for saying "good-bye" in the most loving and caring way possible. This is especially appropriate if the deceased is a child. Sometimes the survivors participate in closing the grave with handfuls of dirt. This, too, is a way of saying "good-bye" and moving toward emotional acceptance of the loss.

The body of the deceased and the final service both play a role in acceptance of death. The funeral service and interment provide opportunities to express the intense feelings that immediately follow the death and help prepare the survivors for grief work. Alternatives to a traditional funeral, such as a memorial service, can also facilitate the grief process.

## Grief Inhibitors

In the belief that people need to be protected, someone may try to keep those closest to the deceased from participating in these tasks. Friends or relatives may encourage survivors-to-be to withdraw from the death scene and to delegate final tasks to others. The survivors may even be deprived of time with the loved one, either during the final moments or immediately after death, in the mistaken belief that witnessing the death or being with the body would be traumatic. No matter how good their intentions, people who influence the family to withdraw from the death scene deprive family members of an experience that facilitates "letting go" and beginning the grief process.

Children, especially, are likely to be excluded. As they observe atypical adult behavior and disruption of the family's normal routine, they may be confused, frightened, or angry. They need explanations about what is happening, much comforting, and a chance to say "good-bye" to the dying person *if they wish to do so.*

Numerous other conditions can inhibit the grief process: a sudden death, an untimely death, the mode of death (accident, suicide, violence), unresolved grief from past losses, past tendency to suppress anger and grief, ambivalent feelings toward the deceased, the use of drugs or alcohol to suppress feelings, resuming normal activities too early, isolation from a death (war in a foreign country), or uncertainty about a death (a plane crash or fire in which the remains are difficult or impossible to identify). The uncertainty created when the body cannot be viewed makes it especially difficult for survivors to accept the death. There is, instead, a tendency to cling to the belief that the victim will come back home some day.

## Condolences

Most people find it difficult to express **condolences** to the bereaved. All too often, statements that are offered as words of comfort or as reassurance actually deny the importance of grief or imply that the person has no right to grieve. The following are examples of such statements:

- "You must be strong" implies that showing one's grief is a sign of weakness.
- "You must be a little man" denies a boy the right to grieve and also implies that, as a male, he is not allowed to cry.
- "It's time to get on with your life" is a way of saying, "I do not grant you any more time for grieving."

Often, the most effective form of condolence is simply silence, accompanied by a hug or kiss if appropriate. Friends and relatives who take time to "be there" for a bereaved person are helpful. Staying in touch, either in person or by phone or mail, keeps the bereaved person believing that you care. Over time, having friends and family who are willing to listen facilitates the grieving process for a bereaved person.

If a year has passed, the person may need professional counseling to facilitate the completion of grief work. But a statement such as, "It's time to get on with your life" is totally inappropriate a month, or even several months, after the death of a loved one. An inappropriate statement may indicate that the speaker does not understand the grief process or its importance to a survivor's future adjustment.

## Uncompleted Grief Work

Some survivors fail to complete the grief process, either because feelings are suppressed or because certain conditions inhibit the grief process. Grief that is not resolved may be indicated by hyperactivity, inappropriate feelings, physical illness (possibly with the symptoms of the deceased, if he or she dies of an illness), changes in relationships with others, hostility, depression, or a lack of feeling. Sometimes the grief reaction becomes chronic; that is, the bereaved becomes locked into the early stages of the process and does not progress toward readjustment.

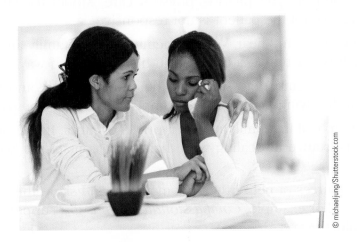

© michaeljung/Shutterstock.com

**FIGURE 16-4 Supportive friends and relatives can contribute greatly to successful grief work.**

Denial of grief at the time of the loss may result in a delayed grief reaction after weeks, months, or even years, usually at the time of another death or when a close friend is grieving.

Supportive friends and relatives can contribute greatly to successful grief work. Professional counseling is needed, however, when a survivor manifests denial or evidence of uncompleted grief work after one year.

## ROLES OF HEALTH CARE PROFESSIONALS

The health care professional is likely to be in contact with relatives of a dying patient before the patient's death, rather than throughout the bereavement period. Because the physician has primary responsibility for providing information about a patient's condition, health care workers must know what the patient, as well as the family, has been told. This can be determined by carefully worded questions and by observation of nonverbal behavior. Active listening is effective for learning what the physician has told the patient and family and identifying where the other person is emotionally.

The health care professional's goal is to help the family, not by giving information or expressing personal opinions, but by helping the other to express feelings and work toward acceptance of the loss at his or her own pace. Various professional workers are prepared to provide skilled counseling for patients and their families. Large hospitals have chaplains and social workers, some of whom have special preparation for helping others cope with a life crisis. Smaller hospitals and most nursing homes rely on community resources to provide this specialized service.

Each death/bereavement situation is unique, so there cannot be a single procedure to guide the health care professional. But there are guidelines that may help the caregiver adapt to each situation.

## GUIDELINES FOR ASSISTING THE FAMILY OF A DYING PATIENT

1. Be available to the family as much as possible. (Do not use the nurses' station as a refuge to avoid interacting with the family.)

2. Use active listening to encourage the expression of feelings.

3. Interact with the patient as you provide physical care. Model for family members the expression of caring, even if the patient is not responsive.

4. Be tolerant of what you see and hear. Various members of the family are at different stages of grieving, and each is reacting to a life crisis in his or her own way.

5. Encourage close family members to stay with the patient, to talk and touch as much as possible throughout the dying process. This is important, even if the patient is comatose.

6. As appropriate, offer to call the family minister, priest, or rabbi. If you observe that a family seems to need assistance in dealing with their grief, contact the hospital chaplain or social worker.

7. Know the available sources of help in your community and share this information with a family as appropriate. For example, *Compassionate Friends* is a support group for parents who have lost a child.

8. Work on your own "unfinished business" related to past losses and on your own fears related to death. Until you have accepted your own mortality and completed your own grief work, you cannot be fully effective in helping others to cope with death and dying.

## ACTIVITIES

1. List significant changes that have occurred in your life, starting with your earliest memories and continuing to the present.

2. Set up a worksheet with three columns with the following headings: EVENTS, GAINS, LOSSES. In Column I, list significant events in the past two years of your life. Beside each event, list in Column II what you gained, and in Column III what you lost, as a result of that event.

3. List three of your possessions that are important to you. How do you think you would react if you learned that these items had been destroyed in a fire?

4. What would be your behavior following the death of your best close friend? Write a description of your feelings, how you would express these feelings, and the people with whom you would share your feelings.

5. Prepare a set of guidelines to help you improve your ways of coping with loss. Be prepared to share these guidelines during a class discussion.

6. Participate in a small-group activity:

   a. Describe reactions to a significant loss that you have experienced or observed.

   b. Which of these examples are healthy reactions to loss?

   c. Which represent an unhealthy reaction to loss?

7. Compare the items below with your list of significant life changes (developed in Activity 1). Add any of these events that have occurred in your life.

   a. Death of a grandparent, parent, brother, or sister

   b. Death of a spouse, son, or daughter

   c. Death of any other relative who was important to you

   d. Death of a friend or classmate when you were a child

   e. Separation, divorce, or end of a long-term sexual relationship

   f. Marriage or establishment of a romantic relationship

   g. Any move—from one neighborhood to another, one city to another, or one state to another

   h. Change of school

   i. Major purchase—house, car, other

   j. Loss of personal possession—theft, foreclosure, fire, other

    k.  New family member

    l.  Pregnancy

    m.  Serious illness of a family member

    n.  Diagnosis of a serious or chronic illness (yours)

    o.  Obtaining a new job; being fired from a job

    p.  Change in job responsibilities or work schedule

    q.  Radical change in financial situation

    r.  Moving out of parents' home

    s.  Your child moves out of your home

    t.  Loss of freedom—confined to your room, not allowed to date or use the car, jail time

    u.  Radical change in lifestyle

    v.  Entered military service, college, other educational program

8. Participate in a class discussion about a health care professional's responsibilities when caring for a patient who attempted suicide.

## REFERENCES AND SUGGESTED READINGS

*Indicates a classic reference that introduced new ideas.

James, John and Friedman, Russell. (2009). *The Grief Recovery Handbook, 20th Anniversary Expanded Edition: The Action Program for Moving Beyond Death, Divorce, and Other Losses including Health, Career, and Faith*. New York: HarperCollins.

*Kübler-Ross, Elisabeth. (1969). *On death and dying*. New York: MacMillan.

*Kübler-Ross, Elisabeth. (1975). *Death: The final stage of growth*. Englewood Cliffs, NJ: Prentice Hall.

*Kübler-Ross, Elisabeth. (1978). *To live until we say goodbye*. Englewood Cliffs, NJ: Prentice Hall.

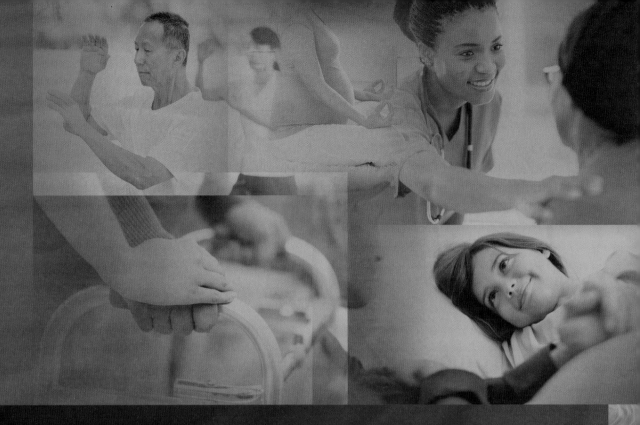

# Death: Attitudes and Practices

## OBJECTIVES

After completing this chapter, you should be able to:

- Contrast past and current practices related to death and dying.
- Define the concept of "death with dignity."
- Describe the purpose of the following: the living will, medical durable power of attorney and advance medical directive.
- Develop a personal philosophy about death and end-of-life care.

## KEY TERMS

Advance medical
  directive (AMD)
Assisted suicide
Bereavement
Conservator

Do not resuscitate
  (DNR) order
Durable power of
  attorney (DPA)
Euthanasia
Living wills

Patient Self-
  Determination
  Act (PSDA)
Proxy
Thanatology

Many people view death as an enemy to be feared and avoided at all costs. A totally different view is reflected in the writings of Dr. Elisabeth Kübler-Ross, who titled one of her books *Death: The Final Stage of Growth*. As a result of her many years of attending dying patients, Dr. Kübler-Ross proposed that the dying process involves a series of emotional/spiritual changes that, ideally, terminate with feelings of peace and tranquility prior to death. The dying process, then, can be an opportunity for emotional and spiritual growth. Some dying people need help to move through this process. Others seem to undergo this growth through their own beliefs, values, and inner resources.

Between these two opposite views of death, there is a wide range of beliefs. These differences are due in part to cultural attitudes and practices in care of the dying, which have undergone a marked change during the past half-century. This chapter reviews those historical changes, examines some influences on beliefs about death, and discusses attitudes and practices related to death and dying.

## PAST ATTITUDES AND PRACTICES

In 1789, Benjamin Franklin wrote, "In this world nothing is certain except death and taxes." His comment reflects an awareness and acceptance of death that was common until the era of modern medicine. Prior to the last century, the leading cause of death was infection. Infant and child mortality rates were high; few families escaped the loss of a child. Death was familiar—a common experience that was highly visible to people of all ages. Illness and death were most likely to occur in the home, with family members and friends gathered around. It was the custom for each member of the family to bid the dying person farewell. In return, the dying person gave his or her blessing to favored relatives. The deathbed scene often included advice and charges to the survivors—to develop certain virtues, care for other survivors, gain honor for the family name.

In some cultures, death was (or still is) celebrated as a release from the troubles of this life and a welcome passage to a happy and trouble-free existence in "the hereafter." Mourning was public, as well as private. A widow was expected to wear black for at least a year following the death of her husband. Men wore a black band on the left sleeve as a public display of mourning for the deceased. The survivors did not participate in social events for many months. There were frequent visits to the cemetery. The gravemarker and subsequent care of the grave symbolized respect for the deceased and the devotion of the survivors. In many other ways survivors demonstrated to relatives and the community their love and respect for the deceased. Until recently, both illness and death were a family affair.

### For Discussion and Reflection

Consider how death was viewed by your family or community of origin. Has your own view of death changed over time?

## CHANGING ATTITUDES AND PRACTICES

Beginning in the early 1900s, infection was brought under control through improved sanitation and immunization. During the late 1930s and 1940s, the sulfa drugs and penicillin were discovered. These changes in the treatment of infection resulted in a dramatic decrease in deaths due to infection, especially among infants and children. As the life span increased, the primary causes of death became heart disease, cancer, respiratory diseases, and accidents. Care of the sick and injured shifted from the home to the hospital. Responsibility for care of the sick was delegated to health care personnel, with family members in the role of bystanders. This trend resulted in isolation of the patient from family members. Children, especially, were excluded from contact with the hospitalized patient. Illness and death ceased to be a family affair.

As a result of this trend, many people today have never been personally involved with serious illness or the dying process. They have never had the opportunity to learn to accept death as a part of the cycle of life. Death is now perceived by many people as a terrible tragedy that "ought not to happen, especially to me and my family."

These changes of the past 50 years have great significance for emotional and mental health. Due to the invisibility of the dying process and the abandonment of many mourning rituals, there is a growing tendency to deny death. In many American subcultures, it is almost as though there is a conspiracy of silence. One just does not talk, or even think, about death until it strikes within one's circle of relatives or friends.

When death does touch a family, there may be a tendency to deny the grief process. Today, the community generally does not provide for bereaved people the kind of long-term support that can facilitate the grief process. Instead, survivors are expected to "pick up the pieces and get on with their lives" soon after the funeral.

In the work setting, life may go on as usual the day after a colleague's funeral, with no one willing to introduce the subject of death into the informal communication channels. The formal communication channel may acknowledge this loss of a member of the organization with a memorandum or floral offering. Otherwise, the work routine continues with minimal recognition that a member is missing.

Within other subcultures, however, a death can bring family members together. Friends and relatives may travel from significant distances to be with the bereaved family. Family members may share meals and spend time sharing memories about the deceased person. This approach is more conducive to healthy grieving and emotional healing than is the conspiracy of silence.

## CURRENT ATTITUDES AND PRACTICES

Changes in infant and child mortality have had a particular effect on societal attitudes toward death as it relates to age. Although death is acceptable for older people (generally age 60 and above), it is viewed as inappropriate for someone under the age of 30 to die. Yet less than a hundred years ago, parents felt blessed if half of their children survived to age 12. Today, we find it especially tragic—unacceptable and terribly unfair—when a child dies.

Changes in the health care system have contributed to changes in societal attitudes toward death. In fact, a highly significant change in attitudes toward death has occurred *within* the health care system. Instead of accepting death as an inevitable outcome of some diseases, death is perceived as an enemy to be conquered with whatever resources the system can offer: new and better drugs, life-support systems, surgical replacement of body parts, heroic measures to restore vital functions. Some physicians believe they have a responsibility to maintain life in the physical body as long as possible, regardless of the patient's potential for recovery or a meaningful existence. Concern for the *quantity of life* has replaced concern for the *quality of life*. When all measures available prove inadequate to keep a patient alive, some personnel view the death as a personal failure ("If only I had made rounds 30 minutes sooner!") or as a failure of the system ("If we had been able to use such-and-such, we could have saved that patient.").

In recent years, however, there is increasing awareness of a need to examine societal attitudes toward death and care of the dying. Some hospitals have modified their policies regarding visitors, some even permitting small children to visit a dying grandparent, parent, or sibling. Hospice and home care of a dying person are increasingly recognized as alternatives to hospitalization. More families now participate in the dying process, thereby permitting the dying person to retain a sense of family membership until the end. These recent trends recognize and respect the *human needs* of the dying person.

## THE EMERGENCE OF THANATOLOGY

During the 1950s a new interest and concern about death and dying emerged, largely due to the work of Dr. Elisabeth Kübler-Ross, sociologists, social workers, and pastoral counselors. Many professionals who were working with dying patients recognized that their educational programs had not prepared them for this role. The concern of these professional workers to meet the needs of patients with terminal illness led to the emergence of **thanatology**, the study of death and dying, and to death education for health care professionals and for the public.

Thanatology involves people from a variety of disciplines: sociology, theology, psychology, counseling, social work, nursing, and medicine. Their work has led to increased awareness of the needs of dying persons, the importance of the grief process, techniques for helping patients and their families cope with death and **bereavement**, and the need for death education.

## THE MEANING OF DEATH

An important aspect of death education is learning to accept one's own mortality. In the past, this important lesson was learned early in life through direct experience with serious illness and death itself, usually in the home. Current practices that isolate dying patients prevent this direct involvement. But death education can help people think through the meaning of death, resolve their fears, reach some level of personal acceptance, and come to terms with their own mortality. In addition, death education can prepare people to accept their feelings as legitimate reactions when they do have to cope with a death crisis. It is especially important that health care professionals who care for dying patients resolve their own fears about dying, because subconscious fears about death influence how one interacts with a person who is dying.

The meaning of death for each person is influenced by cultural background, religious beliefs, and life experiences. Following are examples of beliefs about death:

- Death is the end of existence.
- Death is only the end of physical existence.
- Death is a natural, biological event that concludes life.
- Death is the loss of everything—life itself, the future, loved ones, possessions.
- Death means separation from loved ones.

- Death means a reunion with loved ones who have already died.
- Death is the enemy. It should be fought with all available resources up to the end.
- What follows death is unknown; therefore, it is a fearsome event.
- Death is a test of one's faith; therefore, it must be faced with courage and a willingness to accept pain and suffering.
- Death is a change to another form of existence.
- Death is a transition; the soul moves to another plane of existence.
- Death is the beginning of a new life—perpetual existence in heaven or hell, depending upon Divine judgment of one's deeds on Earth.

Some of these beliefs perpetuate fear of death. Others reflect acceptance of death as natural or as a transition to another dimension of existence.

Death education can help people deal with their fears and clarify their own beliefs about death. It can help them understand that preparing oneself for dying includes grieving for what must be given up: relationships with family members and friends; ambitions, goals, purposes, and dreams for the future; material possessions; and, finally, one's own physical body. Thinking through these losses while in a state of good health usually results in a new perspective on what is important in life.

## DEATH WITH DIGNITY

Increased attention to death and dying has resulted in several trends: the hospice movement, preparation of personnel to provide counseling for dying patients, and advance directives for end-of-life care. The right to die with dignity is inherent in the philosophy of hospice. Death with dignity embodies at least the following:

- The dying person is permitted to retain some control.
- The dying person has the freedom to choose his or her style of dying.
- The dying person is allowed to discuss death openly.
- The dying person is allowed to prepare for dying in his or her own way.
- Human mortality is a biological fact.
- The dying patient's care focuses on maintaining *quality of life*, rather than *quantity of life*.
- Medical intervention that prolongs the dying process, when the prognosis is hopeless, is inappropriate if such intervention violates the patient's wishes.

Death with dignity, then, implies that the highest possible quality of life is maintained and that the dying person's rights and wishes are respected by caregivers. By participating in decisions and being allowed to make choices, the dying person maintains self-esteem and a sense of integrity as a human being. Familiar surroundings help the patient maintain a sense of identity. Those who die at home have the advantage of familiar surroundings and the presence of family members, friends, and even pets. Arrangements that permit the person to die at home can also benefit survivors, though some families are not able to cope with full-time care of a dying person. In any case, dying at home is now recognized as an alternative to dying in the institutional setting.

## EUTHANASIA

The word **euthanasia** is derived from two Greek words: *eu* (good) and *thanatos* (death). Euthanasia is a complex and controversial subject that involves philosophical views of life and death, ethical considerations, religious beliefs, and legal questions. Before taking a position for or against euthanasia, become informed about each of these aspects. With increasing knowledge and exposure to a variety of viewpoints, you will be prepared to formulate an opinion based on information, rather than value judgments alone.

The following discussion is limited to basic information that you, as a health care professional, should know and understand. For that reason, the definition that forms the basis of this discussion is more restricted than that used by authors who present a comprehensive discussion. As used here, *euthanasia is any action, requested by the patient but performed by someone else, that accelerates the dying process.* The request may be made because of intractable pain, loss of bodily control, or a deteriorating condition that will inevitably result in helplessness. The term **assisted suicide** is sometimes used when a physician prescribes lethal medication for a patient to self-administer.

Modern writers differentiate active and passive euthanasia, based on how the death occurs. *Active euthanasia* involves an *intentional intervention* (usually, administration of medication) for the purpose of causing death. *Passive euthanasia* consists of *withholding* and/or *withdrawing treatment*, with the intention of allowing the person to die of the underlying disease process. This definition of passive euthanasia includes withholding or discontinuing life support procedures, such as artificial ventilation, cardiopulmonary resuscitation, and tube feedings.

The primary argument in favor of euthanasia is that present end-of-life care does not provide adequately for relief of suffering. Supporters of euthanasia believe that patients have a right to request to end their lives in situations such as these:

- terminal illness that is causing extreme suffering despite good medical care
- greatly diminished quality of life due to an incurable medical condition
- a physical condition so handicapping that the patient chooses to die rather than live under such conditions

Consideration of a patient's request requires that the patient be a mature adult, the patient has been given full information and can make an informed choice, the condition has existed for some time, and the attending physician has been involved in full discussion of the patient's condition and the patient's request.

### For Discussion and Reflection

Many people have a strong emotional reaction to the topics of euthanasia and assisted suicide. What are your reactions to these topics? As a health care professional, how can you remain true to your own beliefs and values while respecting the rights and decisions of patients?

The danger of euthanasia is *misuse*—someone other than the patient may benefit from the death. Obviously, beneficiaries from the patient's estate should not be allowed to influence the decision, although this is difficult to control when family members are involved in the patient's care. Every effort should be made to ensure that the patient truly desires relief from suffering and has reached that decision independently. Supporters of the right-to-die concept believe that euthanasia should be considered only under clearly defined conditions and with the expressed wish of the patient. The decision should not be left to one doctor and one patient, but should be reviewed by a panel of experts that includes at least two members who have conducted a face-to-face interview with the patient.

## EVOLUTION OF THE RIGHT-TO-DIE MOVEMENT

Euthanasia has been legal in Switzerland since 1942; in Belgium and the Netherlands, it has been legal since 2002. Specific laws and procedures vary, but there are currently a number of nations in which either active or passive euthanasia is legal. In the United States, active euthanasia is illegal, but patients may refuse treatments that would prolong life. As of January 2016, assisted suicide is permitted in the states of California, Oregon, Vermont, and Washington.

In the United States, early right-to-die efforts were spearheaded by Derek Humphry, founder of the Hemlock Society and later the Euthanasia Research and Guidance Organization (ERGO). Other organizations evolved from these early efforts: End of Life Choices, Compassion and Choices, Death with Dignity, Final Exit, First Freedom First, and other right-to-die groups. The World Federation of Right to Die Societies includes 49 member organizations in 22 countries. The efforts of these organizations led Oregon, in 1997, to become the first U.S. state to legalize a patient's right to seek aid in escaping an intolerable health situation. As of January 2016, the following four states have passed legislation legalizing assisted suicide:

- Oregon (Death with Dignity Act, 1997)
- Washington (Death with Dignity Act, 2008)
- Vermont (Patient Choice and Control at End of Life Act, 2013)
- California (End of Life Option Act, 2015)

Supporters of the right to die emphasize the importance of using value-neutral language in discussing assistance with dying, avoiding the use of "suicide," "assisted suicide," and "physician-assisted suicide," using instead the more neutral term "aid-in-dying." In contrast, opponents of the right-to-die movement claim that using euphemisms or value-neutral terminology obscures the reality that an individual is choosing to end his or her own life.

As a health care professional, you will likely meet coworkers and patients who have strong feelings on both sides of the right-to-die debate. Very likely, you will have strong feelings and beliefs of your own as well. Your role is to understand the laws in your state and the policies of your employer, and within the context of those laws and policies, respect the decisions a patient may make.

## SOCIETAL ISSUES RELATED TO CARE OF THE DYING

The availability of life-support technology has given rise to ethical, moral, and legal questions previously unknown to any society. New types of decisions face the physician, the patient, and next-of-kin—decisions that can contribute to guilt feelings, inappropriate procedures, and medical practices based on fear of litigation. It is important for health care professionals to be aware of issues pertaining to the care of dying patients. Issues of particular concern to everyone participating in care of the dying are:

- the definition of death
- quality of life versus quantity of life
- rights of patients and their families

## The Definition of Death

What indicates that a person is dead? This question is especially important now that donor organs are needed for transplants. Each state has a Determination of Death Act that specifies the legal definition of death for that state. The *medical definition* is based on cessation of respiratory or circulatory functions or irreversible coma. In some hospitals brain death is measured in terms of (1) cerebral functions (consciousness, responsiveness to stimuli) and (2) brain-stem functions (control of vital processes). Where both measurements are made, the patient is not declared brain dead unless at least two physicians agree that brain-stem function is absent. The definition of death is especially relevant to the care of young accident victims. It is indeed difficult to give up hope for a young person whose body appears normal, even when tests indicate that there is no brain activity.

Determination of the moment of death is a pressing decision when other patients are waiting for a donor organ. A surgeon waiting to perform an organ transplant is understandably impatient about any delay in pronouncing a potential donor dead. The Uniform Anatomical Gift Act specifies that the physician who declares a patient dead must not be involved with a patient who is awaiting a donor organ. The Uniform Determination of Death Act specifies that both cardiopulmonary and brain function criteria must be met before body organs may be removed. Any state that adopts these statutes, or develops its own statute with clearly stated criteria for determination of death, is providing legal protection for any dying person who is a potential organ donor.

## Quality of Life versus Quantity of Life

Which is more important, the *quality* of life or the *quantity* of life? When the current state of medical practice offers no hope for a patient's recovery, to what extent should life-extending procedures be used? Intravenous fluids, blood transfusion, and tube feedings are used to maintain life, rather than to cure disease. Often such procedures are continued even when a patient's condition is hopeless. Life can be maintained for days, or even weeks, until the body refuses to continue to function. Is the physician or family obligated to "do everything possible" to *extend* life? Or should life-maintenance procedures be discontinued when there is no hope of recovery and the quality of life is nil? Who should make such a decision—a mentally competent patient, the next-of-kin, or the physician? Who should make such a decision if the patient is *not* mentally competent or is comatose?

The right-to-die issue was brought to public attention by the Terri Schiavo case. In 1990, Terri suffered a cardiac arrest; heroic efforts restored heart function, but she remained comatose. Medical procedures indicated that she was brain dead, but she was kept alive by a gastric feeding tube. After Terri had been comatose for 10 years, her husband obtained court approval to discontinue the gastric feedings, but Terri's parents went to court to oppose

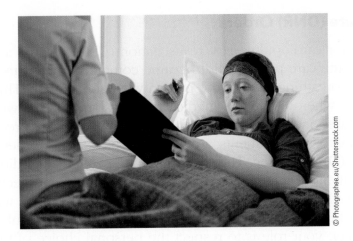

**FIGURE 17-1** Patients have the right to refuse treatment, including life-support measures and resuscitation.

this action. The following seven years of controversy in the courts led to interventions by Governor Jeb Bush and the Florida legislature, then by the U.S. Congress and President George W. Bush. Laws that were enacted to prevent the removal of Terri's gastric feeding tube were declared unconstitutional by the courts.

Terri Schiavo's case aroused a high level of public interest in patients' rights and end-of-life care. This case also raised important questions:

- Should strangers and politicians make decisions about a patient's medical care, especially about dying?

- Is quality of life as important as being kept alive by artificial means?

## Rights of Patients and Their Families

When the recommended medical treatment of a condition has extreme side effects, causes more pain than the disease itself, or involves radical surgery that permanently alters body appearance, does the patient (or the parents, if the patient is a minor) have the right to refuse treatment? Medical opinion is that *any medically approved treatment should be used*. But some patients reject surgery or treatments such as chemotherapy, choosing instead to *let the disease run its natural course*. Although a physician cannot force surgery or chemotherapy on an adult, there have been court judgments that required a child's parents to allow physicians to administer chemotherapy to a child.

Does a patient who is mentally sound have the right to refuse extreme measures for maintaining life? This issue, also, has been before the courts. Judges generally use brain death as the criterion for authorizing a physician to discontinue treatment of a comatose patient. The question is far more complex when a patient is conscious and mentally competent. If the patient has no hope of recovery and does not want to continue to suffer, does that person have the right to say "pull the plug"? Some people view the use of life-support procedures for dying patients as *prolonging death, rather than extending life*. The concept of death with dignity includes the patient's right to reject life-support and resuscitation procedures.

## Do Not Resuscitate (DNR) Orders

After the technique for cardiopulmonary resuscitation (CPR) became an integral part of the curriculum for all health care personnel, it became common practice to "call a code" for any patient who stopped breathing, even if the person was terminally ill. This was especially true in teaching hospitals, where numerous medical students and interns were expected to learn resuscitation procedures, including open-heart massage. When it was recognized that resuscitation is inappropriate for some patients, a new type of physician's order came into being: the **do not resuscitate (DNR) order**. This order is written by the attending physician, often at the request of the patient or a family members designated to make decisions for the patient. As a health care professional, you will likely find yourself in situations where you have a personal opinion about the best option for a terminally ill patient, particularly when a DNR has been signed. However, your role is to respect the personal choice of the patient and family members, even when that choice may differ from your own opinion.

With the development of hospice and a growing trend toward care of a dying person in the home setting, there was need for end-of-life procedures for patients outside the hospital setting. If caregivers called emergency services after the patient died, the paramedics who responded were legally obligated to begin CPR, unless there was a written DNR. There is variation state to state regarding recognition of a non-hospital DNR.

# LEGAL ASPECTS OF THE RIGHT TO DIE

Numerous right-to-die issues have now been addressed by the U.S. Supreme Court, the U.S. Congress, and some state legislatures. In the Mary Beth Cruzan case (*Cruzan v. Director, Missouri Department of Health*, 1990), the Supreme Court ruled that there is a constitutional right to die, but that it is up to the states to define that right. In 1990, Congress passed the **Patient Self-Determination Act (PSDA)**, which mandates that patients be informed about the right to participate in medical decisions regarding their treatment. Laws regarding **living wills** and the **durable power of attorney (DPA)** have now been passed by many states. The living will and medical DPA laws are the result of widespread consumer resistance to indiscriminate use of medical technology that can prolong life indefinitely. Both documents pertain to *self-determination*—the right of a patient to participate in medical decisions and, specifically, the right to refuse medical treatment. An **advance medical directive (AMD)** refers to both medical DPA and the living will.

## The Living Will

The living will permits individuals to indicate their wishes regarding medical care. It is especially valuable when an individual becomes incapable of conveying such wishes to the doctor and family. People who have the foresight to prepare a living will protect their families from having to make painful decisions regarding medical treatment if there appears to be no chance of recovery. Living wills also provide guidance for the physician regarding extreme measures such as life support and resuscitation.

The living will is especially useful in cases of coma or prolonged dying when there is no hope of recovery. Ideally, a living will should be prepared and signed *before* the onset of illness or accident. If a patient wants to sign a living will after being admitted to a health care facility, additional witnesses and safeguards are required. The living will presents the patient's wishes in writing. Some court cases (e.g., Mary Beth Cruzan, Karen Ann Quinlan) have been based on statements the patient made to family and friends indicating that he or she would not want to be kept alive in a vegetative state. In the absence of a living will or other written instructions, lengthy legal proceedings may be required before the patient is allowed to die a natural death by discontinuing life support and/or artificial nutrition.

Everyone who completes a living will and/or a medical DPA should discuss their advance directive(s) with the physician, their families, and especially the **proxy** (the person named as decision maker in the medical DPA). The discussion should be specific about one's beliefs and wishes regarding end-of-life care and about any medical interventions that are not wanted. Without such meaningful discussions at intervals, there is risk that one's wishes will be ignored, even if an advance directive has been completed.

It is not necessary to involve a lawyer in preparing a living will. Each state has a specific form. A living will form should be filled out according to the instructions, signed in the presence of witnesses who are not family members or beneficiaries, and then signed by the witnesses. The original should be filed in a safe place; copies should be provided to members of the family. Upon admission to a hospital, a copy should be added to the patient's chart; *a family member should obtain a receipt from a hospital representative, acknowledging that an AMD for that patient is on file.*

## The Durable Power of Attorney

The medical DPA is a document that designates a specific person to make medical decisions if the patient is unable to do so. The desires of the individual should be made clear to the decision maker at the time the document is prepared. When illness or accident occurs, the decision maker is responsible for seeing that the patient's wishes are carried out. Some DPA forms include statements pertaining to life support, resuscitation, and artificial feeding, so that specific instructions are included in the legal document. The advance health care directive may refer to a living will, a durable power of attorney, or both.

## The Patient Self-Determination Act

Under the PSDA, any hospital, nursing home, hospice, or health maintenance organization (HMO) that receives federal funding (Medicare and Medicaid) must inform patients about their rights, specifically the right to refuse certain types of treatment. This federal law also prohibits health care professionals from discriminating against a patient who elects to forgo life-sustaining procedures. The PSDA specifies that any patient who enters a hospital or nursing home must be informed about:

- The right to make decisions about medical treatments
- The right to refuse a treatment (medical or surgical)
- The right to prepare an AMD if the patient does not already have a living will or medical DPA
- The procedure in that institution for preparing an AMD
- The right to have an AMD made part of his or her medical record

This law resulted from the proliferation of court cases regarding the right to die. A number of families have experienced emotional trauma and incurred tremendous legal

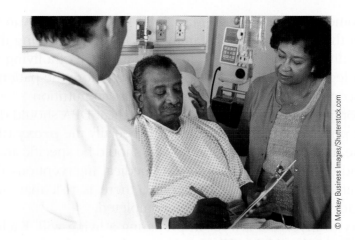

**FIGURE 17-2 As a health care professional, your role is to provide information about the patient's rights and choices, not to influence the patient's decision or discuss your personal beliefs.**

expense in the effort to allow their loved one, in a state of irreversible coma, to die. Health care professionals, regardless of their own opinions, must respect the wishes of patients that have been stated in an AMD. Box 17-1 shows some of the requirements of the Patient Self-Determination Act.

As a health care professional, you may encounter situations in which a patient asks your opinion or advice about treatment or end-of-life care, such as whether to accept or refuse a treatment or whether to sign a DNR. Keep in mind that your role is to provide information about the patient's rights and choices, but not to influence the patient's decision or discuss your personal beliefs.

## Involvement of the Courts in Health Care Decisions

Increasingly, the legal system is becoming involved in health care decisions. This is most likely to occur when (1) relatives of a comatose person believe life support should be discontinued, but there is no advance directive, (2) an advance directive is ignored by health care personnel, or (3) the family wants to do "everything possible" for their loved one, even though the physician and hospital believe life support/nutrition should be discontinued.

In the first situation, the courts use one of two standards for determining whether or not life support may be discontinued. The "substituted judgment" standard recognizes that many individuals have not prepared advance directives and that their loved ones can best decide that individual's preference for end-of-life care. The "clear and convincing evidence" standard requires that the patient's preferences have been clearly stated to relatives or friends prior to the patient becoming unable to make medical decisions personally.

The second situation is discussed under the topic "A Dilemma for Health Care Professionals." The third situation is less common, in that most families of a comatose patient accept the recommendation of the physician. If a family does demand that treatment continue, even though there is no hope of improvement in the patient's condition, the hospital or physician may request that the court appoint a **conservator**. The responsibility of the conservator would be to evaluate the situation and recommend a course of action based on what the patient probably would choose, if able to express those preferences.

BOX 17-1

## The Patient Self-Determination Act

Provisions of the PSDA apply to all health care agencies that receive federal funds (Medicare and Medicaid reimbursement).

Each health care institution will:

- Provide written information to each patient regarding:
    a. The right to make decisions concerning medical care, including the right to refuse medical or surgical treatment.
    b. The right to prepare AMDs.
    c. The institution's policies concerning the implementation of such rights.
- Document in the patient's medical record whether or not the individual has completed an advance directive yet.
- Provide care without discrimination against the patient who has completed an advance directive.
- Establish policies and procedures to ensure compliance with state law regarding advance directives.
- Provide educational activities for staff and the public on the matter of advance directives.

The Department of Health and Human Services will:

- Provide a national public education campaign.
- Develop written materials explaining patients' rights, to be distributed by health care facilities.

## A DILEMMA FOR HEALTH CARE PROFESSIONALS

Sometimes health care personnel choose to ignore an AMD, believing that they are obligated to do everything possible to keep a patient alive. This behavior involves conflict between the health care professional's philosophy of health care and the legal rights of patients. The conflict may extend beyond the staff, involving hospital policy and established procedures.

### Liability for Performing Unwanted Treatment

Performing heroic measures to restore breathing or a heartbeat can be enormously satisfying. As conveyed on television, it is an exciting part of being a health care professional. But keeping someone alive who has provided written instructions that prohibit life-support measures not only violates the patient's rights but is also illegal. Ignoring a DNR can result in prolonged suffering, further medical expenses for the patient and family, and possibly litigation against health care professionals and the hospital. Every health care professional should understand the legal aspects of AMDs; knowing which patients have advance directives is the responsibility of each caregiver.

## Preparation for Death-and-Dying Situations

You may or may not be preparing for a role in health care that includes the care of dying patients. Regardless of your expected role, you should take the following steps to prepare for participation in a life-or-death situation, either in your career or in your personal life:

- Know the provisions of federal laws and the laws of your state pertaining to the rights of patients and their families,
- Know the policies of your employing health care agency.
- Be aware of your own beliefs about death and dying.

The concept of death with dignity, knowledge about AMDs, and awareness of the provisions of the PSDA should help you accept that patients have a right to participate in decisions about end-of-life care. You should also learn to accept the inevitability of death, the limitations of medical science, and the inappropriateness of heroic measures in some situations. *It is especially important that you develop your own philosophy about death, which includes facing your own fears about death and accepting your own mortality.*

Thoughtful consideration of the following questions will help you clarify your beliefs and develop your own philosophy of death:

- What do I believe about death?
- What do I believe about my own death?
- What fears do I have about dying?
- What would I have to give up if I were dying?
- What work do I want to complete before I die?
- What relationships do I want to mend before I die?
- What do I want to say to my loved ones before I die?
- What do I want to say to a loved one before he or she dies?
- Who should dispose of my possessions following my death? Who is to receive what?

By developing your own personal philosophy of death, you will have clearer beliefs about the care of a dying patient. If the health care professional role you expect to assume does not involve caring for dying patients, you may be tempted to ignore this exercise. But you cannot be sure what the future holds—in your career or in your personal life. So consider the following in terms of "What do I believe about the care of a patient who . . .":

- Does not want to be resuscitated if a cardiac arrest occurs?
- Refuses intravenous fluids or tube feedings during the final stages of an illness?
- Refuses dialysis, even though the kidneys are not functioning?

### For Discussion and Reflection

1. Consider one or more of the questions listed above. What actions you can take within the next month based on your answers to the questions?
2. Identify a time when a child or teen in your community has died. What were your reactions? Do you react differently to the death of a young person than to the death or an older person?

- Refuses chemotherapy, even though the oncologist insists there is a 20 percent chance it will help?
- Begs the doctor, "Just let me die."?
- Begs the doctor, "Just put me out of my misery."?

Inadequate management of pain is the reason some patients wish for death or consider suicide. The expression of a wish for death, then, may mean that the patient needs improved management of pain. However, many dying patients have accepted death and are ready—mentally, emotionally, and spiritually—even before the physical body ceases to function. Be sensitive to the needs of such patients, and especially to a patient's readiness for death.

As a health care professional, you may experience a range of emotions when a patient dies. Although you are expected to remain professional, it is not necessary or advisable to "keep a stiff upper lip" and deny all feelings of grief. A brief statement of sincere grief or compassion can be very meaningful to the family of the deceased.

## Ethics Committees

The Karen Ann Quinlan court decision included a recommendation that ethics committees, rather than the courts, should handle controversial patient care situations. In 1995, the Joint Commission on Accreditation of Health Care Organizations began requiring that health care facilities set up a code of ethical behavior. As a result, most hospitals have established ethics committees to review patient care conflicts. Some ethics committees involve patients' families in hearings, thereby ensuring that all viewpoints will be heard and increasing the probability that a decision will be acceptable to the hospital, the physician, and the family. In other hospitals, the ethics committees exclude families from the hearing, relying on reports of the medical staff for rendering a decision. The latter approach carries the risk of having the patient's end-of-life choices ignored in favor of aggressive medical treatment.

Ideally, ethics committees would always protect the patient's well-being and respect the expressed wishes of the patient and family for end-of-life care. Ethics committees can and

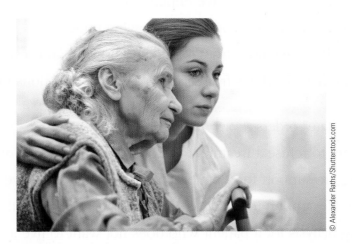

© Alexander Raths/Shutterstock.com

**FIGURE 17-3** By developing your own personal philosophy of death, you will have clearer beliefs about the care of a dying patient.

should encourage staff training in the legal and ethical issues most often involved in patient care/institutional conflict.

Numerous issues have been addressed in the medical community, the mass media, and the courts: definition of death, when life support may be discontinued, when artificial feedings for persons in a persistent vegetative state may be discontinued, the right of a patient to choose accelerated death, culpability of a person who assists a patient to commit suicide, and the moral/ethical/legal aspects of euthanasia. Some legal issues may be resolved within the next several years. In the meantime, everyone involved in end-of-life care must resolve for themselves the ethical and moral issues related to the dying process.

## ACTIVITIES

1. Draw a line that represents your life span. It can be any shape or length. The beginning represents birth; the end, death. Mark several significant losses at points along the line. Study your life line. What was your reaction to each loss? Is your reaction different now that time has passed?

2. Consider your losses if you were to die in an accident tomorrow:

   a. List the relationships you would lose.

   b. List the possessions you would be giving up.

   c. List uncompleted tasks you would leave behind.

3. Refer to your list of relationships and your list of possessions. Decide how you would want your property distributed. Prepare instructions to guide your survivors in carrying out your wishes:

   a. Disposition of your body

   b. A funeral or memorial service

   c. Disposition of your property

   d. Care of your survivors, if you have dependents

4. Participate in a class discussion about the following topics:

   • Withholding artificial feedings from a patient who is in an irreversible coma

   • Withholding artificial feedings from a patient who is conscious but approaching death

   • "Do not resuscitate" orders

   • A patient's right to refuse a treatment the doctor wants to administer

   • Discontinuing life support for a patient in a persistent vegetative state

   • Discontinuing life support for a conscious patient who requests that it be discontinued

   • Discontinuing dialysis for a patient who does not want to live as a quadriplegic

5. At the top of a blank sheet of paper, write "What I believe about death." List your present beliefs.

6. At the top of a blank sheet of paper, write "What I believe about care of a dying patient." List your present beliefs.

7. Obtain a copy of the legal document used in your state for AMDs. Read through the document. Is it a living will? Is it a medical DPA? What rights does it give the patient? What rights does it give the family?

8. Use the Internet to learn about one of the following cases: Terri Schiavo, Mary Beth Cruzan, Karen Ann Quinlan, Brittany Maynard. Share your findings with a classmate.

## REFERENCES AND SUGGESTED READINGS

Bruenig, E.S. (2015). How to think about your right to die. *New Republic, 246*(9/10), 13–15.

Gawande, A. (2014). *Being mortal: Medicine and what matters in the end.* New York: Metropolitan.

Schencker, L. (2015). Assisted-suicide debate focuses attention on palliative, hospice care. *Modern Healthcare, 45*(20), 22–25.

Voorhees, J.R., Rietiens, J.C., van der Heide, A., & Drickamer, M.A. (2014). Discussing physician-assisted dying: Physicians' experiences in the United States and the Netherlands. *Gerontologist, 54*(5), 808–817.

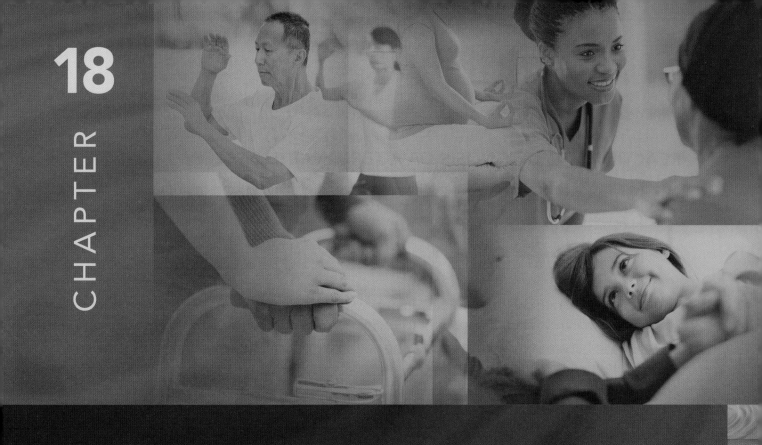

# CHAPTER 18

# Caring for the Dying Person

## OBJECTIVES

After completing this Chapter, you should be able to:

- Describe the fears commonly expressed by a dying person.
- List the five stages of dying, as proposed by Dr. Elisabeth Kübler-Ross, as well as limitations of Kübler-Ross's model.
- Discuss personal, family, and medical issues related to the care of a dying person.
- State guidelines for meeting the needs of a dying patient.
- State the primary focus of palliative care.

## KEY TERMS

Hospice                    Palliative

As a result of current practices in the care of terminally ill patients, many people today have had little or no personal contact with a dying person. Their experience with death is limited to occasional attendance at a funeral. There is a universal tendency to fear the unknown, so death and dying are taboo topics of conversation for most people. But diagnosis of an illness for which there is currently no cure brings a patient and family members face to face with the reality of death. The reaction to such news includes fear—fear of the unknown and fear of death.

## REACTIONS TO DIAGNOSIS OF A TERMINAL ILLNESS

As a health care professional, you are likely to encounter patients and their families who are experiencing these fears. Counselors who work with dying patients have identified a number of fears expressed by many patients:

- What happens after death? What lies beyond death?
- Will I be forgotten?
- Will my loved ones be cared for adequately without me? If they can get along without me, does that mean I was not important to them?
- What will become of my work, my lifelong efforts to accomplish something? Will my work be continued by someone else? Will someone else take credit for my work?
- What will happen to my property? Will my possessions be cared for? How will they be distributed?
- Will I become dependent on others?
- Will I be a burden? Who will pay my medical bills?
- Will I lose my mind?
- Will I lose control of my life? Who will make important decisions that affect me?
- Will I have more pain than I can bear?
- Will I be left to die alone?

A major responsibility of caregivers is to recognize manifestations of fear and encourage a patient to verbalize them. Expressing fears about death to an understanding listener facilitates the dying process. For example, the following behaviors may indicate that a patient is afraid:

- Being withdrawn or avoiding contact and conversation with others
- Refusing to see family and friends
- Refusing to eat, resisting medication
- Negative comments and behaviors toward health care staff

## STAGES OF DYING

In 1969, Dr. Elisabeth Kübler-Ross published her book *On Death and Dying*, in which she proposed that a dying person goes through five stages, beginning with denial and ending with acceptance that death is approaching. Kubler-Ross's model has been widely used by counselors, therapists, and health care professionals who work with individuals who are dying. Each stage is described below. Understanding these stages can help health care professionals and family members understand a patient's emotions about a terminal illness as well as cope with their own emotions about death.

## Denial

The first stage of dying involves denial—"No, I am not dying. It just isn't true." This reaction seems to occur regardless of whether or not a person is told directly that he or she has a terminal illness. Denial may be manifested in many ways: changing doctors several times, continuing one's daily routine as though nothing is wrong, refusing to talk about the illness, refusing treatment, or embarking on a search for any and all treatments.

Denial serves a useful purpose. As a defense mechanism, it gives the patient time to deal with the shock of knowing that life is coming to an end. Denial may recur at intervals throughout the dying process. As a health care professional, you should not "push" a patient to talk about death when he or she does not want to, but you can invite patients to talk whenever they feel ready.

## Anger

The second stage of dying is characterized by anger. As the patient begins to face the reality of terminal illness, the reaction is, "Why me? Why not somebody else?" During this stage, the patient may direct anger at anyone and everyone. It is a difficult time for health care professionals as well as the family. The caregivers, it seems, cannot do anything right during this period. The patient's behavior is easier to tolerate if one remembers that this patient is in the process of learning to face his or her death.

As a health care professional, you may experience expressions of anger from a patient. It is important to remain professional and not to take angry comments personally. You can validate a patient's feelings with a comment such as "You seem to be angry about having to be here." It is never acceptable for a health care professional to show anger in return. If a patient's angry behavior persists or makes you uncomfortable, you can use I-statements to respond, set limits (discussed in Chapter 14), or consult your supervisor.

## Bargaining

In the third stage of dying, the patient begins to bargain—with God, fate, the doctor or nurses, or the family. This bargaining may be unknown to the caregivers, or it may be shared. Perhaps the patient prays to stay alive until some particular event—the birth of a grandchild, a wedding, a child's graduation. Perhaps the patient promises to change behavior or lifestyle, if he or she can have a second chance: "If only I can be well again, I'll never take another drink." Bargaining may take the form of being a "good" patient—cheerful and cooperative regardless of annoying treatments or pain.

## Depression

The fourth stage is marked by depression. With increased symptoms, especially pain or weakness, the patient can no longer maintain denial; bargaining seems pointless; anger gives way to sorrow over impending losses. Dr. Kübler-Ross believes that this period involves two different types of depression: (1) a *reactive depression* to the impending losses faced by the patient, and (2) a *preparatory depression* related to the impending separation.

## Acceptance

The fifth stage is one of acceptance. *Provided the patient has enough time and is helped work through the previous stages*, this stage represents several accomplishments:

- The patient is neither depressed nor angry.
- The patient has grieved for the many losses.
- The patient is tired and/or weak and dozes frequently for short periods.

The stage of acceptance is not a happy stage. It is more likely to be, according to Dr. Kübler-Ross, devoid of feeling. But the patient is at peace.

Kübler-Ross's stages provide a framework for a compassionate understanding of grief and loss. The five stages of grief are still widely used by many counselors and therapists. At the same time, some experts in the field of thanatology have suggested that Kübler-Ross's stages of grief have limitations:

- People who are grieving do not always move smoothly from stage to another.
- The idea that people need to reach a state of acceptance or closure may be unrealistic. In some instances, people may continue to grieve a loss for many years, and doing so is not necessarily a sign of pathology.
- Though based on Kübler-Ross's clinical experience, the stages have not been empirically validated.
- The Kübler-Ross model does not account for cultural differences in how people experience grief.

Keeping these limitations in mind, you may find that Kübler-Ross's stages provide a helpful way to understand the emotions and behaviors of patients and family members as they come to terms with dying. However, keep in mind that each patient's experience is unique. Kübler-Ross's or any other model should be viewed as a tool for understanding, not a rigid process that every person must follow.

## DYING AS A GROWTH PROCESS

When death is viewed in light of the many losses involved, it is difficult to think of dying as an opportunity for growth. Viewed in terms of the emotional changes and the *transformation* that may occur as the dying process is completed, both spiritual and emotional growth become evident.

The dying person has a choice: to withdraw in despair, to suppress negative emotions, or to reach out to others. It is through the third option that growth occurs. Growth requires commitment to experiencing self, becoming aware of one's own identity, communicating one's experience to others, and accepting that one's life had purpose and meaning. These changes are facilitated by a support network of loving and caring people, who also have the opportunity for growth as they share in the dying experience.

### For Discussion and Reflection

Think about your first experience with death. How old were you? Was the deceased an important person to you? Did you participate in or witness any part of the dying process?

Many people need the help of a skilled counselor to work through the negative aspects of life experiences. The goal of helping a person work through the dying process is to have the individual achieve emotional adjustment and live life to the fullest during whatever time remains. Arrival at the stage of acceptance with a sense of peace indicates successful resolution of the emotions of the dying process. Once the dying person can deal with the notion of having an illness for which there is no cure, the person can enrich the time remaining through a series of activities:

- Review one's life—various experiences and relationships and the meanings of each.
- Visit places and people that are important.
- Review memories with friends and relatives.
- Make up for missed opportunities.
- Resolve old conflicts.
- Think through and talk over with loved ones such questions as "What will happen to my survivors?" and "How will my place be filled?"

Although these activities may be painful, there will also be joy as these experiences are shared with others who have been a part of one's life experience. The following conditions contribute to successful adjustment of dying patients:

- Supportive relationships with relatives, family, and clergy
- Relatively good adjustment and past patterns of successfully coping with problems
- Willingness to talk about the illness and approaching death
- Control of pain, because pain interferes with adjustment

In addition to striving for emotional adjustment, the patient must face a number of challenges. The illness and impending dependence on others necessitates changes in lifestyle and relationships. For those who have a high level of independence, certain changes in self-concept are difficult, but necessary:

- From "I am an independent person" to "I must let others do some things for me."
- From "I am self-directing, capable, and in control of my life" to "I must let others have control over some aspects of my life."

In addition to these changes in self-concept, there must be a change in planning. Instead of thinking "Some day I will . . .," a dying person must think, "Today I will . . ." It is also important that the dying person continue to feel that life has meaning.

## PERSONAL AND FAMILY ISSUES RELATED TO CARE OF THE DYING

When a person is diagnosed with an incurable illness, certain decisions must be made. What treatments should be used? Should drugs or treatments that are known to have serious side effects be used? Should experimental drugs or procedures whose effects are not fully known be used? Should the patient find another physician? Another clinic? Another medical center that may have "a new cure"?

If the patient's condition is deteriorating or the patient is in the terminal phase of illness, questions about care must be decided. Should the patient be in a hospital or nursing home?

Should the patient be at home? Who will provide care? Can this responsibility be rotated among family members? Or will one person have to provide around-the-clock care? Is there a home health service that could provide skilled care as needed? Is there a hospice in the community? The most important questions are:

1. Where does the patient want to be during his or her final days?

2. If the patient wants to die at home, is the family willing and able to undertake the care of a dying person at home?

3. If the patient or family members request counseling to assist them in coping with the emotions involved in the dying process, what resources are available in your community? In many communities, grief counseling is available through hospice.

## HOME CARE

In *Coming Home: A Practical and Compassionate Guide to Caring for a Dying Loved One*, Deborah Duda states that dying at home is "the old, natural way which most of the world never questioned." She describes advantages of dying at home as well as conditions under which this decision would not be appropriate. Among the advantages she lists are that the dying person feels wanted, can influence surroundings, has more freedom and control, maintains respect and dignity, can enjoy home-cooked food, has the opportunity to express feelings to various relatives and friends, and the familiar setting is conducive to family support as the patient does the inner preparation for death. Another advantage, not included in Duda's list, is privacy; the patient's last days are family-centered, with minimal intrusion by outsiders. Also, the monetary cost of dying at home can be much less than the costs of intensive care and life-maintenance procedures commonly used in hospitals during the final days of a patient's life.

Dying at home is *not appropriate*, according to Duda, when either the patient or the family actively prefers institutional care. Some families are not able to provide care, either because of their own limitations or because the patient's needs cannot be met in the home setting. If family members cannot handle the emotional drain, the physical demands of caring for someone

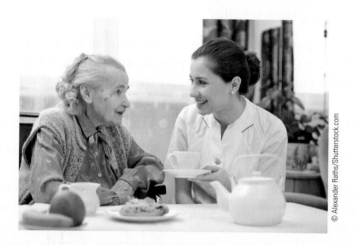

**FIGURE 18-1** For some patients, home health care is a positive alternative to institutional care.

who is terminally ill, or the overall stress of such a situation, then choosing to die at home would not be appropriate. If the patient has arranged to be an organ donor and the specific terminal illness does not preclude use of the organs, then the patient's death should occur in the hospital setting, with a surgical team on call to harvest any usable organs as soon as the patient is pronounced dead.

Arranging for someone to die at home requires careful planning. The family should contact hospice and home health services to arrange for assistance and consultation services as needed. Roles should be discussed and agreed upon; the primary caregiver should be selected, with others agreeing to assume care at specific times. This may draw family members closer together as they share the common goal of providing loving care for the person they will soon lose. Or the family may become divided by disagreements and unequal division of responsibilities, with one or two persons carrying most of the burden. Careful advance planning may prevent the latter situation and allow the patient to spend his or her final days in a harmonious family setting.

## HOSPICE CARE

**Hospice** care can be provided as home care or, if available, as residential care. According to the National Hospice and Palliative Care Organization, roughly two-thirds of patients receiving hospice care in 2013 did so in their place of residence (which might include a private residence or a nursing home), while about a fourth of hospice recipients received care in an inpatient facility. Home care with the supportive assistance of hospice personnel is an appropriate choice if the patient does not need or want hospitalization. Hospice care is provided by a team: the patient's physician; nurses to assess the patient's needs, develop a care plan, and provide skilled nursing care as needed; home health aides to provide personal care and, in some cases, assist with household needs; a social worker to provide emotional support and direct the family to community resources as needed; a chaplain and/or the patient's religious advisor; trained volunteers to provide visitation, companionship, and emotional support. Other benefits of hospice care include providing periods of respite for the primary caregiver and, later, offering bereavement counseling for the survivors. Compared to the hospital setting, hospice provides a more caring and comfortable way for a patient to live out his or her final days and also provides support and guidance for family members.

## PALLIATIVE CARE

**Palliative** care is the field of medicine focused on managing pain and symptoms of patients who have a serious illness, regardless of the diagnosis or prognosis. The primary focus of palliative care is *comfort*, both physical and psychological, rather than *cure*. Effective palliative care provides relief from such physical symptoms as pain, shortness of breath, and nausea. For patients who are dying, palliative care also includes emotional support to relieve anxiety, accept the dying process, grieve for impending losses, and to say "good-bye" to loved ones.

Family and close friends are an important part of palliative care. Their presence may relieve a patient's fear of abandonment—of dying alone. Frequent visits by the person designated as "agent" in an advance medical directive may provide reassurance that end-of-life decisions will be honored. Many patients who have prepared an advance medical directive do not want "high-tech" interventions, believing that *such measures prolong dying, rather than living.*

Many physicians, with a strong commitment to prolonging life, recommend such measures as additional chemotherapy, mechanical ventilation, artificial feeding, or dialysis, even when the patient is in the final stages of dying. The patient, the family, and the "designated agent" should question the benefit of such recommendations and keep in mind the patient's right to refuse treatment.

## MEDICAL ISSUES RELATED TO CARE OF THE DYING

Diagnosis and prescription of therapy are responsibilities of the physician. When the diagnosis of a fatal disease is confirmed, the physician faces several difficult questions:

- Does an adult patient have a right to know the diagnosis?
- Does an adult patient have a right to decide who should be given information about his or her condition?
- Does a physician have a duty to inform a patient that he or she is dying?
- How much information should the patient be given?
- How and when should the patient be told that he or she is dying?

Past medical practice has been to tell the family that the patient is dying, but "protect" the patient by telling him or her as little as possible. This is a departure from ethical practices related to confidentiality. Does a dying patient have less of a right to confidentiality than one who is not dying? Several studies have revealed that (1) many physicians do not make a practice of telling patients that they are dying, and (2) most people believe they would want to be informed.

*How* the information is given is important. It is possible to convey in a tactful and caring manner that the illness will be fatal. People listen selectively, so patients are likely to deal consciously only with as much of the message as they are able to handle at that moment. There are several reasons why patients should be informed:

- A patient who is not told that she is dying is deprived of opportunities to talk about the illness and dying. This "conspiracy of silence" results in the patient feeling isolated.
- A dying patient needs to get her affairs in order. This pertains to everyone, not just the wage earner or a businessperson. Getting one's affairs in order includes personal as well as business and financial decisions.
- Many dying patients want to deal with spiritual matters in preparation for dying.
- Lack of correct information may lead the patient to seek help from one practitioner after another, until financial resources have been exhausted. A second opinion often is desirable, but a fruitless search for a nonexistent cure may be avoided by honest communication.

Some patients want to have full information about their disorder, the treatment options available, and the probable course of the illness. In general, defense mechanisms provide some protection against being overwhelmed. The patient focuses on some aspects of the illness and ignores others, according to her capacity for coping. Other patients do not want to be told and are willing to delegate control and all treatment decisions to the physician. It would be destructive to try to force such a patient to "face the truth." On the other hand, such patients are likely to ask questions that indicate a need for reassurance. These patients usually suspect

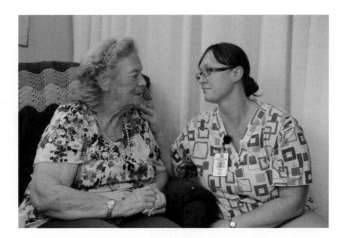

**FIGURE 18-2 Many patients find comfort in talking about their illness and dying with a sensitive caregiver.**

the truth, and their questions indicate a need to talk. Active listening may reveal underlying fears and anxieties for which the patient needs reassurance that she will be cared for and that pain will be alleviated.

Many physicians provide information to their patients gradually and try to balance bad news with something positive. Later, they give additional information according to the patient's readiness. How much to tell the dying patient must be decided by each physician, based in part on each patient's situation and emotional stability.

Health care professionals involved in care of a dying patient should know what the physician has told the patient so they can respond appropriately to questions from the patient and family. Many patients find comfort in talking about their illness and dying with a sensitive caregiver. Frequent contact with caring people who *listen* results in the patient coming to terms with the illness. When there is good communication with family members, relationships improve. Good communication with health care personnel increases the patient's trust.

### For Discussion and Reflection

With a classmate, discuss whether, when, and how a patient should be told that he or she is dying. Now imagine that the patient is a close friend or family member. Would your opinion change if the person dying is someone to whom you have a close connection?

## RIGHTS OF THE DYING PERSON

Some issues discussed in previous chapters pertain to rights of patients. Patients' rights issues are also concerned with truth, informed consent, control, choices, and protection of personal dignity. A patient who signs an agreement to undergo surgery or certain other treatments should do so only after being given full information:

• What is the probability that the surgery or treatment will help?
• What are the possible side effects?

- Will irreversible body changes result?
- Are alternative treatments available?
- What is the cost of the recommended treatment?

Some patients prefer to delegate decisions to others; that choice should be respected. Many patients wish to retain some degree of control and to participate in decisions; this, too, should be respected. Choices regarding life-maintenance procedures and advance medical directives have already been discussed. Some other choices of patients, especially during the final days, include:

- Solitude versus being surrounded by significant others
- Remaining at home versus being in the hospital
- Remaining alert versus being sedated

Choices made by the patient or family members may conflict with what a health care professional considers to be "best" for the patient. This is a conflict of values. If the patient and family have arrived at acceptance of impending death, and if they are concerned about death with dignity, health care professionals may feel frustrated that various available procedures are not being used to prolong life (or prolong the dying process, depending upon one's view). It may help the health care professional to keep in mind that the Patient Self-Determination Act, advance medical directive legislation, and informed consent statutes all resulted from practices that forced unwanted procedures on dying patients.

Each individual's experience with death is unique. While the guidelines in this chapter will help prepare you for assisting a patient who is dying, each patient's needs will be individual. Ultimately, the patient has the right to make decisions based on personal preferences, values, and financial needs.

## ROLES OF HEALTH CARE PROFESSIONALS

Terminal illness by definition results in death. The goals of care for terminally ill patients, therefore, are different from the goals for patients who have the potential to regain physical well-being. It is difficult for many health care professionals to accept any goal other than "getting better." Working with dying patients requires that a health care professional be able to *substitute palliative goals for curative goals*. Palliative goals include keeping the patient comfortable, being available to listen, providing comforting touch as appropriate, accepting the patient's choices, and respecting the patient as a human being, even if comatose and nonresponsive.

The stages of dying proposed by Dr. Kübler-Ross can help health care professionals to understand and accept some of the behaviors manifested by a dying person. For example, anger directed at a caregiver is more easily accepted if it is viewed as one manifestation of a specific stage of the dying process. But attempting to "place" a patient in one stage or another does not serve the patient's needs. Rather, effective care demands the utmost in caring, always keeping in mind that this patient's emotional needs are paramount.

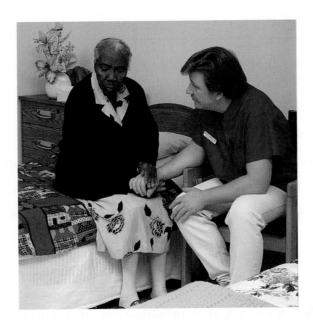

**FIGURE 18-3 Effective care requires keeping the patient's emotional needs in mind.**

## GUIDELINES FOR CARE OF A DYING PERSON

These guidelines can be useful as you strive to provide *humane* care consistent with the choices and needs of a dying patient:

- Reassure the patient as needed that you will be there and that you will do all possible to provide comfort. Then keep your word.
- Be aware of the patient's emotional state. Respect the patient's unique way of reacting to the illness and dying.
- Allow the patient to talk about dying; do not deny the fact that the patient is dying with statements such as "Oh, you have lots of time left."
- Allow the patient to express feelings. Anger, crying, remorse, and similar feelings help the patient to deal with the impending loss of life.
- Do not make promises that you cannot keep. Such expressions may make you feel better, but deny the reality of the patient's dying process.
- Let the patient know that you care. Use touch as appropriate and be with the patient as much as your other duties permit.
- Listen—a patient provides clues to her specific needs.
- Do not force your feelings or your beliefs on the patient.
- Whenever appropriate, allow the patient to express a preference about her care.
- Respond to a patient's request for prayer, a religious reading, ritual, or service. Call the hospital chaplain or the patient's spiritual advisor as appropriate.

By keeping these guidelines in mind, the health care professional can become the patient's ally in dealing with the process of dying.

## ACTIVITIES

1. Participate in a class discussion to identify various ways health care professionals could meet the following needs of a dying person:

    a.  Relative freedom from pain and discomfort.

    b.  Maintaining as much independence as possible.

    c.  Satisfaction of any remaining wishes ("things I wish I had done").

    d.  Maintenance of self-esteem when it becomes necessary to yield control to others.

    e.  Achievement of emotional adjustment, acceptance of impending death, and a state of inner peace.

2. In a class discussion, consider the following questions:

    a.  How can the rights of a comatose patient be protected?

    b.  What are the rights of a dying patient whose organs could be used as transplants for patients in the same hospital?

3. List things you have been wanting to do "some day." If you learned today that you have a terminal illness, which of these would you try to do before you die? Set a date and plan to do one of the things on your list.

4. Write out a set of guidelines for your next of kin describing the care you wish to receive if you are terminally ill.

5. Locate contact information for the Hospice agency in your community, if applicable, and for other agencies that can provide counseling and support for a person who is terminally ill.

## REFERENCES AND SUGGESTED READINGS

Committee on Approaching Death. (2015). *Dying in America: Improving quality and honoring individual preferences near the end of life*. Washington, DC: National Academies Press.

Duda, Deborah. (2010). *Coming home: A practical and compassionate guide to caring for a dying loved one*. Austin, TX: Synergy.

Jahner, J. and Wolff, B. (2015). Palliative care: Patient-centered assessment and communication to improve quality of life. *New Mexico Nurse, 60*(4), 4–6.

National Hospice and Palliative Care Organization (2014). *NHPCO's facts and figures; hospice care in America; 2014 Edition*. Alexandria, VA: National Hospice and Palliative Care Organization.

Parkes, C. M. (2013). Elisabeth Kübler-Ross, On death and dying: A reappraisal. *Mortality, 18*(1), 94–97. doi:10.1080/13576275.2012.758629.

Prosch, T. (2014). *AARP the other talk: A guide to talking with your adult children about the rest of your life*. Columbus, OH: McGraw-Hill Education.

# SECTION VI

# Trends in Health Care

Health care in the United States is changing rapidly. As a health care professional, you should be informed about current trends and issues, especially those that affect roles and relationships of health care personnel.

Much of the public is now well-informed about health matters; with increasing knowledge, many people want to participate in health care decisions. Lifestyle and stress management are widely recognized as major factors in both treatment and prevention of illness. And more people are using alternative (nonmedical) approaches to health care.

Some patients enter the health care system with a passive attitude: "I'm sick. Fix me. Make me well." These patients are not likely to refuse treatments or seek alternative therapies. But there is a new breed of patient who asks questions and expects answers, may refuse an invasive procedure or specific treatment, and may even question whether or not orthodox medicine can help with his or her health problem. Inadequate answers or a judgmental attitude on the part of a health care professional interferes with establishing rapport or, worse, may alienate the patient. It is essential, then, that health care professionals understand and accept those patients who wish to assume more responsibility and actively participate in decisions about their health care.

Section VI is designed to help you learn about selected trends in health care as a basis for working with today's patients and for expanding your understanding of holistic health, healing, and the role of stress management in health maintenance.

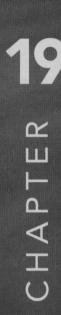

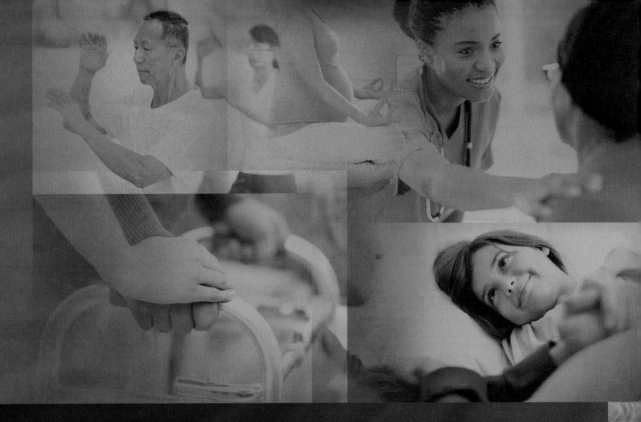

# Health Care Through the Ages

## OBJECTIVES

After completing this chapter, you should be able to:

- Discuss reasons that some innovations in science and medicine are initially rejected or labeled as quackery.
- Describe beliefs about sickness (or a sick person) that were common in early cultures.
- List scientific or medical advances during the past 400 years that provided the foundation for current health care practices.
- Compare and contrast holistic and orthodox health care.

## KEY TERMS

Allopathic
Alternative therapy
Complementary therapy
Dolorology
Empirical

Herbalism
Holistic health care
Neurotransmitters
Psychoanalysis
Psychopharmaceuticals

Scientific method
Synergism
Variables

The history of science and health care includes numerous examples of innovative ideas that were rejected initially by those in power at the time. Many of these innovative approaches were eventually accepted by orthodox medicine. Some innovations were premature—they required changes the culture was not yet ready to accept. Innovations—new ideas—may conflict with existing beliefs and may be perceived as a threat by current practitioners. Many scientists who proposed a new idea or a new method have been subjected to criticism, ridiculed, or even persecuted. Yet some of those innovators who suffered persecution are now recognized as heroes of medicine or a particular field of science. Understanding how health care has evolved throughout history will provide a context to help you understand current innovations and new developments in health care.

## HEALING IN EARLY CIVILIZATIONS

For thousands of years the healing practices of each culture were handed down from one generation to the next. The role of healer was highly respected; possession of the secrets of healing conveyed power second only to the power of the ruler. The priests and priestesses performed religious services and were also guardians of healing secrets. The role of *healer* was a *power role*.

### Greece and Rome

Although early Greek mythology attributed illness to supernatural causes, it was the Greeks who eventually separated healing from religion and the role of physician from that of priest.

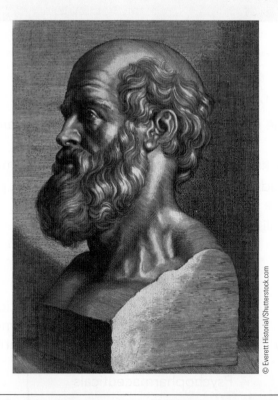

© Everett Historial/Shutterstock.com

**FIGURE 19-1 The Greek physician Hippocrates established a systematic approach to diagnosing illness based upon careful observation and collection of information.**

Hippocrates, a Greek physician who lived during the period 460–377 BCE, is known as "the father of modern medicine." Hippocrates insisted upon careful observation and the collection of factual information, thereby establishing a systematic approach to diagnosis of illness. His treatments included diet, fresh air and sunshine, and healthful personal habits and living conditions—what we today refer to as "a healthful lifestyle." Hippocrates demonstrated that illness results from natural causes, rather than from evil spirits or the anger of the gods. This established medicine as the healing profession. Thereafter, religion was the domain of priests and care of the sick was the domain of physicians. Hippocrates also emphasized a code of behavior for physicians—the beginnings of medical ethics. The Hippocratic oath is still used by many medical schools as part of the graduation exercise for medical students.

### Early Judeo-Christian Period

Jews and early Christians believed in a divine cause for illness and divine intervention as the basis for healing. The Greeks and Romans, with their many gods, could attribute illness to the wrath of one god and healing to the kindness of another god. Jews and Christians, however, believed in one God. This raised an important question: How could the same being who causes illness also heal the sick? This dilemma was resolved by associating illness with sin. If a person became sick, then certainly that person had sinned and was being punished. These beliefs are reflected in some religions today; a current example of this is the view of some people that acquired immune deficiency syndrome (AIDS) is divine punishment for homosexuality, sexual promiscuity, or drug abuse.

## EVOLUTION OF MODERN HEALTH CARE

The Middle Ages (also known as the Dark Ages) lasted over 1,000 years, from the fall of the Roman Empire to the Renaissance. Throughout this period, epidemics and plagues recurred, especially in crowded cities. But there was no organized health care system as we know it. Many monasteries had gardens in which various therapeutic herbs were cultivated; the monks performed simple healing procedures. In communities far from a monastery, an older man (the village "wise man") or woman (the village "crone" or "wise woman") served as healer for the community. Perhaps these healers possessed natural healing abilities. It is likely that they possessed secrets of healing that had been passed down from one generation to the next. Eventually, the influence of the wise healer was perceived as a threat to the power of the local priest. A healer who was especially successful might be condemned as a heretic or witch. Many were tortured and then executed via such methods as hanging or burning at the stake. Persecution of healers who were neither priest nor physician continued up to the 1800s. Once a system of medicine had become established, natural healers were then condemned as "quacks."

The Renaissance (a French term meaning "rebirth") followed the Dark Ages and lasted about 400 years. There was renewed interest in science, art, music, and literature and less emphasis on religion. This was a period of discoveries, of new insights and theories, many of which provided the foundation for the **scientific methods** that are an integral part of modern medical research.

### Developments in Science

During the 1500s, Andreas Vesalius (1514–1564) studied the human body and made accurate anatomical drawings. Existing beliefs about human anatomy were based on dissection of animals, because it was illegal to dissect a human body. Therefore, in order to obtain cadavers for his anatomical studies, Vesalius removed bodies from the gallows at night. As a result of these secret studies of human anatomy, Vesalius corrected many misconceptions about the structure of the human body. Vesalius was ridiculed by his colleagues for proposing that their beliefs about human anatomy were erroneous, but today he is credited with establishing anatomy as a science. His book of anatomical drawings is a classic.

Just as dissection of human bodies was necessary to identify internal structures, the development of the microscope was a necessary prelude to the discovery of bacteria, the study of cell and tissue structure, and the identification of chromosomes and genes—the basis for modern genetic research. Zacharias Janssen is thought to have invented the compound microscope around 1590. But it would be over 200 years before refinements in lens-making made it possible to magnify objects without distortion. Meanwhile, Anton van Leeuwenhoek (1632–1723) used a simple microscope to study a wide variety of subjects, including various body fluids. As an amateur scientist, van Leeuwenhoek systematically recorded his observations and made detailed drawings. His work provided the foundation for the science of microbiology, even though he was widely criticized when he first published his observations.

## The Germ Theory and Antisepsis

It was not until the 19th century, less than 200 years ago, that handwashing was proposed as a means of preventing infections. A Hungarian physician, Ignaz Philipp Semmelweis (1818–1865), noticed that women who were assisted in childbirth by doctors who had just come from the autopsy room invariably developed "childbed fever." He proposed that doctors should wash their hands after completing an autopsy, to protect their patients. For making this suggestion, Semmelweis was persecuted by his colleagues to such an extent that he eventually suffered a nervous breakdown.

Ironically, in 1865, the year of Semmelweis's death, Joseph Lister (1827–1912) introduced antisepsis to the practice of surgery. The beginning of surgical asepsis was a major event in the history of medicine. Dr. Lister was such a renowned surgeon that his innovation was accepted, and he did not experience rejection and persecution by unconverted colleagues. Lister's use of antisepsis introduced control of infection as an integral part of medical practice. It is noteworthy that Lister's introduction of antisepsis preceded any proof of the existence of microorganisms. Two other scientists, working separately, were to provide proof that microorganisms are present on hands and all objects, thus providing the scientific basis for both handwashing and medical asepsis.

Robert Koch (1843–1910), a German scientist, was responsible for a scientific breakthrough that we now know as the *germ theory*. Through his study of microorganisms, Koch determined the specific cause of several infectious diseases, including tuberculosis. He also established the rules for proving that a specific organism was the cause of a particular infection; this provided the foundation for the field we know today as bacteriology. Development of the germ theory was a major event that established the scientific basis for asepsis, immunization, and modern sanitation.

Many scientists had observed microorganisms under a microscope, but it was Louis Pasteur (1822–1895) who established that those tiny objects were living things that reproduced themselves. He demonstrated that wine could be preserved by destroying the microorganisms present. The process he used is known as "pasteurization" and is still used today to ensure that milk and various other foods are safe.

Later, Pasteur developed a vaccine to prevent rabies in people who had been bitten by a rabid animal, thus sparing them a horrible death. Pasteur's contributions are numerous, yet he, too, was subjected to ridicule by his colleagues, even though he was a highly respected scientist. His contributions were recognized prior to his death, however. The Pasteur Institute, founded in 1888 in his honor by the French government, continues to conduct research on the causes, treatment, and prevention of disease.

## Control of Infectious Diseases

The work of Koch and Pasteur led to the development of vaccines to protect people against certain diseases, especially the group of infections known as "childhood diseases." But three of the most devastating diseases are caused by viruses, rather than bacteria: smallpox, poliomyelitis, and, currently, AIDS.

In 1796, an English physician by the name of Edward Jenner (1749–1823) developed a method of protecting people from smallpox, a serious disease with a high mortality rate. Smallpox victims were seriously ill for two to three weeks. Those who survived had numerous small scars, known as pockmarks. Widespread use of the smallpox vaccine eliminated the disease in Europe and North America by 1950, but epidemics killed thousands of victims in other parts of the world. Between 1950 and 1970, intensive worldwide efforts to vaccinate the total population of any country where smallpox occurred resulted in eradication of this disease. Because the disease was considered to have been eradicated, vaccinations were discontinued except for persons traveling to remote areas where exposure was a possibility. Meanwhile, the smallpox virus was kept alive in various laboratories, presumably for the purposes of scientific research. Unfortunately, terrorists now threaten to use these stores of smallpox virus as a weapon of mass destruction. With two generations of unvaccinated populations in Europe and the Americas, the potential for a worldwide epidemic now exists.

Up until the outbreak of AIDS, the viral scourge of the twentieth century was poliomyelitis, also called "infantile paralysis" because children were very susceptible and many were left with permanent paralysis. During the 1940s and 1950s, polio epidemics occurred with increasing frequency, especially during the spring and summer months. The mortality rate was high; many survivors were handicapped by paralysis. In 1953, Dr. Jonas Salk's vaccine became available. The Salk vaccine was widely administered and is now required in some states for admission to the public schools. Polio has not been completely eradicated, but cases are now relatively rare. Jenner and Salk made it possible to protect entire populations against two serious viral infections.

Another modern-day threat is the influenza virus. Each year a different strain of the flu emerges, with epidemics occurring in certain regions, especially Asia. During 2008–2009 the emerging flu virus was identified as H1N1, the strain that caused the deadly 1918–1919 flu pandemic that claimed the lives of millions of victims. Once the H1N1 virus was identified, public health officials became concerned about the possibility of another flu pandemic. The public was urged to practice good health habits, especially handwashing, covering the nose and mouth when sneezing or coughing, and wearing a face mask when in areas where flu cases are numerous.

## The Discovery of Radiation

Two physicists in France, Pierre (1859–1906) and Marie (1867–1934) Curie, laid the foundation for radiation therapies. Together they studied radioactive substances and identified two previously unknown elements: radium and polonium. After her husband's death, Marie Curie discovered that radium had created an image of a nearby key on a piece of film. This discovery revealed what is now basic knowledge—namely, that radioactive materials give off invisible rays that affect nearby substances.

Marie Curie and her daughter, Irene, then only 17 years old, took a portable X-ray machine to the front lines during World War I to make X-rays available to doctors treating wounded soldiers. After the war, Irene did research on radioactive substances with her husband and her mother for many years. The contributions of the Curies are basic to various diagnostic and therapeutic procedures in current medical use.

Concurrently with the work of the Curies in France, a German physicist by the name of Wilhelm Konrad Roentgen (1845–1923) accidentally discovered X rays. After conducting some experiments that involved passing an electric current through a special type of glass tubing, Roentgen noticed that some nearby photographic plates had become fogged. His investigation of the cause led to further experiments that resulted in the identification of invisible rays that could pass through soft tissues, but not through bone or metal. This discovery revolutionized diagnostic practices in medicine. Again, the dangers of radiation and X rays were not known in the beginning. Many radiologists died of leukemia before it was recognized that health care professionals must have adequate protection when they are working around any type of radiation.

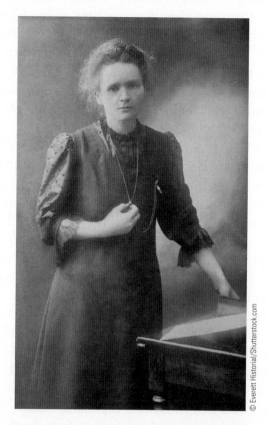

**FIGURE 19-2 Physicist Marie Curie won two Nobel Prizes for her research on radiation and radioactivity.**

## The Beginnings of Psychiatry and Psychosomatic Medicine

The pioneers just discussed all contributed to medicine as it pertains to physical health. Psychiatry, the medical specialty concerned with mental illness, began with the work of Sigmund Freud, an Austrian physician who first recognized the power of subconscious memories to affect health. Freud developed **psychoanalysis**, a technique for helping patients explore the unconscious part of the mind. Although many of Freud's theories are not accepted by modern practitioners, his writings and those of his students provided the foundation for psychotherapy. He was truly a pioneer, daring to explore territory that had never before been explored by physicians. Freud made the mind and emotions a concern of medicine, which had previously limited its focus to the physical body.

> **For Discussion and Reflection**
>
> 1. Discuss one of the historical developments in health care described above. How has this development influenced health care today?
> 2. Which historical development in health care was most interesting to you? What did you find interesting?

**Brain Chemistry** The division between physical illness and mental illness has been clouded further by the discovery of a biochemical factor in several mental illnesses, especially unipolar disorder, bipolar disorder, and schizophrenia. Several chemicals, known as **neurotransmitters**, are produced by certain cells within the brain. These chemicals affect mental alertness, memory, ability to concentrate, thought processes, judgment, mood, sleep patterns, sexual behavior, irritability, energy, and other factors that influence the ability to perform one's daily activities. An increase or decrease in certain neurotransmitters may have a profound effect on behavior. The discovery of differences in certain neurotransmitter levels of psychiatric patients versus "normal" individuals has led to the development of a new class of drugs. These **psychopharmaceuticals** influence either the production of a specific neurotransmitter or its transmission from one cell to another. The availability of psychopharmaceutical drugs has had a radical effect on the psychiatric field. Many psychiatrists have abandoned "talk therapy" and now limit their practice to diagnostic evaluations and prescription of one or more psychopharmaceutical drugs to manage a patient's symptoms.

Psychologists, clinical social workers, and counselors now provide most of the psychotherapy, often in conjunction with a psychiatrist who prescribes psychopharmaceutical drugs. Individual therapy is often combined with group therapy sessions, which seem to be especially beneficial for those patients who need the interaction and support that group sessions can provide.

**The Genetic Factor** The line between "physical" and "mental" illness has also been clouded by sociological studies and gene research that demonstrate a genetic tendency toward certain mental illnesses. These findings give weight to the hereditary aspect. At the individual level, biorhythms, exposure to light, sleep patterns, REM (rapid eye movement) sleep, and dreams have been found to differ from "normal" in psychiatric patients. One relatively common problem, seasonal affective disorder (SAD), occurs during the winter months, when daylight hours are decreased and cloudy days occur frequently. This disorder is a depressive state precipitated by the seasonal decrease in light. Victims of SAD tend to become depressed in the late fall, then improve as winter draws to an end and spring approaches. These individual patterns and environmental factors further cloud the question of what a "physical" illness is and what a "mental" illness is.

**Multiple Causation** The previous discussion indicates the fallacy of the "mental illness stigma," still pervasive in American society. That bias is no more justified than a bias against diabetes, a disorder involving faulty sugar metabolism. But diabetes, hypertension, autoimmune disorders, and many other physical illnesses are now considered to have an emotional and/or stress-related component. Even the infectious diseases, once blamed on the causative bacteria or virus, are now viewed in terms of numerous factors that impact an individual's immune system.

## ALLOPATHIC, ALTERNATIVE, AND COMPLEMENTARY MEDICINE

The literal meaning of **allopathic** is "utilizing drugs." Orthodox medical practice in the United States relies primarily on drug therapy and surgery. *Allopathic medicine* is used in current literature on health care to refer to orthodox medicine as practiced in this country. In this textbook, the terms *conventional* and *orthodox* are used interchangeably, with *allopathic* used to refer to the existing system of medical practice in the United States. The terms **alternative therapy** and **complementary therapy** refer to a wide variety of nonmedical therapies, many of them based on a holistic concept of health and health care. Because "alternative therapy" implies a therapy that is used *instead of* medical care, the more inclusive term *complementary therapy* is preferred by many practitioners, most of whom have clients who are also receiving some type of allopathic care.

A complementary therapy may be provided by someone with a professional level of educational preparation (college degree plus professional training), someone with formal educational training leading to a certificate and/or licensure, or someone who has been trained in a specific therapeutic technique. **Holistic health care** takes into consideration the patient's total being (physical, mental, emotional, spiritual, life context, nutrition, lifestyle) and uses a variety of therapeutic techniques, according to the specific needs of each patient.

Some of these complementary therapies are "innovative" only from the perspective of health care in the United States. The Chinese have been using acupuncture for at least 5,000 years. Homeopathic medicine has been practiced throughout Europe for 200 years. Chiropractic techniques were developed in the early 1900s. Being over 90 years old, chiropractic no longer qualifies as "innovative." It is a form of therapy now widely accepted by the American public and by many physicians.

## HOLISTIC MEDICINE

With increasing evidence of multiple causation of disease, the allopathic approach to treatment of symptoms is being replaced by emphasis on removal or treatment of causes. The search for causes leads naturally to a holistic approach to the care of each patient as an individual with a particular lifestyle, stressors related to occupation and family dynamics, and behavior patterns developed over a lifetime. Any of these could be contributing to the current health problem.

A new treatment emphasis is emerging, calling for treatment of *causes* of illness, rather than management of symptoms. Holistic practitioners focus on the total patient. They insist that treatment must include the mental, emotional, and spiritual aspects of the person, as well as the physical aspects. Holistic medicine requires taking time to identify and deal with causes, rather than treating symptoms only. A holistic approach requires taking a detailed history—both family and individual—and conducting a lifestyle inventory to address some or all of the following:

- Genetic clues to the patient's illness may be found in the family history.
- Individual clues may be found in the individual's own history, such as abuse or neglect on the part of the primary caregiver, or the existence during childhood of attention deficit hyperactive disorder.
- A description of the patient's home life and work situation may yield clues about whether or not stress is a contributing factor.
- The patient may experience additional symptoms, such as sleep disturbances.

Holistic treatment of the patient can begin even before a final diagnosis has been established. Holistic health care utilizes the skills of many different therapists; it includes the techniques of allopathic medicine as appropriate, but extends the role of the physician into areas beyond orthodox medical practice. Consider the following examples:

- If stress is obviously a causative factor, the patient can be taught stress management techniques.
- If emotional factors are revealed, appropriate therapy for constructive expression of emotions can be planned.
- Assertiveness training can be recommended to help a patient learn to cope with life problems effectively.
- If faulty dietary habits are revealed, instruction in healthful eating may be given.

Thus, each possible causative factor is dealt with in order to *heal the total patient*.

## INNOVATORS AND MODERN MEDICINE

Increasingly, the powerful influence of emotions and stress on health is being recognized. The onset of diseases such as cancer is most likely to occur when the immune system is depressed. It is well known that disorders such as ulcers and high blood pressure have an emotional component, but the emotional component may be the result of long-term stress. Several physicians who acknowledged the roles of stress and emotional factors in the onset and course of illness provided the early foundation for holistic medical practice. They believed that strategies for managing stress and resolving emotional factors must be incorporated into the therapeutic protocol. Their contributions led to changes in cancer therapy, pain control, management of hypertension, and the use of medical intuitives in diagnosis.

### Cancer Therapy

Dr. O. Carl Simonton is an oncologist who noted that the cancer patients who met with him regularly for group counseling seemed to "hold their own" better than cancer patients who did not participate in the group sessions. Some members of the group actually improved. In 1976 the Institute of Noetic Sciences sponsored a project in which Dr. Simonton and his wife,

Stephanie (a counselor), provided psychological counseling to cancer patients who had been labeled "terminal" by their own physicians. Only patients who had received orthodox medical therapies for their cancer were accepted into the project. In addition to participating in counseling sessions, each patient was encouraged to write three sets of objectives, one set for three months in the future, one set for six months, and one set for twelve months. Each set of objectives had three components:

1. Meditate for 20 minutes at least twice a day
2. Exercise for 20 minutes five days each week
3. Have one hour of play per day, seven days per week

Play time could not be accumulated; if a patient played two hours on Saturday, there still must be an hour of play on Sunday. Time spent watching television could not be counted as play time. Patients had to specify their play activities in writing. In regard to exercise, the patient would choose something he or she was capable of doing safely. One patient might be able to walk a mile. Another, confined to bed, might be limited to flexing and extending the fingers and arms periodically. Dr. Simonton helped his patients *program themselves for living*, as opposed to programming themselves (or allowing others to program them) for dying.

Long-term follow-up of these patients indicated that about one-third lived longer than expected, some experienced complete recovery, and those who did not survive experienced a higher quality of life up until the time of death. "Higher quality" means less pain, increased activity, slower decline, and increased participation in family and community life, as opposed to lying in bed helpless and in pain for weeks prior to dying. According to Dr. Simonton, the patients who improved the most were those who were willing to get in touch with any negative aspects of their lives during the counseling sessions.

Publication of the results of this therapeutic approach met with skepticism and criticism from the medical community. Does this rejection of an innovative treatment sound familiar? Some of the historical figures discussed earlier did not live to see their innovations accepted into common practice. The Simontons are more fortunate. Their approach emphasizing psychological factors was premature. Medicine was not yet ready to give up the notion that cancer is a *physical* disease or to accept the powerful influence of mind and emotions on physiological processes. But within 10 years, numerous physicians had accepted the Simontons' approach and were incorporating purposeful, regular counseling into the treatment protocol for cancer patients.

## Pain Management

Dr. C. Norman Shealy is a neurosurgeon who practiced the conventional methods of his specialty until he became aware that many of his patients gained only temporary relief of symptoms, even from extensive surgical procedures that were supposed to correct the problem. Dissatisfied with these results, and especially concerned about the number of neurosurgical and orthopedic patients with chronic pain, Dr. Shealy searched for more effective methods. Collaborating with a young electrical engineer, he spent two years designing a low-voltage electrical unit

### For Discussion and Reflection

In your view, how do thoughts and emotions affect the prognosis or quality of life of an individual with cancer or another life-threatening illness?

that could short-circuit pain by preventing the pain sensation from traveling up the spinal cord to the brain. This research led to a device now known as the transcutaneous electrical nerve stimulator, or TENS. It is widely used for control of acute temporary pain and also for long-term, chronic pain. When this technique was first developed, it was an example of "alternative medicine." Because Dr. Shealy was able to demonstrate the effectiveness of TENS to the satisfaction of other neurosurgeons, this example of "alternative medicine" quickly assumed a place within conventional medical practice. Dr. Shealy, the first physician to specialize in management of pain, coined the term **dolorology** for this new medical specialty. (*Dolor* is the Latin word for "pain.")

## Management of Hypertension

Dr. Herbert Benson, a professor at the Harvard Medical School, became concerned about increasing evidence that heart attacks, strokes, and hypertension are now occurring in men approximately 13 years earlier than in their fathers. Believing the stress of modern life to exact a high price, both psychologically and physiologically, he studied approaches to stress management outside conventional medicine's use of tranquilizers and/or sedatives. Drugs can control some symptoms related to stress, but do not eliminate *sources* of stress, reverse the physiological effects of prolonged stress, or correct an underlying psychological problem.

Harvard research studies have shown that control of involuntary body processes, such as blood pressure, heart rate, and flow of blood to a specific part of the body, may be learned through the use of biofeedback. After reviewing research related to conscious control of body functions, Dr. Benson raised the question, "Can we influence our own physiological reaction to stress through individually controlled mental practices?"

Dr. Benson began his search for a practical, *easily learned* means of physiological control. He found that people who used Transcendental Meditation experienced certain body changes within a few minutes after achieving the meditative state. These changes were different from the physiological changes that occur during sleep and hypnosis. Eventually, Dr. Benson and his research team demonstrated that hypertensive patients could lower their blood pressure by using a simple meditative technique twice a day. Many patients were able to discontinue their blood pressure medication and maintain a normal blood pressure simply by incorporating meditation into their daily routines.

Three modern medical pioneers—all seeking more effective therapy for their patients—concluded that meditation, practiced at least twice a day for 20 minutes, has therapeutic effects. Dr. Simonton found that this simple practice benefitted cancer patients, even those considered to be terminal by their own physicians. Dr. Shealy found that meditation could be used to manage pain, especially chronic, long-term pain. And Dr. Benson demonstrated that meditation enabled many hypertensive patients to control their blood pressure. Each of these physicians used an alternative practice to enhance the therapeutic benefits of conventional medicine for his patients. Their findings are widely accepted now; in fact, many health care agencies now offer wellness programs that include meditation instruction.

These innovators influenced the practices of some physicians and the breadth of services offered within some health care agencies. The effect on the roles of various health care professionals remains to be seen, however. Ultimately, each health care professional's open-mindedness will determine whether or not he can adapt successfully to the role changes required by a holistic approach to health care.

## The Scientific Model

Today, the scientific model is considered by the medical community to be *the method* for proving the effectiveness of a specific technique, drug, or procedure. Complementary procedures are criticized by members of the medical community because they have not been "proven effective" by the scientific method. Yet many current medical practices have never been subjected to rigorous scientific research. At present a double standard exists, in which complementary practices are rejected or viewed with suspicion by members of the scientific community because of a lack of rigorous research, but certain long-standing medical practices that have never been subjected to such research are accepted without question.

The scientific model requires an approach in which the experimental treatment is administered to certain subjects (the experimental group), whereas an ineffective treatment is administered to other subjects (the control group); sometimes, there is a third group that receives no treatment. The experiment is called a "double-blind study" if neither patients nor caregivers know which subjects are in the experimental group and which are in the control group. A blind study prevents patients' and caregivers' expectations from influencing the outcomes of an experiment.

Studies on the effects of drug therapy have shown that the expectations of those conducting an experiment influence the results. For example, the health care professional who knows

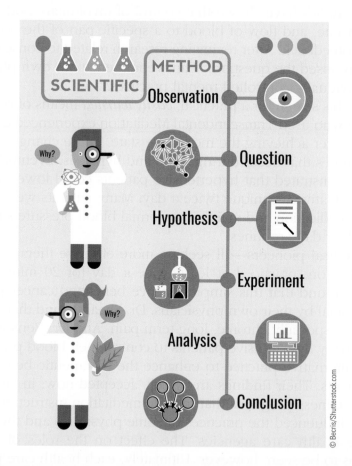

**FIGURE 19-3** The scientific method is used to prove the effectiveness of a specific drug, technique, or procedure.

that a patient is being given the experimental drug expects it to help the patient. This expectation can affect the patient's response to the drug. Factors that influence the outcome of an experiment are known as **variables**.

**For Discussion and Reflection**

How might researchers measure the influence of emotions and attitudes on health and recovery? What are the challenges of measuring emotions and attitudes?

The scientific model requires that only one or two variables be manipulated, while all other influences are carefully controlled. After treatment, the experimental subjects (those receiving a specific treatment) are compared with subjects in the control group (who did not receive the treatment). A treatment is considered effective only if there are significant differences between the treatment group and the control group. Research findings are considered valid (proven correct) only if other researchers can repeat the experiment and get the same results.

It is relatively easy to measure and record the effects of a precise amount of a drug on blood pressure. It is more difficult to measure an emotion such as fear and prove that minimizing a preoperative patient's anxiety results in faster postoperative recovery. It is impossible to see or measure a patient's "will to live." Yet emotions, belief systems, and factors such as intention (to get well or to escape one's present life situation by dying) are known to be powerful influences on the course of illness. Health care professionals often see two patients who have the same diagnosis and are receiving the same treatment. One recovers, but the other declines and dies. The big question: What made a difference in the outcome of these two patients? The "difficult to measure" variables are ignored by researchers who are committed to the scientific model—that is, precise measurement (quantitative data) of the effects of the specific variable being studied. Some members of the scientific/medical/healing community who are open to alternative approaches are now designing studies that adapt the scientific method to the study of intuitive diagnosis and influences on healing, such as prayer and Healing Touch. No one, however, has devised a method for measuring such powerful factors as the will to live, expectation, or intention.

## Empirical Evidence

**Empirical** refers to experience and observation; *empirical data* are observations collected without the rigorous design of the scientific method. Many alternative therapies involve counseling, meditation, massage, and other procedures that affect the emotional state, tension level, and perhaps even the beliefs of the patient. Practitioners who use various nonmedical therapies have accumulated a large body of empirical data, but their methods are criticized by members of the scientific community who demand numerical data obtained through research procedures that fit the scientific model. In spite of the difficulties, researchers are now making progress in designing such experiments.

Meanwhile, more and more physicians, seeking better results for their patients, are sufficiently impressed by the empirical data to include certain nonmedical techniques in their practice. Yet most physicians continue to practice allopathic medicine without an awareness of or interest in the potential value of complementary therapies. Thus, allopathic medicine and holistic medicine represent *two very different belief systems* that have a profound effect on each practitioner's approach to patient care.

## Dilemma of the Health Care Professional

A health care delivery system in the process of significant change presents something of a dilemma for members of the health care team. What is the appropriate response for you, a health care professional, to a patient who is using a complementary therapy in addition to medical treatment? Should you question the legitimacy of the treatment? Should you tell the physician that the patient is not complying with the medical regimen prescribed? Does compliance mean that the patient must follow the medical protocol and forgo any other type of therapy? These questions are less relevant to the average hospitalized patient than to a patient with a chronic health problem, long-term illness, or life-threatening disease. The probability of your caring for such a patient depends on your role, the particular health care setting in which you perform your role, and the extent to which you interact with each patient.

## ISSUES IN HEALTH CARE

The conflict between orthodox medical practice and complementary therapies is especially evident in several areas: pharmaceuticals versus natural remedies, herbal remedies, nutrition, and nutritional supplements. A full discussion of each of these topics is beyond the scope of this book, so the following paragraphs are intended only to introduce each topic as an area of concern for health care professionals. Many books and journals are available to those who want to become informed about any of these topics. Because of the wealth of information now being published, ongoing study will be necessary to keep up with new developments.

## Pharmaceutical Drugs

Pharmaceutical companies constitute a multibillion-dollar industry. The industry justifies the high prices of drugs in the United States on the basis of costs involved in research and obtaining approval from the Food and Drug Administration (FDA). Yet those same drugs sell for much lower prices in other countries. Some cost factors that pharmaceutical companies do not reveal to the public include incentive programs (all-expenses-paid trips, hospitality rooms at professional meetings) to influence doctors' prescription choices, financial support to researchers in university settings, payments to public figures to promote a particular drug, and the costs of advertising. Company representatives visit doctors' offices regularly with gifts for doctors and the office staff, as well as literature and free drug samples.

In addition, drug companies now promote specific drugs to the public, with the FDA's approval. Television commercials and full-page advertisements with beautiful, smiling people tout the benefits of specific drugs for common ailments, such as arthritis and osteoporosis. The risk of side effects is presented with rapid-fire dialogue on television or in the fine print of an advertisement. The purpose of advertising is to sell drugs—by priming patients to pressure their doctors for a specific drug prescription.

Many drugs available today save lives, control symptoms, and prolong life. But the long-term effects of many new drugs are

### For Discussion and Reflection

In your personal experience or prior study, what conflicts have you observed between orthodox and complementary health care? Could this conflict be resolved through innovations, or new approaches, in health care?

unknown; most drugs receive FDA approval on the basis of short-term research. Thousands of deaths per year are due to prescription drugs: unexpected side effects, incorrect dosage, drug interactions, allergic reactions, or damage to vital organs, especially the heart, liver, or kidneys. For example, the diabetes drug Rezulin was approved by the FDA in 1997; it was withdrawn from the market in 2000 after being linked to numerous fatalities due to liver damage. With increasing public awareness of these problems, many people are using herbs, natural remedies, homeopathic remedies, nutritional healing, and other alternatives to pharmaceutical drugs.

## Herbalism

**Herbalism**, the medicinal use of plants, is perhaps the oldest form of healing. Healers throughout the ages have used the roots, stems, leaves, flowers, nuts, and fruits of plants to treat illnesses and injuries. This knowledge was passed down from generation to generation by word of mouth, although certain ancient cultures recorded their healing practices on papyrus or clay tablets.

Plants contain many different components that work together. Even when the active ingredient has been identified, it is probable that other components of the plant support and facilitate the effects of the primary active ingredient. The enhancement of an effect by a combination of ingredients is known as **synergism**, which is considered by herbalists to be a major advantage of herbs over prescription drugs.

## Nutrition and Health

Traditionally, nutrition education has focused on the components of a balanced diet—proteins, fats, and carbohydrates—and the major food groups from which they are derived. As the health movement developed over recent decades, with its emphasis on exercise and healthful eating, greater attention has been directed to other components of the diet: vitamins, minerals, trace minerals, amino acids, and fiber.

- Vitamins are organic nutrients that serve numerous functions in the body; a severe deficiency results in a medically recognized condition, such as scurvy or rickets, but symptoms of a mild or moderate deficiency may not be recognized and correctly diagnosed.

- Minerals are inorganic substances that the body needs in relatively large amounts (e.g., calcium); trace minerals are those the body needs in tiny amounts (e.g., copper).

- Amino acids are the building blocks of the body; there are 20 amino acids, of which 8 are essential and 12 are nonessential. An essential amino acid must be obtained from foods, whereas a nonessential amino acid is one the body can synthesize from other nutrients.

The body must have an adequate supply of these various components in order to build and repair tissues—an ongoing process throughout life—and to carry out various body processes.

Nutrition has recently become a national concern. Obesity and diabetes are epidemic, indicating that large numbers of people do not eat healthful meals. Instead of a home-cooked dinner, prepared from homegrown vegetables, many people eat at fast-food restaurants or serve a dinner of convenience foods. Corporate farming provides stores with fruits and vegetables of questionable nutritive value and, possibly, contamination with chemical herbicides and pesticides. The food industry is using chemical additives whose effects on health are unknown. Many meats contain antibiotics and hormones. These and numerous other factors contribute to growing concern about practices within the food industry that alter or modify a food from its natural state.

Anyone who wishes to have a healthful diet must find a source of organically grown foods or grow their own. Free range chickens and eggs and organic meats are available, although more expensive. The grocery shopper must read labels to avoid foods that contain chemical additives, usually as preservatives, artificial ingredients, unhealthful forms of fat, or dyes. These choices are not convenient or affordable for everyone. Nor are most people concerned enough to focus on healthful eating. So the adverse effects of unhealthful eating have significance for health care professionals. Holistic practitioners consider diet to be an important factor in health, and possibly a contributing cause of any chronic illness. But healthful eating may require more than wholesome food.

Healthful eating is a primary requirement for maintaining health and for treating illness, but diet alone may not be enough to protect one's health against stress and the many pollutants to which we are all exposed. Full protection and a therapeutic plan for healing requires supplementation.

## Nutritional Supplements

Although obstetricians and pediatricians have recommended vitamins to their patients for many years, most allopathic practitioners do not. Naturopathic schools and chiropractic schools emphasize nutrition in accordance with their holistic philosophy. Nutritionists who are associated with holistic health centers are more likely to counsel patients about all aspects of nutrition, including the use of supplements, than dietitians in an allopathic agency. Anyone seeking guidance about nutrition should find a qualified counselor and/or embark on a self-education program. If *nutrition therapy* is needed, then professional consultation is essential.

Vitamin, mineral, and amino acid supplements are all available as tablets, capsules, and powders. Natural products sold in health food stores and holistic centers are preferable to the synthetic products marketed through chain stores. For example, vitamin C made from rose hips is preferable to ascorbic acid (the chemical name for vitamin C), for the same reason that herbal products differ from pharmaceutical drugs—the whole is better than a single primary ingredient. A multivitamin is preferable to taking several vitamins separately, which can lead to an imbalance. The B vitamins should be taken in the form of B complex, again because the ratio of the different vitamins should be balanced.

As a health care professional, you will find it beneficial to become knowledgeable about nutrition, healthful eating habits, and supplements. This will help you maintain a high level of wellness and enable you to protect yourself against health risks to which you may be exposed in your work. It will not be within your role to prescribe, but it will be appropriate to suggest sources of information if a patient asks you about nutrition or supplements. You may occasionally have an opportunity to suggest a change in eating habits that could enhance a patient's nutritional status.

## STAYING INFORMED

Many issues now confront society and the health care system:

- Abortion
- AIDS

- Genetically modified foods
- Organ transplants
- Prolonged use of life-support systems
- Patients' rights (including the right to refuse treatment), a patient's right to die, and advance medical directives
- Malpractice litigation

**For Discussion and Reflection**

Which if the topics listed above is of most interest to you? What personal experience or prior knowledge do you have about this topic? Where on the Internet might you find reliable, unbiased information about this issue?

Some of these are moral and ethical issues; some have direct implications for certain roles, and therefore are of special concern to health care professionals. Many of these issues are highly emotional; the proponents of one side or the other may base their arguments on catch phrases that arouse strong emotional reactions in the listener.

A full discussion of these issues is beyond the scope of this book; they are mentioned here because every health care professional should be informed about them. Being informed makes it possible to avoid emotionalism and examine an issue thoughtfully. Read, attend meetings, consider various viewpoints, and use every opportunity to become informed; then decide what *you* believe instead of blindly adopting the opinion of someone else. Strive to keep an open mind, combined with a healthy dose of skepticism.

For a large segment of the population, the major issues in health care are *accessibility* and *cost*. For professionals of health services, the major issue relates to the patient-physician relationship and *who should make decisions about health care options*. For third-party payers (insurance companies), the major issue is maintaining greater income (through insurance premiums) than is paid out for health care services—*making a profit*. The Affordable Care Act, passed in 2010, was designed to improve access to health care. While many individuals have benefitted from the opportunity to purchase low-cost health insurance, other individuals have seen the cost of insurance rise as a result of the act. Health care costs and access continues to be a hotly debated political topic, one that raises the following questions:

- Who is entitled to health care?
- What is *essential* health care and what is *nonessential*?
- Who should decide whether a specific service for a specific patient is essential or nonessential?
- What is a reasonable cost for each type of service?
- What is a reasonable income for each health care professional?
- Who will pay for essential services?
- Who will pay for services that are deemed nonessential, but are desired (or demanded) by a patient?

The issues of accessibility and cost are of personal concern to you and your family, even though you, as a health care professional, will probably have ready access to health care. These issues are of great concern to many of your patients, however. As you interact with a patient who is dissatisfied with his health care plan, you may be the object of that patient's displaced anger. Do not take it personally. Be a good listener, and be aware that the

**For Discussion and Reflection**

Describe your experience with health insurance. Have you been successful in finding affordable coverage for yourself and your family? What challenges have you or your family personally experienced regarding the costs of health care?

complaints you are hearing may be all too true. Meanwhile, we can all hope that eventually everyone will have access to affordable health care.

## THE HEALTH CARE SYSTEM— TODAY AND TOMORROW

You are preparing to assume an important role in today's health care system. But that system exists because of the many significant contributions of scientists, physicians, and others throughout history. Some of those contributions were initially rejected and their proponents ridiculed. Today, health care innovations and new theories, or new viewpoints regarding accepted theories, are appearing frequently. Some are rejected by orthodox medicine as quackery or, at best, "not scientifically proven." Some are tried by the more open-minded members of the orthodox medical establishment and, upon proving to be clinically effective, are incorporated into an established medical practice.

What is the appropriate attitude toward such innovations for you in your role as a health care professional? What is an appropriate attitude toward an innovative therapy that is provided by someone whose practice is not under the immediate direction of a medical doctor? Eventually you will need to deal with these questions and decide what will be your attitude toward innovative therapies.

### Technological Advances

Today's health care system is a dynamic (i.e., ever-changing) system. Many current innovations are technological—new, sophisticated equipment for laboratory tests, new techniques for identifying and mapping physical changes in the patient's body, modifications in therapeutic devices, complex machines for maintaining vital functions. These technological innovations tend to be readily accepted into the existing system, though the high cost of some equipment may limit its use to large facilities. Some technological innovations require additional training for health care professionals. The expanded role or time-saving feature of some innovations results in ready acceptance. This is especially true of equipment and techniques that contribute to diagnosis.

### Emerging Therapies and Roles

Other innovations—primarily therapeutic approaches—are less readily accepted. Rejection by medical personnel often is based on the fact that a particular technique is performed by someone who is not under the direction of a physician. Techniques such as acupressure, Shiatsu, Structural Integration, therapeutic massage, and craniosacral therapy require highly specialized training. Others, such as acupuncture and chiropractic techniques, require completion of a lengthy formal educational program. In addition, professional counselors such as psychologists, social workers, and counselors are assuming a greater role in patient care. Many of these have completed a doctoral program (i.e., Ph.D., Ed.D., D.C.) as lengthy as medical education.

Some of these nonmedical practitioners are required to be licensed by the state. But education or training, certification, or licensure do not guarantee acceptance by all allopathic physicians.

Because public acceptance of these complementary therapies is increasing, you are encouraged to keep an open mind, listen to patients, and withhold judgment until you have enough information to make a rational evaluation.

## ACTIVITIES

1. Participate in a discussion of one of the following topics:

   a. Beliefs about the causes of illness and recovery.

   b. Innovations that have been introduced into your local health care system within the past five years.

   c. A complementary therapy that you have heard someone label as "quackery."

   d. A complementary therapy that someone you know is using.

2. Participate in a role-play where you are a health care professional; your patient has just told you that she is enrolled in a class to learn how to meditate.

3. Use the Internet to research the Affordable Care Act, which was passed in 2010. How has access to health care changed as a result of the act? As much as possible, try to sort through the different political viewpoints surrounding this act and focus on facts.

## REFERENCES AND SUGGESTED READINGS

Almgren, Gunnar. (2013). *Health care politics, policy and services: A social justice analysis,* 2nd ed. New York: Springer.

Brill, Stephen. (2015). *America's bitter pill: Money, politics, backroom deals, and the fight to fix our broken healthcare system.* New York: Random House.

Matthew, Dayna Bowen. (2015). *Just medicine: A cure for racial inequality in American health care.* New York: NYU Press.

Pickering, Clifford. (2012). *The medical book: from witch doctors to robot surgeons, 250 milestones in the history of medicine.* New York: Sterling.

Werth, Barry. (2014). *The antidote: Inside the world of new pharma.* New York: Simon & Schuster.

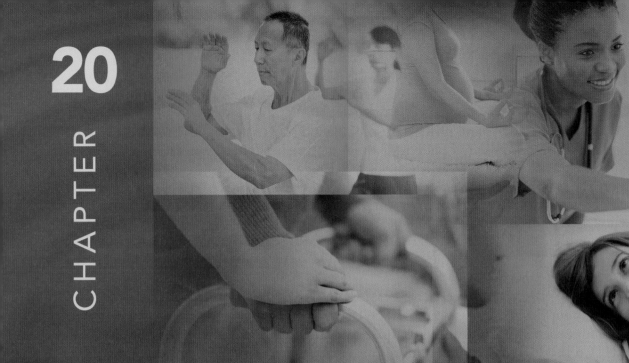

# What Is Healing? Who Is the Healer?

## OBJECTIVES

After completing this chapter, you should be able to:

- Explain *placebo effect*.
- Describe the relationship of emotional states to the immune system.
- Discuss characteristics of patients who survive despite diagnosis of a life-threatening condition.
- Describe the holistic view of health and healing.
- Explain the importance of stress management to health.

## KEY TERMS

| | | |
|---|---|---|
| External locus of control | Internal locus of control | Placebo effect |
| Integrative medicine | Nocebo effect | Psychosocial |
| Intention | Placebo | |

Every health care professional has wondered at times why one patient recovers from a serious illness, while another patient with the same disease and therapy slowly declines and eventually dies. What triggers the healing process in some patients, even when the prognosis is grim? What is the relationship between a patient's attitude and beliefs and the outcome?

## THE IMMUNE SYSTEM—PROTECTOR AND DEFENDER OF THE BODY

Also puzzling is the fact that in an epidemic, some people get sick and others, even members of a victim's family, do not contract the infection. This raises questions about the immune system. Why does it protect sometimes, but not always? How do both attitudes and genetics influence health outcomes?

It is now known that all of us have cancer cells in our bodies, but certain components of the immune system destroy those abnormal cells with great efficiency until . . . what? Why does the immune system stop destroying those abnormal cells? What change permits those cancer cells to reproduce and form a tumor? Can internal factors such as emotions and stress or external factors in the environment trigger this process?

These questions have led to a number of discoveries about what affects the immune system. Physicians in ancient cultures observed that a grieving person was likely to develop cancer within a year or two following a significant loss. But at that time, the existence of the immune system was completely unknown. Modern clinicians and researchers have established the validity of that ancient observation. Certain emotional states, especially grief, depress the immune system and render it less capable of destroying abnormal cells present in the body. The result is a favorable climate for the growth of cancer cells.

This particular body/mind/emotions relationship is now widely accepted. Yet much research on cancer still involves searching for an external intervention. This type of thinking denies the powerful mind/body relationship, clinging instead to the "old" way of attributing both the cause and the cure of disease to external influences. Even though today's research techniques enable scientists to study the immune system more effectively, there are still many unanswered questions.

## THE PLACEBO EFFECT

Another puzzle is the **placebo effect**—improvement or recovery when the "drug" administered to a patient is actually a **placebo**, an inert substance such as a sugar pill. This phenomenon is also called *placebo response*. Researchers use placebos in studies of new treatments to determine whether the treatment produces better outcomes than the inert substance. However, research shows that patients may improve even when given a placebo because of expectation and conditioning—they expect to feel better following treatment, and they have been conditioned to experience an improvement in symptoms following the administration of treatment or consultation with a doctor.

Why does the patient improve, even though the "treatment" administered is not medically acknowledged as having therapeutic value? Studies of placebo effect have led to recognition that expectation may influence the outcome of

### For Discussion and Reflection

In your opinion, does a person's state of mind influence his or her physical health? For example, do emotions, attitudes, and stress levels contribute to health or illness?

treatment. Expectation applies to both patients and health care professionals; if either or both believe that a treatment or drug is going to cure the patient's illness, improvement is more likely to occur. Placebo effect is a problem for researchers who are trying to test the effectiveness of a new treatment, because it is difficult to control. This is why double-blind studies are used to test the effectiveness of a new drug.

The placebo effect can be seen as a puzzling variable in medical research, but it can also be viewed as further evidence of the role of emotions, intention, and expectation on the healing process—in other words, the mind/body connection.

## THE MIND/BODY HEALING SYSTEM

Mind-body medicine is an approach to health that acknowledges the interconnection between mind, body, and spirit. Emotions and beliefs, including unconscious beliefs, influence a person's physical health. Psychologist Suzanne Little (2013) describes mind-body medicine as "the interplay of mind, emotions, and physical processes in health and illness" (p. 37). This approach incorporates findings from "disciplines as diverse as neurobiology, developmental psychology, behavioral medicine, and spiritual healing" (p. 37).

Mind-body medicine also includes a number of different therapies and treatment modalities. These various modalities all emphasize the mind-body connection, but the treatment itself might primarily focus on the physical (acupuncture), the mental (hypnosis), or both (yoga) (Little 2013). According to Little, research has shown mind-body techniques to be promising in treatments of the following illnesses, to name a few:

- Hypertension
- Coronary artery disease
- Headaches
- Gastrointestinal disorders
- Chronic pain
- Anxiety
- Cancer

One of the benefits of most mind-body techniques is that they can be used alone or in conjunction with conventional medical treatments. The practice of combining mind-body or alternative treatments with conventional treatments in order to achieve the best outcome for patients is known as **integrative medicine**. Integrative medicine will be discussed in greater detail in Chapter 21.

## WHO GETS SICK? WHO GETS WELL?

Some clinical practitioners and researchers are proposing new ways of looking at the causes of disease. One theory is that there are *several* contributing causes in any illness, rather than a single cause. Some of the causative factors lie *within* the individual:

- Immune system function (specifically resistance and susceptibility)
- Emotional states, which we now know to have powerful effects on the immune system

- Physiological changes due to chronic stress
- Subtle factors—beliefs, attitudes, will to live, and, possibly, an unconscious desire to escape one's life situation
- Lifestyle factors, including diet, exercise, and substance use

According to the Centers for Disease Control and Prevention (CDC, 2014), lifestyle changes could significantly reduce death rates from the top five causes of deaths in the United States:

- Heart disease
- Cancer
- Chronic lower respiratory disease
- Stroke
- Unintentional injuries

The CDC recommends the following lifestyle changes to reduce an individual's risk:

- Avoid tobacco
- Increase physical activity to 150 minutes per week of moderate activity or 75 minutes per week of vigorous activity
- Eat a healthy diet by increasing fruits, vegetables, and whole grains and reducing consumption of red meat and processed meats
- Limit exposure to sun and UV rays
- Limit alcohol consumption

All of the above contributors to illness or injury involve *choices*, and the choice each individual makes is based on a combination of beliefs, values, and attitudes that influence behavior. From a holistic perspective, persons who choose unhealthful practices are also choosing to be sick or injured at some time in the future.

## THE THERAPEUTIC ENVIRONMENT

As a health care professional, you need to provide a therapeutic environment that will facilitate the healing process. You have already learned that a therapeutic climate includes physical comfort and correct technique in performing procedures, but is something else required for a truly therapeutic climate?

Perhaps you have noticed that the patients of some physicians and some therapists seem to recover more readily than the patients of other physicians and therapists. Perhaps the same surgery was performed, the same drugs prescribed, the same therapeutic techniques used. What makes the difference in results? Does the difference lie within the patient, or can it be attributed to some characteristics of the health care professionals?

Recently, researchers have acknowledged that all medical treatment occurs in a **psychosocial** context. Many factors can influence the patient's treatment experience and likelihood

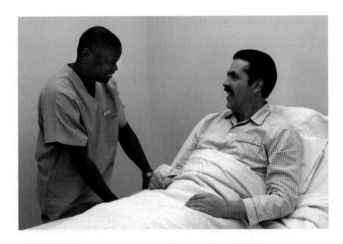

**FIGURE 20-1** **When the therapeutic environment helps to instill a sense of trust and being cared for, the patient is more likely to develop a positive expectation regarding treatment.**

of recovery. Some of the factors that contribute to the psychosocial context around the patient and the therapy include the following (Bendetti 2013):

- Personal beliefs and expectations of the patient
- Interaction with other patients
- Memories about previous therapies
- Words of doctors and medical personnel
- Sight of health professionals, hospitals, and medical instruments
- Color, shape, smell, and taste of medications
- Being touched by needles and other devices

When the therapeutic environment helps to instill a sense of trust and being cared for, the patient is more likely to develop a positive expectation regarding treatment. On the other hand, when a patient has a negative experience with health professionals, whether in the past or the present, the patient's expectation can be negative. When a patient experiences stress, side effects, or increased pain as a result of negative expectations or perceptions, this is known as the **nocebo effect**.

## INTENTION

Current thinking, then, emphasizes both the role of the patient and the role of positive, supportive relationships in determining the outcome of illness. This presents a *new dimension* to the role of health care professional. Patient care that consists of carrying out the physician's orders or performing assigned procedures is a limited role. The challenge to health care professionals is to perform patient care with the *conscious **intention*** of helping the patient to heal. This does not require additional time or effort. It does require concentration—*giving full attention to the patient* and *focusing on caring, positive thoughts throughout a procedure* for the purpose of providing a healing climate.

Would this make a difference? A wealth of literature provides extensive evidence that *intention does make a difference.* Each health care professional must make a personal decision about whether or not to strive for creating a truly healing climate in each contact with a patient. Be aware also that healing occurs only if the patient has the *intention* to get well. Intention, in turn, is affected by such factors as belief systems, faith, and will to live. A newly recognized challenge for health care professionals is acceptance—*nonjudgmental acceptance*—of a patient who does not intend to get well.

## WHO SURVIVES?

"When you are hit by adversity or have your life disrupted, how do you respond? Some people feel victimized. . . . Some shut down. They feel helpless and overwhelmed. . . . A few, however, reach within themselves and find ways to cope with the adversity" (Siebert, 2010, p. 1). With these words, Dr. Al Siebert, a psychologist, introduces his book *The Survivor Personality.* Dr. Siebert believes that survivors differ from other people only in their ability to "*reach within themselves and find ways to cope.*" For many years, he has studied people who survived various types of life crises, including the diagnosis of an incurable disease. Dr. Siebert discusses the reluctance of the medical profession to acknowledge that some patients survive despite medical predictions of imminent death. As noted earlier, when such patients improve and no longer exhibit symptoms of their "fatal" illness, most doctors label the improvement as "spontaneous remission" and make no effort to determine the factors that may have contributed to the patient's improvement.

Dr. Siebert's research led to the identification of several common factors in the stories of people who survived medical diagnosis of a terminal illness; such patients:

- Develop their own strategy for survival after finding that they cannot get guidelines for survival from their physicians.

- Recognize that they must search and experiment to find the survival strategy that is unique to their own situation.

- Perceive their health crisis as a wake-up call—something in their lifestyle is contributing to the illness, and survival requires change.

- Accept that survival may require modifying one's belief system.

- Decide to make changes in ways of living, relationships, thought patterns, beliefs, and/or expression of feelings in order to improve the quality of life.

A factor that Dr. Siebert believes differentiates survivors is a psychological concept known as locus of control. People with an **external locus of control** believe that their lives are controlled by factors external to themselves: illness is caused by some outside force (germs, an accident, punishment for one's sins), and any cure will also be an external force (e.g., the physician, a drug, a special treatment). This type of person looks to the doctor to make her well or, if that is not possible, to manage her illness. She does not want advice about what she can do for herself.

People with an **internal locus of control** feel responsible for what happens to them; consequently, they are likely to seek ways of dealing with any adversity, including a serious illness. This type of person seeks information and wants to know what worked for others. People characterized by a strong internal locus of control want to participate in treatment decisions and may seek complementary types of therapies, learn to meditate, and make extensive changes in lifestyle. Also, they are likely to view the adverse situation as a learning

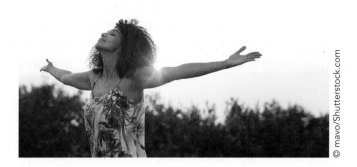

**FIGURE 20-2 People with an internal locus of control are more likely to seek ways of dealing with any adversity.**

experience or "wake-up call." Some survivors refer to a past adversity as "the best thing that ever happened to me," meaning that the experience led them to examine their life situation and make significant changes in their lives.

## THE HOLISTIC APPROACH TO HEALTH CARE

You have learned about many of the factors that influence a person's health, including individual choices. The belief that illness is the result of outside influences (e.g., germs, accidents that "just happen") affects the choices people make. Thinking, "Other people get sick or have accidents, but I don't," may result in carelessness. How people feel about themselves influences their choices and self-care. Behaviors that indicate lack of self-care and unhealthy choices include:

- Being a workaholic
- Not allowing oneself time to play (not using leisure time for recreating oneself)
- Eating "on the run" or eating mostly convenience meals
- Ignoring bodily sensations that may be early warning signs of illness
- Ignoring the effects of stress on the body, mind, and emotions
- Ignoring safety precautions in the workplace
- Driving fast or recklessly
- Not wearing a seat belt

Life choices are increasingly recognized as contributing causes of illness or accident. Modern living exposes us to many stressors not known by earlier societies. Each day we encounter air pollution, food additives, building materials and home furnishings that give

**For Discussion and Reflection**

Have you, or has someone you know well, survived a serious illness or injury? If so, consider what factors supported recovery.

**For Discussion and Reflection**

List the responsibilities you currently have—for example, parenting, taking classes, and working part time. How do you balance these responsibilities with self-care?

off toxic fumes—the list is almost endless. But the greatest stressors for many people are time pressures and interpersonal relationships.

Job responsibilities plus home responsibilities plus commuting time plus errand-running leave little leisure time for many people. Time pressures interfere with the development of satisfying and mutually supportive relationships, even within a family setting. Relationship problems may continue for years because "there just isn't time to work on it." People are risking their health when they fail to make time to cope with stress and improve relationships.

## Characteristics of Holistic Health Care

The holistic philosophy recognizes that each individual is unique. Health, sickness, and healing are related to a balance or imbalance among body, mind, emotions, and spirit. The holistic philosophy also emphasizes that disease is the result of multiple factors, not just one. When a patient's treatment is based on a single cause and other contributing factors are ignored, the patient is likely to experience a sequence of illnesses.

## Diagnosis and Therapy from a Holistic Perspective

Preventive medicine recognizes *unmanaged stress as a major contributor to illness.* It also recognizes that *healing* in modern society requires the learning of stress management techniques. From the holistic perspective, several approaches emerge as essential to healing:

1. Concern for the patient's total being: emotional, mental, and spiritual, as well as physical aspects

2. Having the patient participate in a planned program of health care, including lifestyle changes

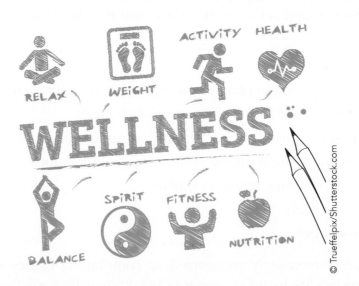

**FIGURE 20-3 The holistic approach to health care emphasizes making healthy life choices.**

3. Teaching the patient stress management techniques

4. Helping the patient face and resolve emotional issues

5. Helping the patient assume responsibility for his or her illness, health, and well-being

It may take weeks or months to make all the changes needed, to deal with emotional issues that may underlie the illness, or to experience the full benefits of therapy. Many patients are not willing to take responsibility for their own health, and therein lies the problem: Even those who are willing to take some responsibility may find it hard to change their lifestyle, deal with painful issues, or even to persist in a long-term plan until the benefits become apparent.

There is also a problem from the standpoint of health care delivery. The holistic approach is time consuming. It requires going beyond the physical examination and related diagnostic studies to study the "whole patient" and the life context within which that patient lives and works. It involves *teaching people*, rather than providing a quick cure. It requires patience and persistence to help people identify underlying causes of illness and make significant lifestyle changes. It also requires that health care professionals maintain a loving, caring attitude toward their patients.

## CONCLUSION

Regardless of the delivery system, it is desirable that health care encompass the holistic concepts that (1) each patient is an individual who lives and works within specific settings that impact that person's health, and (2) therapy must address all dimensions of that individual's being: emotional, mental, and spiritual as well as physical. In addition, the information provided in this unit makes it apparent that stress management must become an integral part of health care for prevention and health maintenance, as therapy for chronic conditions, and as a significant part of the treatment protocol for persons recovering from serious illness or injuries. Because of growing recognition of the importance of stress management within the medical community, Chapter 22 is designed to help you, as a future health care professional, learn several techniques for managing stress. *Only as a practitioner of stress management will you be prepared to help others learn about the importance of managing their own stress.*

But there will always be patients who prefer orthodox medical care to holistic care, and there will be health care professionals who find greater job satisfaction in one system than in the other. As a health care professional, you may eventually have the opportunity to pursue your career in either type of health care setting. Your own beliefs about health and healing should be considered when you are faced with such a choice.

## ACTIVITIES

1. Participate in a class discussion of one or more of the following statements:

   • Love, including self-love, is essential to health and well-being.

   • Harmony among body, mind, emotions, and spirit is essential to health and well-being.

   • Life choices can increase the probability of illness.

- Life choices can increase the probability of an accident.

- Life choices can promote health and well-being.

2. The next time you encounter a difficult situation involving a patient (or coworker, teacher, friend, family member), consciously project positive feelings for that person. Continue to think and feel positively as you deal with the situation. Afterward, when you are no longer in that person's presence, consider the following questions:

  a. What was the effect on you of your positive thinking? Were you calmer, less angry than you might have been? What was your physical condition—relaxed or uptight?

  b. What was the effect on the other person? Was there an improvement in attitude or behavior as you projected positive feelings?

3. Drawing on your personal experience (relatives, friends, acquaintances) and your clinical experience, list examples of people who:

  a. Recovered from a life-threatening illness, contrary to the expectation of their physicians.

  b. Recovered from a serious illness through medical intervention, such as surgery, only to develop symptoms of another serious illness within a year.

  Refer  to one of the examples you listed above and consider what factors may have contributed to recovery. What traits characterize that person?

4. List several routine stressors that you have experienced or can expect to experience over the next year.  Examples could include a reduction in work hours, a speeding ticket, an unexpected home repair, or a breakup with a significant other. Although it is normal to feel frustrated or angry when events like these occur, how can you take a positive approach to each of the situations you listed rather than dwelling on the negative?

5. Use the Internet to research the mirror box, which is used to reduce phantom pain following an amputation. Describe how the use of the mirror box illustrates the mind-body connection.

## REFERENCES AND SUGGESTED READINGS

Abrams, D.I. & Weil, A. (2014). *Integrative oncology,* 2nd ed. New York: Oxford University Press.

Benedetti, Fabrizio. (2013). Placebo and the new physiology of the doctor-patient relationship. *Physiological Reviews, 93*(3), 1207–1246. doi:10.1152/physrev.00043.2012.

Centers for Disease Control and Prevention. (2014). Potentially preventable deaths from the five leading causes of death—United States, 2008–2010. *Morbidity and Mortality Weekly Report.* (May 2, 2014). Atlanta, GA: Centers for Disease Control and Prevention.

Little, Suzanne. (2013). Mind-body medicine. In B. Kliger & R. Lee (Eds.), *Integrative medicine: Principles for practice* (pp. 37–69). New York: McGraw-Hill.

Siebert, Al. (2010). *The survivor personality.* New York: Perigee.

Turner, K.A. (2015). *Radical remission: Surviving cancer against all odds.* New York: HarperCollins.

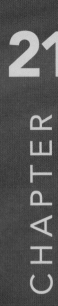

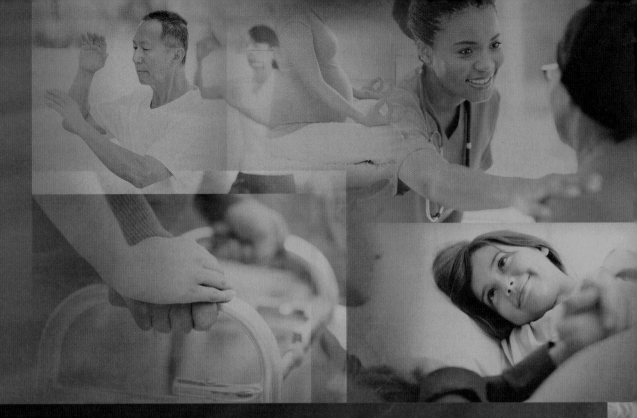

# Alternative, Complementary, and Integrative Medicine

## OBJECTIVES

After completing this chapter, you should be able to:

- Distinguish between a legitimate health care professional and one whose practice and/or qualifications are questionable.
- State the focus of psychoneuroimmunology.
- Describe examples of alternative or complementary therapies.
- Discuss therapies that are used frequently in integrative medicine.
- Describe how a health care professional might respond to someone who asks advice about an alternative or complementary therapy.

## KEY TERMS

Ayurveda
Chiropractic
Holism

Homeopathy
Integrative medicine
Naturopathy

Osteopathy
Psychoneuroimmunology
(PNI)

Increasing numbers of people are using alternative and complementary therapies to assist in stress reduction or to alleviate a specific health problem. An *alternative therapy* refers to treatment used instead of orthodox treatment. For example, a patient may choose to use herbal medicine or a homeopathic remedy rather than taking a prescribed pharmaceutical drug. A *complementary therapy* is treatment used in conjunction with orthodox treatment. For example, a patient might take prescribed medication to treat hypertension while also practicing meditation to reduce stress. **Integrative medicine** is a patient-centered, holistic approach in which orthodox and alternative treatments are used together in an effort to treat the whole patient.

In the past, alternative and complementary therapies were viewed with great skepticism by most allopathic physicians, although both alternative and complementary therapies have long been used effectively by many cultures outside the United States. In recent years, with the rise of integrative medicine, both the medical community and American society as a whole have become more open to the idea of using complementary therapies alongside orthodox treatments. As a health care professional, you should keep an open mind when learning about alternative therapies, but you should also carefully evaluate the evidence for the therapy's effectiveness.

## WHAT IS LEGITIMATE THERAPY?

A legitimate health care professional does not make false promises. A legitimate health care professional employs appropriate therapies and encourages each patient, even in the presence of serious illness, to maintain hope and a positive attitude. On the other hand, one should be suspicious if practitioners:

1. *Promise* a "cure."
2. Claim to have a *secret method* not available to other practitioners.
3. Demand a large payment "up front."
4. Become defensive or evasive about their qualifications.

Recognizing unrealistic claims of curative power is the first line of defense in protecting oneself from a fake healer. The second line of defense is determining the qualifications of the practitioner.

### Education and Credentials

Many roles in health care services require formal education. Qualified *professional* practitioners display in their offices at least two college or university degrees and a license from the state or a certificate from a recognized professional organization. Qualified practitioners of a complementary therapy also have documentation. Educational programs that prepare a specific type of practitioner issue a certificate or diploma to those who successfully complete the program of study. In some states, certain complementary practitioners must be licensed by the state.

If such documentation is not displayed, ask to see written evidence of a practitioner's qualifications. A potential client has the right to know the qualifications of a practitioner, especially when a fee is involved. If questions regarding licensure, certification, or educational

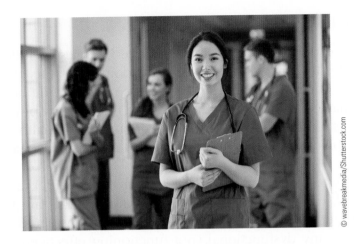

**FIGURE 21-1 Legitimate practitioners are licensed or credentialed.**

preparation make the practitioner defensive, evasive, or even uncomfortable, seek help elsewhere.

## Implications for Health Care Professionals

As a health care professional, you may be asked for a recommendation or opinion about an alternative therapy or a particular practitioner. Exercise caution in responding to such a request. Your best and safest approach is to help that person obtain the information needed for (1) evaluating the proposed therapy or practitioner, and then (2) making his or her own decision. Do not make such a decision for someone else. Instead, point out the educational, licensure, or certification requirements for the therapy being considered. You should also know what constitutes a legitimate title. Anyone may call themselves "counselor," "therapist," or "healer." But the terms *licensed* and *certified* can be used legally only if the practitioner has been granted that title by the state, an educational program, or a professional association.

Each person who considers the services of a nonmedical therapist has a responsibility to evaluate the qualifications of the practitioner, then make a *conscious decision* based on information about that specific therapy and that particular practitioner. After a reasonable trial period, another *conscious decision*—to continue or not continue—should be based on whether or not the therapy is beneficial. The need for careful evaluation of a therapy and professional is less critical if the therapy is offered through a holistic health center headed by a physician or other health-related *professional* practitioner. The employing agency has a responsibility to check credentials and determine if the practitioner is competent.

As a health care professional, your role is to provide information, not opinions, if a patient asks about an alternative or complementary therapy. Opinions are subjective based on your own ideas and experiences. However, by providing facts and information, you can empower patients to make their own informed decisions about a particular course of treatment.

### For Discussion and Reflection

If you were considering a complementary therapy, what information would you get before receiving treatment?

# HOLISTIC MEDICINE

Changes in health care during the past two or three decades include changes in medical practice and roles. Health care was once the sole domain of the medical doctor and the dentist, but numerous other professional practitioners now provide health care. The growth in holistic medicine has contributed to greater involvement of nonphysicians (psychologists, counselors, nutritionists, and various other practitioners) in health care, with increasing emphasis on responsibility of the patient to participate in decisions regarding his or her health care program.

A holistic approach to healing requires that the patient's mental, emotional, and spiritual aspects be considered, in addition to the physical functions that are the focus of orthodox medical practice. Further, the patient's total life situation is considered, with special attention to stress factors and to any dysfunctional (not functioning effectively) attitudes and beliefs. Treatment includes whatever orthodox medical interventions are indicated, plus measures to decrease the effects of stress and to correct any dysfunctional attributes that have been identified. The total treatment plan may include one or more complementary therapies provided by nonmedical practitioners. Note that the patient's willingness to assume responsibility for his or her health is viewed as essential to healing.

A startling wake-up call to orthodox medicine was delivered when a special article of *The New England Journal of Medicine* was printed in the January 1993 issue. A group of health professionals associated with several medical schools and major hospitals conducted a survey during 1990 to determine the extent to which the American public was using unconventional therapies. The findings clearly indicated that the American public was seeking and using numerous unconventional therapies, either in conjunction with medical care or as an alternative. Some of the major findings of this study include:

- *One in three* U.S. adults used an unconventional therapy in 1990.
- Visits to providers of unconventional therapies *exceeded* the number of visits to primary-care medical doctors nationally.
- Out-of-pocket expenditures for unconventional therapies were comparable to out-of-pocket expenditures for all hospitalizations.
- About one out of every four Americans under the care of a medical doctor for a *serious health problem* also used an unconventional therapy.
- Of unconventional therapy encounters, 7 out of 10 *occurred without the knowledge of the medical doctor.*

This article in a prestigious medical journal received much attention in the medical community and was brought to the attention of the public by articles in the mass media. Subsequently, a number of significant changes began to occur. Some medical practices and health care agencies broadened their scope to include one or more complementary therapies as an option for patients. The U.S. Congress directed the National Institutes of Health to establish an Office of Alternative Medicine. Journals of alternative medicine were established. Numerous books by physicians and other professionals with a holistic perspective have been published. Newsletters that emphasize the holistic approach and/or the use of natural remedies are now available.

The remainder of this chapter is devoted to preparing you to understand and accept some of these changes: several emerging areas in medicine, some nonmedical systems of therapy, and specific therapeutic techniques. Some were among the "unconventional therapies" included in the 1990 survey; all would be included, or at least accepted as having potential value, in a holistic health care system today.

## PSYCHONEUROIMMUNOLOGY

It has long been accepted in conventional medicine that emotional factors may affect various body functions, even to the point of changing body structure, as in an ulcer. There is now compelling evidence that mental/emotional states affect the immune system. The "mind/body connection" is being studied extensively by researchers such as Dr. Pelletier, Dr. Joan Borysenko, and her husband, Dr. Myrin Borysenko, an immunologist. This area of research is called **psychoneuroimmunology (PNI)**, an interdisciplinary field involving such disciplines as psychology, biophysics, biophysiology, and medicine. PNI includes the study of mental factors (i.e., attitudes, thoughts, beliefs) and stress on the immune system. PNI research is also identifying neurochemicals that are released in association with anger, hostility, guilt, and other negative emotional states.

## OSTEOPATHY

The first school of osteopathic medicine was established in Missouri in 1892. Originally, **osteopathy** was fiercely opposed by the medical establishment but was widely accepted by the public. The basic theoretical foundation for osteopathic practice is that musculoskeletal disorders, especially any changes in the vertebral column, interfere with circulation of blood, flow of body energies, and other functions essential to good health. Osteopathic technique originally consisted of manipulations to relieve tension around the spinal column. The educational preparation of osteopaths was gradually extended until it became as lengthy as medical education, the primary difference being instruction in manipulation of the spine as a therapeutic tool. Eventually, osteopaths were accepted by teaching hospitals for specialization in such areas as surgery and obstetrics. Most general hospitals now grant staff privileges to osteopaths. In addition, there are 180 osteopathic hospitals in the United States; some general hospitals have an osteopathic wing. There are now 15 colleges of osteopathic medicine. All states and Canada have licensure requirements for osteopaths. The osteopathic physician uses the legal title "D.O." (doctor of osteopathy) instead of "M.D." (doctor of medicine).

## CHIROPRACTIC

The basic theory underlying the practice of **chiropractic** is that any *subluxation* of a vertebra creates pressure on one or more nerves where they emerge from the spine. A subluxation may involve rotation of a vertebra to the right or left or dislocation of the vertebra in a posterior or anterior direction. This pressure interferes with proper function of the nerve, which then affects the functioning of the body part served by that nerve. The purpose of a chiropractic treatment, then, is to remove pressure from the nerve by restoring each vertebra to its proper alignment.

### For Discussion and Reflection

Are you familiar with any doctors of osteopathy who practice in the area where you live?

A chiropractor uses X-ray films, various tests of body movement and muscle strength, measurements (e.g., length of the legs, level of the hips, level of the shoulders), and palpation to locate problem areas.

A subluxation may result from normal daily activities. Sitting for long periods of time, poor posture, and poor body mechanics when bending or lifting have an adverse effect on spinal alignment. Any fall, a car accident, even a sudden stop, can result in a subluxation or damage to the soft tissues surrounding the spine. The most frequent symptoms are low back pain, headache, pain in the temporomandibular joint (TMJ), and pain that radiates down a leg or down one arm. The injury known as whiplash involves the muscles of the neck and shoulders; once the swelling and pain of whiplash have subsided, subluxation of one or more cervical vertebrae may be found.

The underlying philosophy of chiropractic is that correction of any problem that interferes with nervous system functioning enables the body to heal itself. Chiropractic treatment consists of adjustments at specific points to correct subluxations and relieve nerve pressure, plus a number of other techniques as needed by the individual patient: traction, cold, heat, massage, acupressure, ultrasound, or electromagnetic stimulation.

Chiropractic education is a four-year postbaccalaureate program, so it is equal in length of time to medical and osteopathic education. Licensure, required in every state, is based on a National Board Examination. Some states permit chiropractors to use acupuncture; other states limit acupuncture to medical practitioners. The legal title for a chiropractor is "D.C." (doctor of chiropractic). Chiropractic care has gained acceptance in recent years, with many major medical insurance policies now covering chiropractic treatment.

## NATUROPATHY

**Naturopathy** is a healing system that evolved from the popular spas of Germany and Austria, which used water, fresh air, sunshine, and exercise to promote health and healing. Naturopathy was introduced in the United States around 1890 and was widely practiced, with emphasis on nutrition added to the other natural approaches to therapy, until the 1930s. At that time, new drugs and advances in surgical techniques overshadowed naturopathy and became the predominant forms of health care for several decades. In the 1960s there was a resurgence of interest in naturopathy, and it is now widely practiced.

The basic belief of naturopathy is that the body has "vital force," the power to heal itself. The naturopathic physician searches for causes of a client's health problem and develops a plan for stimulating the body's own vital force and restoring a state of homeostasis, or balance. Diagnosis includes assessment of the client's physical condition, emotional status, and lifestyle. The vital force can be weakened by unhealthful diet, lack of exercise, inadequate rest and sleep, stress, emotional issues, negative attitudes, and exposure to pollutants. When the vital force has been weakened, the individual is susceptible to infectious agents and allergens. Symptoms such as fever are indications that the body is attempting to heal itself; therefore, symptoms should not be suppressed. Instead, the body should be supported in its self-healing effort.

Naturopathy uses two different approaches. Cleansing the body of toxic buildup may require a period of fasting, a juice fast, detox teas or foods, and perhaps a special procedure, such as a liver flush. Following the cleansing procedures, the focus is on strengthening the vital force with a nutritional diet, supplements as indicated, plus healing practices such as breathing exercises, relaxation techniques, and physical exercise. The naturopathic physician performs therapeutic interventions such as acupressure and is qualified to prescribe both herbal and homeopathic remedies. In some states, naturopathic physicians may qualify to perform acupuncture. Naturopathic physicians often refer clients for massage therapy, reflexology, chiropractic adjustments, or to a class for learning yoga, meditation, or movement therapy. If the patient's condition indicates a need for a pharmaceutical drug or surgery, the naturopathic physician would refer the patient to an allopathic physician.

## PSYCHOTHERAPY/COUNSELING

The area of practice known as *psychotherapy* originated with the work of Sigmund Freud (1856–1939), beginning around 1880. Freud's concern with the mind—a radical new approach in medicine—eventually resulted in a new medical specialty, psychiatry. Initially, the specific concern of psychiatry was mental illness. During the last 40 years, however, the *human potential movement* has emerged. People have become aware that developing their full potential was being hindered by such problems as poor adjustment, lack of assertiveness, inability to cope with life problems, poor interpersonal skills, and addiction. The demand for services to help people deal more effectively with their life situations led to rapid growth of the mental health field.

As a result of this expansion, mental health ceased to be the exclusive domain of the psychiatrist. Professional counseling emerged as a field of practice, related to but different from psychiatric practice. Most psychotherapists work with clients who are not mentally ill, but need help in learning to cope with some type of life problem: to release suppressed emotions, correct faulty thought patterns, improve interpersonal skills, or modify the dynamics within a family or work setting.

Mental health is now an interdisciplinary field involving psychologists, social workers, counselors, ministers, recreation therapists, occupational therapists, music therapists, and art therapists. Often, mental health providers prescribe both medication and counseling or therapy to help patients manage mental health conditions.

The educational preparation varies from about six years (for a master's degree) to eight or more years (for a doctorate) in such fields as psychology, social work, pastoral counseling, family therapy, and counseling. Titles of professional workers in the field include licensed clinical psychologist, licensed clinical social worker (LCSW), licensed marriage and family therapist (LMFT), certified rehabilitation counselor (CRC), and certified addiction counselor (CAC). If a practitioner uses a term such as "licensed counselor" or "certified counselor" rather than one of the above legal titles, it would be wise to ask: (1) Licensed (or certified) by whom? and (2) What is the special area of licensure (or certification)? Unless a license was issued by the state or a certificate was issued by an educational program or professional association, the term *counselor* is meaningless.

## HOMEOPATHY

**Homeopathy** was developed as a therapeutic system by Samuel Hahnemann (1755–1843), a German physician who had become dissatisfied with medical practices of the early 1800s. The basic principle of homeopathy is that "like cures like." For example, the tears and runny nose of a new cold are like the tears and runny nose produced by close contact with raw onions. Therefore, allium (Latin for "onion") in *very small* doses could be used to treat a cold. Over a period of many years, Dr. Hahnemann used volunteers to determine the effects of a large amount of many substances—plant, mineral, and animal. He then matched these effects to the symptoms of various disorders and experimented to find the dilution (i.e., the minimal amount) of that substance that would control those specific symptoms. Determining the effects of a specific substance is known as a "proving." After many years of research and clinical trials, Dr. Hahnemann's use of homeopathic remedies was so effective that he developed a large following of patients and physicians throughout Europe.

Homeopathy has been practiced in Europe and India for over 200 years. In England, there are two levels of homeopathic medical practice: At one level, the homeopathic physician has been trained in diagnosis and treatment according to the methods of Dr. Hahnemann and his followers; at the other level, the homeopathic physician has completed orthodox medical training, then chosen to specialize in homeopathy. Homeopathic hospitals were included in the British National Health Service when it was established in 1947. The royal family of Great Britain has used homeopathic physicians for several generations.

Homeopathic remedies are prepared according to very precise measurements and procedures. The original solution, usually an alcoholic extract, is diluted repeatedly to produce the dilution used as a remedy. *The more dilute a remedy is, the more powerful its effects.* This is known as *potentiation*. The extreme dilution of homeopathics is the basis for rejection of homeopathy by many allopathic physicians. Extreme dilutions are the basis for desensitization procedures used by allopathic physicians to treat allergies! The manufacture of homeopathics is regulated by the Food and Drug Administration (FDA). The *Homeopathic Pharmacopoeia of the United States* is the official source of detailed information about every homeopathic medication.

Homeopathics are available without a prescription. Consultation with a homeopathic physician is the preferred approach to using homeopathics, but this is difficult to obtain in many communities.

Homeopathy was popular in the United States during the 1800s. In 1900, there were 22 homeopathic colleges and 56 homeopathic hospitals. There were also homeopathic sanitariums, mental asylums, and children's hospitals. Increasing opposition from conventional medicine during the early 1900s led to the decline of homeopathy; the last homeopathic college closed in 1930 (Campbell, 1996). Currently, there is renewed interest in homeopathy in the United States. The National Center for Homeopathy teaches postgraduate courses for physicians, so acceptance and use of homeopathy is slowly spreading throughout the medical community. The National Center for Homeopathy also offers workshops for anyone interested in learning about homeopathy, either for personal and family use or as the introductory phase of a career path.

The practice of homeopathic medicine is regulated by the states. Most states allow the use of homeopathy by licensed health care professionals: medical doctors (M.D.), osteopaths (D.O.), naturopaths (N.D.), dentists (D.D.M. and D.D.S.), chiropractors (D.C.), and veterinarians (D.V.M.). Interestingly, because homeopathic remedies are inexpensive, safe, and easy to use, a layperson can learn to select appropriate medications for many common illnesses. Homeopathy is an inexpensive therapy, but its effectiveness depends upon *selection of the best remedy* for a specific health problem and *correct use* of homeopathic substances. Obviously, any acute illness or an illness that does not respond to home treatment should be evaluated by a licensed health practitioner.

## AYURVEDIC MEDICINE

**Ayurveda** has been practiced in India for several thousand years. *Ayurveda* is a Sanskrit word that means "science of life," and the focus of this approach to health care is on various factors that affect one's life: diet, *prana* (the breath), exercise, spiritual practices, and one's relationship to nature based on body type (*dosha*).

Doshas are three types of vital energy that exist throughout nature: *vata*, *pitta*, and *kapha*. Each dosha is a combination of two of the five elements: ether, air, fire, water, and earth. Each human body is primarily one type of dosha, but may also exhibit some characteristics of one or both of the other two doshas. In the human body, doshas are affected by foods, the time of day, seasons, emotional states at any given time, stress, and the elements of that specific dosha. *Prana* refers to life energy that is taken into the body through breathing and food.

Imbalance in the dosha or any blocks to the flow of prana result in a toxic condition and illness. Ayurvedic healing emphasizes detoxification of the body. A cleansing routine is followed by specific therapeutic modalities: strict dietary regimen that includes a prescribed eating schedule appropriate to the patient's dosha, herbs, and various approaches to improving the flow of prana, such as massage, yoga, meditation, and specific exercises. Therapy is designed to restore balance to the dosha and improve the flow of prana.

## TRADITIONAL CHINESE MEDICINE

Traditional Chinese medicine (TCM), which is becoming popular in the United States, differs from Western medicine in many ways. The licensure designation for the U.S. practitioner is doctor of oriental medicine (O.M.D.). Many practitioners are trained in both oriental medicine and Western medicine and integrate these two systems into their practice. TCM, the prevalent form of medicine throughout Asia, uses a wide range of remedies, with herbalism being the predominant therapy. In China, some larger hospitals have two sections, one for TCM and the other for Western medicine; patients choose the type of care they wish to receive.

TCM is based on the concepts of **holism** (i.e., wholeness) and balance of *yin* and *yang*. The basis of yin/yang theory is that everything is either yin or yang and is balanced by its polar opposite. Yin embodies feminine characteristics: the moon, night, passivity, coldness, blood, and body fluids. Yang is masculine: the sun, day, activity, heat, energy, growth, and metabolism. Both yin and yang embody some degree of the other; the ideal is perfect balance, but the relationship is flexible. Perfect balance leads to health, wholeness, and harmony.

A problem in one part of the body affects the whole, so treatment must restore the body to a state of wholeness. The perfect balance of yin and yang is disturbed when either yin or yang becomes excessive; each organ is either yin or yang. Excessive yang is indicated by acute pain, spasms, and headaches; excessive yin is indicated by coolness, dull aches and pains, and fatigue. Illness is viewed as evidence that a state of imbalance exists, so treatment is aimed at restoring balance.

For the U.S. public, the best-known aspect of Chinese medicine is acupuncture, a technique that is at least 5,000 years old.

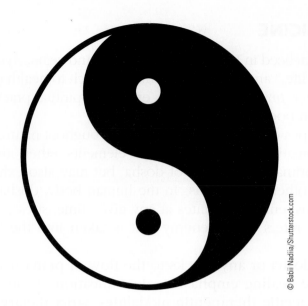

© Babii Nadia/Shutterstock.com

**FIGURE 21-2** Traditional Chinese Medicine is based on the concepts of wholeness and the balance of yin and yang.

## ACUPUNCTURE

Acupuncture is based on the theory that life energy, known as *chi*, flows through channels located throughout the body. Twelve major channels, known as meridians, are associated with specific internal organs. There are numerous branches and connections, so that the cells in every portion of the body receive this flow of energy. Any blockage in the flow of energy results in disease until such blockage is removed or clears up spontaneously. Each meridian has its own pulse, which is different from the arterial pulses of the circulatory system. The acupuncturist uses these 12 pulses to locate any blockage in energy flow. The location of the blockage determines what organ or body part is affected.

Modern researchers are now using sensitive electronic equipment to trace these energy pathways and locate the points of energy concentration, thus using scientific methodology to validate the underlying theory of acupuncture. Such research is a major focus of "energy medicine," an emerging specialty in medicine. The energy pathways and significant points located throughout the body provide the basis for a number of complementary therapies, such as Shiatsu, kinesiology, acupressure, trigger point therapy, and reflexology.

## ACUPRESSURE AND SHIATSU

Acupressure is widely practiced throughout China and has now gained followers in this country. Acupressure is a noninvasive alternative to acupuncture for relief of pain or muscle tension and for boosting one's energy level. When acupressure successfully stimulates the flow of energy (i.e., relieves a blockage), it stimulates self-healing by the body. Acupressure may be learned and used by anyone, may be self-administered, and is safe. The technique involves using the fingers, knuckles, or even an elbow to apply pressure at specific locations. Points that are relevant to the problem are tender. After locating a tender point, the acupressurist applies pressure for several seconds, then releases. The pressure-release sequence is repeated for several minutes until tenderness at that point disappears.

There are numerous books from which one may learn acupressure. There are also several centers where health practitioners may learn advanced techniques. The practice is not regulated, meaning that a practitioner does not have to be licensed. Those who complete a course or workshop are awarded a certificate from the school or center that offers such training. Word-of-mouth recommendations and personal experience are about the only means of determining the effectiveness of the procedure or a particular practitioner.

Shiatsu is the Japanese adaptation of acupressure. In Japanese, the word *shiatsu* means "finger pressure." Shiatsu consists of a rhythmic application of pressure at specific points, using the thumbs, fingers, or palms. Detailed charts show the points at which pressure should be applied for a specific purpose. For areas above the neck, pressure is applied for no more than three seconds. In other areas, pressure is applied for seven seconds. If a particular point is painful, pressure should be light; every few minutes, pressure can again be applied to the painful spot. The point becomes less painful with each application of pressure until, eventually, deep pressure can be applied. Shiatsu can even be self-administered to relieve a headache, toothache, or other pain in a specific area. Performed by a therapist, Shiatsu is a form of whole-body therapy. Many massage therapists use selected Shiatsu points to enhance the effectiveness of a therapeutic massage.

## REFLEXOLOGY

Reflexology uses specific pressure points on the hands and feet that correspond to specific organs or body areas. For example, a line along the arch of the foot corresponds to the spine. A person with neck pain has tender points toward the front of the arch; one with low back pain, toward the heel end of the arch. The reflexology points have been mapped; charts show

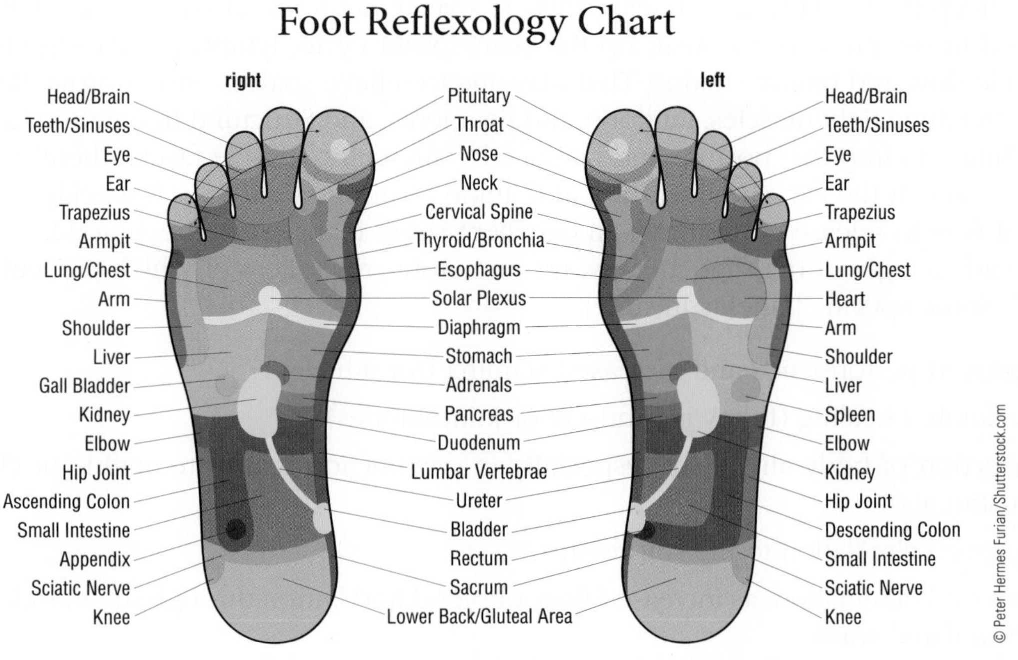

**FIGURE 21-3  Reflexology uses specific pressure points on the hands and feet that correspond to specific organs or body areas.**

the points on the feet and hands that correspond to specific body areas. The illustration on this page shows reflex points on the feet from the therapist's view (i.e., the left foot is on the right side of the diagram).

Reflexology may be used therapeutically, but it is especially effective if used once a week as a preventive measure. At the end of a reflexology session, the client is usually completely relaxed.

Massage schools include reflexology in their curriculum. Although learning the basics of reflexology from a good textbook may be adequate for self-use or for working on friends and family, anyone who claims the title "reflexologist" should be certified by an educational program. States do not regulate the practice of reflexology.

## THERAPEUTIC MASSAGE

Massage is an ancient therapeutic technique. Swedish massage, probably the best-known type, consists of several basic techniques and specific procedures for manipulating the soft tissues. Swedish massage was originally developed as a medical treatment, performed only by a masseur (male) or masseuse (female) with extensive training. At one time, massage was the primary technique used by physical therapists; today, however, most physical therapists use a variety of techniques but very little "hands-on" massage.

Most massage therapists use some of the basic techniques encompassed by Swedish massage. Some massage therapists incorporate polarity therapy and pressure point therapy into the massage routine. A neuromuscular massage therapist also uses pressure at certain points to stimulate nerve function, which then improves muscle activity in the area. Certain techniques are especially effective for specific problems, such as sports injuries, tension headaches, whiplash, or muscle spasm. Swedish massage utilizes long strokes, kneading, and friction to relax the superficial layer of muscles and improve circulation. Variations on this basic technique include deep tissue massage to release muscle spasm; neuromuscular massage that uses concentrated finger pressure to break up the pain/spasm cycle; lymphatic massage to increase lymphatic flow and remove toxins; Thai massage to relieve spasms and improve flexibility by gently stretching tight muscles, tendons, and ligaments; and Structural Integration (also known as "Rolfing") to improve posture and balance by stretching muscle fascia, thereby realigning the body so that the ear, shoulder, hip, and ankle form a straight line. A weekly massage is a pleasant way to release tension and an excellent stress management technique.

The advantages of massage therapy are numerous, regardless of which particular method is used. Some specific benefits include:

- Improved performance and increased stamina (for athletes)
- Accelerated healing (following muscle or joint injuries)
- Correction of body alignment (especially in conjunction with osteopathic or chiropractic adjustments)
- Improved circulation to the soft tissues
- Improved elimination, as increased flow of blood and lymph through the muscles removes accumulated waste
- Improved balance and coordination as posture, alignment, and muscle function improve
- Decrease in anxiety, as excess lactic acid is removed from muscles and blood

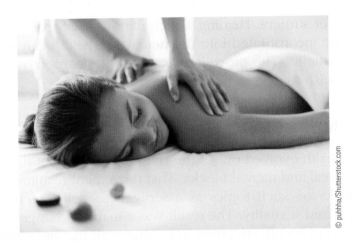

**FIGURE 21-4** **Massage therapy can improve circulation, reduce pain, and promote relaxation.**

- Release of suppressed emotions that may be the basis of long-term muscle spasm
- Increased energy as muscle tension is released, because tight muscles tend to trap energy
- Relief of pain and/or muscle spasm associated with such conditions as arthritis, chronic neck or back pain, asthma, multiple sclerosis, and other chronic disorders

A certified massage therapist (CMT) has completed a formal course of instruction. Available courses vary in length from about 100 hours to several thousand hours. A legitimate massage therapist is completely professional and respects the modesty of the client at all times. The massage therapist does not diagnose or prescribe, but does need information about any existing health problem and the reason for seeking massage therapy.

Licensure requirements vary from one state to another. In those states that do not require a license, learn the educational qualifications of any practitioner you are considering as a therapist. Qualified massage therapists are willing to discuss their educational preparation. The best recommendation for a massage therapist (or any health care professional) comes from satisfied clients.

## HEALING TOUCH

Healing Touch is an energy-based system of therapy developed by Janet Mentgen, RN (1938–2005), who began practicing in 1980. The goal of Healing Touch is to facilitate self-healing by restoring harmony and balance in the body's energy system. A clear energy field and balanced flow of energy through the body have both relaxing and energizing effects. Healing Touch is effective in treatment of chronic illness, acute illness, and injury, often as an adjunct to allopathic medical care. Surgery patients benefit from receiving energy work either preoperatively or postoperatively; the ideal is to have energy work before surgery

**For Discussion and Reflection**

Of the complementary therapies described above, which were already familiar to you? Which were new? Have you or a family member experienced one of these therapies?

and as soon as possible after surgery. Healing Touch is now used extensively in all clinical areas of nursing and can be incorporated into the practice of health care professionals who are in direct contact with patients. The procedures can also be learned by persons without a medical background who wish to develop their healing abilities.

## THE SELF-HELP TREND

Public interest in holistic health evolved out of the self-help movement that focused on freeing oneself from psychological and mental blocks. That movement resulted in a flood of "pop psychology" self-help books on such topics as assertiveness, self-esteem, communication, interpersonal relationships, and sexuality. The result was a marked change in attitudes toward responsibility for increasing one's effectiveness in coping with life situations and improving relationships. Various health organizations began to emphasize exercise and a healthful diet, further encouraging individual responsibility for health and well-being.

The current interest in complementary therapies seems to be a natural outgrowth of these earlier movements. Also, more and more people recognize that modern life involves high levels of stress. One can seek escape from stress and life problems through such crutches as tranquilizers or alcohol. Or one can utilize stress reduction techniques and modify lifestyle to eliminate some sources of stress. If a chronic health problem exists for which allopathic medicine offers only symptomatic relief, one can choose that approach or seek an appropriate complementary therapy.

The person who is seeking techniques for self-help probably has already assumed some degree of responsibility for health management. That does not mean that the individual fully understands all that is involved in achieving optimal health. If you have the opportunity to help such a person, encourage the individual to learn about wellness rather than to seek help for a single problem. That means considering lifestyle, stressors in the life situation, stress management techniques, nutrition, exercise, and any mental/emotional factors that may be affecting physical health. By now you surely recognize that this is the holistic approach. High-level wellness (and, in the case of chronic diseases, recovery) cannot be achieved without a holistic approach. The goal for every patient should be true healing, so that optimal health, whatever that might be *for that individual,* can be achieved.

### For Discussion and Reflection

1. In your opinion, what are the advantages and disadvantages of the self-help trend described above?
2. With health information readily available online, do you think many patients have researched symptoms and treatments before they visit a health care professional? What are the advantages and disadvantages of using the Internet to research health information?

Some self-help techniques can be learned from books and articles. Others, such as identifying emotional factors that need to be resolved, may be accomplished more readily with professional help. The person who begins a self-help program alone may experience improvement, then become aware of the need for help. Whatever the approach, most of the following will contribute to improvement in one's overall health:

- Awareness of choices that affect health
- A *conscious* choice to modify lifestyle
- Daily use of a stress management technique

- Self-study, workshops, and/or counseling to release feelings related to old traumas, unmet needs, and/or unresolved conflicts
- One or more techniques for directing the flow of body energies and releasing blockages

## INTEGRATIVE MEDICINE

In their book *Integrative Medicine,* David Rakel and Andrew Weil (2012) suggest that the once widely-used terms *complementary medicine* and *alternative medicine* are no longer necessary. These terms "serve only to detract from a therapy by making it sound second class." Rakel and Weil suggest that therapies such as nutrition and spirituality "are hardly of lesser significance than conventional therapies" (p. 5). Currently, there is an increasing move toward integrative medicine, in which conventional treatment and therapies which were once considered complementary or alternative are used together. For example, a cancer patient might undergo chemotherapy, a conventional treatment, but also participate in a support group and use visualization or meditation to relieve pain and aid healing.

Rakel and Weil define integrative medicine as follows: "Integrative medicine is healing-oriented and emphasizes the centrality of the physician-patient relationship. It focuses on the least invasive, least toxic, and least costly methods to facilitate health by integrating both allopathic and complementary therapies" (p. 6).

In *Integrative Medicine: Principles for Practice*, Kligler and Lee (2013) identify the following therapeutic modalities, many of which have been described in this chapter:

- Botanical Medicine
- Integrative Approach to Nutrition
- Chiropractic and Osteopathic Care
- Acupuncture and East Asian Medicine
- Ayurvedic Medicine
- Movement and Body-Centered Therapies
- Homeopathy
- Physical Activity and Exercise
- Spirituality and Health

By selecting the treatments most suited to a patient's needs, integrative medicine offers a more holistic, patient-centered model of medical care than orthodox medicine alone has traditionally offered. As integrative medicine continues to evolve, Kliger and Lee (2013) suggest that "ultimately, the point at which integrative medicine will achieve its greatest success will be when this constellation of modalities is no longer referred to as integrative medicine but rather as good medical practice" (p. 21).

## ROLE OF THE HEALTH CARE PROFESSIONAL

Increasingly, medical doctors are open to holistic health care and some complementary therapies. Numerous medical doctors are writing books about their expanded approach to therapy, some providing anecdotal reports of their patients' healing experiences. Some patients are writing about how they took responsibility for their own healing and recovered from a supposedly irreversible disease.

As a health care professional, you have a responsibility to encourage patients to believe in their doctors and in their prescribed therapies. Inevitably, however, you will encounter a patient, relative, or friend who asks your advice about a complementary therapy. It would be appropriate for you to help such a person obtain information, but that person should make the decision to use or not use a specific therapy. Use your best judgment in each situation without exerting influence in either direction. An open mind combined with healthy skepticism is a good combination. Do not deny someone the potential benefit of a complementary therapy simply because you are ignorant about it or because it is not offered in your particular health care agency at this time.

## ACTIVITIES

1. Participate in a class discussion about how a health care professional should respond to a request for advice about using a specific complementary therapy for a chronic problem.

2. Participate in a class discussion in which those who have experienced a complementary therapy may share their experiences.

3. As a class project, planned with your instructor, find out what complementary therapies are available in your community. Present findings to the class as oral reports or, with the approval of your instructor, invite an alternative therapist to speak to the class and demonstrate one or more therapeutic techniques.

## REFERENCES AND SUGGESTED READINGS

Kligler, Benjamin and Lee, Roberta. (2013). *Integrative medicine: Principles for practice*. New York: McGraw-Hill.

Kreitzer, Mary Jo and Koithan, Mary (Eds.). (2014). *Integrative nursing*. New York: Oxford University Press.

National Center for Complementary and Integrative Health. (March 2015). *Complementary, alternative, or integrative health: What's in a name?* Retrieved from https://nccih.nih.gov/health/integrative health.

National Center for Complementary and Integrative Health. (January 2015). *How to find a complementary health practitioner*. Retrieved from https://nccih.nih.gov/health/howtofind.htm.

Rakel, David (Ed.). (2012). *Integrative Medicine*, 3rd Ed. Philadelphia, PA: Elsevier.

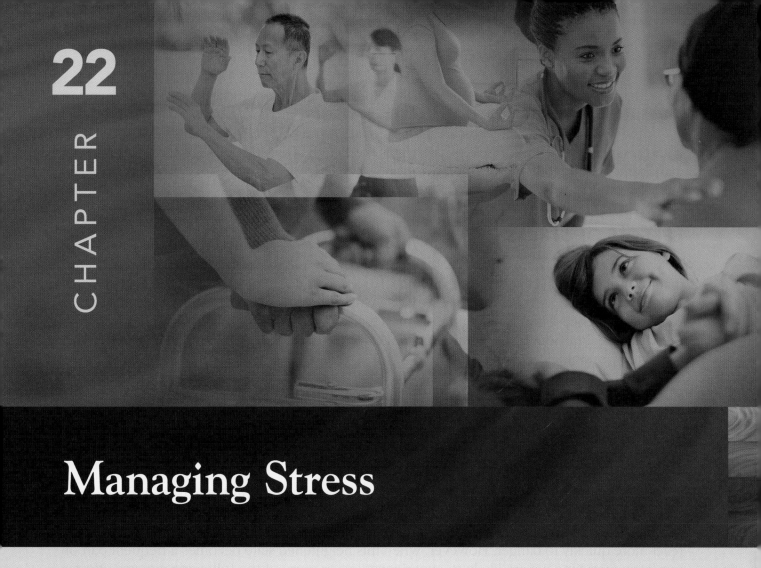

# Managing Stress

## OBJECTIVES

After completing this chapter, you should be able to:

- Identify internal and external causes of stress.
- Describe the physiological changes that occur as a result of stress.
- Describe the physiological changes that occur as a result of relaxation.
- Discuss how *self-talk* can contribute to stress and to stress management.

## KEY TERMS

Mental chatter          Relaxation response
Mindfulness             Stress management

You have now learned that most health care professionals acknowledge the role of stress and psychosocial factors in the onset of illness. It is not within the role of nonphysician health care professionals to prescribe **stress management** for a patient, because diagnosis and prescription of a therapeutic plan are the domain of medicine. In some circumstances, however, it is appropriate for any health care professional to talk with a patient about the importance of stress management. Your participation in helping a patient learn about stress management is more likely if you are working with a holistically oriented medical practitioner.

In the meantime, as a health care professional, you have a responsibility to yourself and your family to maintain the best possible state of health. That includes learning about stress management and modifying your daily routine to include one or more specific stress management techniques.

## EFFECTS OF STRESS

As you have learned, stress is a physiological and emotional response to thoughts or events that an individual perceives as threatening or overwhelming. For most people, just thinking about a threatening event, whether real or imagined, produces a reaction much like they would experience if the threatening event actually occurred. This "fight or flight" response prepares the individual to respond to danger—even if the danger is only imagined. The following physiological changes occur:

- Heart rate and respiratory rate increase
- Muscles tighten
- Adrenalin and cortisol are released
- The mind may begin to "race" with fearful or distressing thoughts

When these changes occur, it is much more difficult for an individual to think clearly, make a rational decision, and process information.

In an actual emergency, these physiological changes enable us to run faster, fight harder, or react more quickly to danger. However, when this heightened state becomes a frequent part of our lives, over time we are likely to experience one or more of the following adverse effects:

- Chronic headaches or stomachaches
- Digestive problems, including heartburn, diarrhea, or constipation
- Difficulty sleeping
- Cardiovascular problems
- Weight gain, due to high levels of the stress hormone cortisol
- Reduced immune system functioning (Morey *et. al.,* 2015)

Sexual and reproductive functioning are also impacted by high levels of stress over time:

- In men, chronic stress affects testosterone levels, sperm production, and may contribute to erectile dysfunction and impotence (APA 2016).
- In women, chronic stress may contribute to irregular menstrual cycles, increased PMS symptoms, and lowered sexual desire (APA 2016).

### For Discussion and Reflection

Would you rate your current level of stress as low, medium, or high? If you selected medium or high, what are the main causes of stress in your life right now? How many of these are in your control?

# MANAGING STRESS

Our goal is not to avoid stress entirely. A certain amount of stress is inevitable in life, and in small doses, stress is beneficial, providing a burst of energy that can help us handle a specific situation more effectively. Research suggests that in moderate doses, short-term stress can stimulate memory and brain function (Sanders 2013). However, when stress becomes chronic, or ongoing over a period of time, we increase the risk of facing the adverse effects described earlier.

Various external factors can chronic stress. Examples include the following:

- A job that involves dangerous or challenging situations on a regular basis
- A relationship that involves frequent disrespect, conflict, or abuse
- Local or national events such as natural disasters, military conflict, or economic problems

Internal factors such as emotional and behavioral patterns contribute to stress as well. Some examples include the following:

- Recalling painful events from the past over and over
- Worrying about the future or about "what might happen".
- Expecting events to go a certain way, and becoming frustrated when they do not
- "Finding fault" with others because they do not behave as we would like
- Repeatedly blaming, criticizing, or negatively labeling ourselves

The first step to managing stress is to reflect and identify the external and internal situations which cause our stress. For most people, there may be several causes. Once the causes of stress have been identified, consider whether the *situation* needs to be changed or whether *your reaction to the situation* needs to change. For example, if your job has become increasingly challenging, you may decide to look for other employment. On the other hand, you may decide that by changing your attitude and taking more time for self-care, you can handle the challenges of your job without as much stress.

*Stress management* refers to various techniques you can use to counter the physiological effects of stress. These techniques help promote the **relaxation response**, which is the opposite of the stress response. When you relax, your heart rate and breathing slow down, your blood vessels dilate, and you can think more clearly.

There are many ways of coping with stress. Some people have a daily exercise program that significantly reduces their stress level. Others participate in a sport at least once a week. Sports may or may not reduce stress, depending upon one's level of competitiveness. If winning is important, then losing a game may increase stress, rather than reduce it.

Certain activities that people think of as "relaxing" do *not* have stress management value. For example, watching television, partying, going to the beach, a weekend skiing trip, and other such recreational activities are diversions—escapes from the daily pressures of the job and home responsibilities. Though pleasant and possibly self-renewing, recreational activities do not bring about the physical and psychological changes that are essential to managing stress effectively.

Three approaches that have proven useful for managing stress are relaxation, exercise, and mindfulness. For each of these approaches, there are a variety of practices and techniques that can be used.

## RELAXATION

Relaxation techniques are designed to consciously evoke the body's relaxation response, which includes slower breathing, a slower heart rate, relaxed muscles, and a sense of peace, calm, and well-being. The National Center for Complementary and Integrative Health (2016) describes the following relaxation techniques:

- *Autogenic Training* teaches you to focus on feeling warm, heavy, and relaxed in each part of your body.

- *Biofeedback-Assisted Relaxation* uses electronic devices to measure heart rate, muscle tension, or other body functions and provide feedback so you can learn to control these functions.

- *Deep Breathing or Breathing Exercises* use long, slow, deep breaths to promote relaxation.

- *Guided Imagery* includes imagining pleasant scenes such as a beach or mountain stream to create feelings of peace and relaxation.

- *Progressive Relaxation* involves tightening and then relaxing one muscle group at a time throughout the body.

- *Self-Hypnosis* teaches people to relax in response to a cue or "suggestion."

Often, two or more of these techniques can be combined and used together. Many professional counselors teach relaxation techniques, and many books and websites also provide instructions for relaxation. Although relaxation techniques should not be used as a substitute for medical care when you have a medical condition, the techniques are considered safe for almost everyone and can often complement other types of treatment.

## EXERCISE

When you exercise, your body releases *endorphins,* chemicals which block pain and promote a sense of well-being. Endorphins are responsible for the well-known "runner's high." Unless you are a serious athlete, however, low- to moderate-intensity exercise, rather than high-intensity exercise, is recommended for stress management.

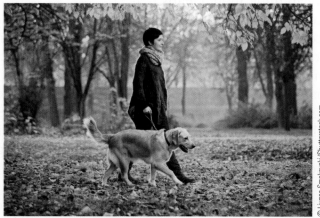

© Ljupco Smokovski/Shutterstock.com

**FIGURE 22-1 Non-competitive activities such as walking, swimming, yoga, and tai chi are generally more effective than competitive activities for stress reduction.**

Non-competitive activities such as walking, swimming, yoga, and tai chi are generally more effective for stress reduction than competitive activities in which players are focused on winning. Notice that exercising for stress management is different than "working out" to increase your fitness level. A ten-minute walk in the park may not help you reach your target heart rate for cardio training, yet it can release tension and provide a sense of calm and well-being.

---

**For Discussion and Reflection**

Do you exercise regularly? What type of exercise do you enjoy? Have you noticed a difference in your level of stress after exercising?

---

## MINDFULNESS

**Mindfulness** refers to the practice of giving our full attention to what is happening at the present moment. Most people pay only partial attention to the present as they go throughout the day. Their attention is divided between what they are doing, such as driving, cooking dinner, or attending class, and listening to an ongoing stream of **mental chatter** that runs in the background of their thoughts.

Stored memories provide the content for mental chatter; it may be factual or psychological, useful or destructive. When mental chatter arouses negative feelings associated with a past experience, we relive a bad experience that cannot be changed. Thus, mental chatter may be the source of ongoing stress. Mental chatter can be so engrossing that a person is out of touch with what is happening at the moment. By taking conscious control, however, an individual can learn to avoid stressful feelings associated with past experiences and anxiety related to some anticipated future event.

Mindfulness can be practiced both in everyday activities and through *meditation.* As you move through your day, practice focusing your full attention on what you are doing at the moment. If you are driving, notice the vehicles around you. Notice the color of the sky, the flowers growing beside the highway, and so on. If you are talking to someone, look directly at the person and focus on what they are saying. While there are times when we all need to "multi-task," look for opportunities throughout your day to put away distractions, turn off the mental chatter, and give your full attention to the task at hand. When you give your attention to the present situation, you are more effective in your daily activities and less likely to be drawn into a cycle of worry by your mental chatter.

Meditation is a practice which combines breathing and mindfulness, allowing you to clear your mind of thoughts and focus your attention on your breath, a lit candle, a specific word or phrase, or some other calming focal point. Although many ancient spiritual traditions include meditation, you do not have to practice a specific religion, or any religion at all, to meditate. According to the National Center for Complementary and Integrative Health (2016), there are many ways to practice meditation, but they have four common elements:

- A quiet location free from distractions
- A comfortable body position such as sitting or lying down
- A focal point for the attention
- A non-judgmental attitude, letting thoughts come and go without judging or holding on to them

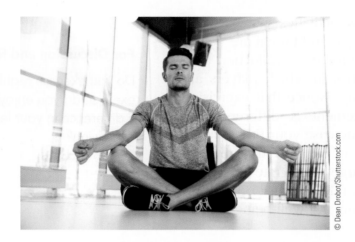

**FIGURE 22-2 Meditation combines breathing and mindfulness, allowing you to clear your mind of thoughts and focus your attention on your breath or other calming focal point.**

Many people learn meditation from a counselor, therapist, or other practitioner, but others teach themselves using books, recordings, or online videos. When practiced over time, meditation has been shown to produce positive changes in the body and brain. Like relaxation, meditation should not be used as a substitute for medical care, but research has shown that it often complements medical treatments.

In addition to its physical benefits, meditation has profound psychological benefits when practiced over time. People who meditate regularly often report the following experiences:

- Changes in perception of self, others, and life events
- Reevaluation of values and beliefs
- A freeing of emotions, especially suppressed emotions
- Greater compassion
- Increased capacity for self-love and love for others
- Greater readiness to accept love
- Improved ability to cope with life situations
- Increased awareness of "self"

## USING POSITIVE AFFIRMATIONS

To combat the effects of mental chatter described above, many people use *affirmations,* or positive statements that provide an alternative to negative self-talk. An affirmation should be short, positive, and related to feelings or beliefs. It should be stated in the present tense: "I am . . ." rather than "I will be . . ." The affirmation can be repeated silently during relaxation or in a quiet moment at the beginning or completion of a meditation. The affirmation can also be written on a card that you carry with you, tape to your mirror, or place in any location where you will see it frequently. Repeat your affirmation mentally at intervals throughout the day to maintain a positive state of mind and reinforce the positive feeling or belief. Examples of affirmations include the following:

- I am happy, healthy, and joyful.
- I am strong, courageous, and confident.
- Today I let go of old habits and choose to create new ones.

You have now learned several methods for managing stress. As students in a health care educational program, you experience the stress of assignments and tests. As you carry out clinical assignments, you experience the stress of the health care setting, which may be somewhat overwhelming to you at first. In addition, you experience the stress associated with your other life roles. Recognize that you are subject to many stressors and be good to yourself. Eat right, sleep right, take time to play, and use a stress management technique at least once each day!

## ACTIVITIES

1. For one week, list the stressors you experience in class, in the clinical area, at home, and in your various relationships. For each stressor you listed, note whether the stressor is within your control, partly within your control, or outside your control.

2. For one of the stressors you listed as being within your control, describe changes you could make to reduce stress in the future.

3. To become aware of your mental chatter, complete the following exercise:

    a. Settle into a comfortable position, note the time, close your eyes.

    b. For three minutes, be aware of any thoughts that occur to you.

    c. Notice how one thought leads to another, in endless procession.

    d. Begin to label each thought as it occurs: a memory, expectation about a future event, a judgment about an event or someone, something you like or dislike.

    e. Become aware of any feelings that arise as certain thoughts occur: fears, anxieties, anger, guilt, pleasure.

    f. For the next two minutes, count the thoughts that occur. Open your eyes and note the position of the second hand and the minute hand. Now, give your full attention to your breathing, excluding all thoughts of any type. As soon as a thought occurs, note the positions of the second hand and minute hand. How long were you able to focus on your breathing without any thought occurring? You probably maintained the focus on your breathing for only a few seconds, certainly for less than a minute. This illustrates the power of mental chatter.

4. To learn how mindfulness can control mental chatter:

    a. Observe your breathing—the movement of air in and out of your nostrils, the movement of the chest wall, or the expansion and contraction of the abdomen during inspiration and expiration.

    b. When a thought occurs, be aware that your attention has shifted from focusing on the breath to focusing on mental chatter. Without trying to control it, just quietly observe your mental chatter. *Note that as you observe without getting involved,* your body becomes more relaxed.

c. Gently return to focusing on the breath. Each time a thought occurs, repeat these two steps. The length of time you can maintain your focus on the breath will increase with practice. Now, you should also be more aware of how mental chatter automatically controls your attention, *unless you take conscious control.*

## REFERENCES AND SUGGESTED READINGS

American Psychological Association. (2016). *Stress effects on the body.* Retrieved from http://www .apa.org/helpcenter/stress-body.aspx.

Morey, J.N., Boggero, I.A., Scott, A.B., & Segerstrom, S.C. (2015). Current directions in stress and human immune function. *Current Opinion in Psychology, 5*(October 2015): 13–17.

National Center for Complementary and Integrative Health. (2015). *5 Things To Know About Relaxation Techniques for Stress.* Retrieved from https://nccih.nih.gov/health/tips/stress?nav=chat.

National Center for Complementary and Integrative Health. (2016). *Meditation: In depth.* Retrieved from https://nccih.nih.gov/health/meditation/overview.htm.

National Center for Complementary and Integrative Health. (2014). *Relaxation techniques for health.* Retrieved from https://nccih.nih.gov/health/stress/relaxation.htm?nav=chat.

Sanders, Robert. (2013). Researchers find out why some stress is good for you. *Berkeley News,* April 6, 2013. Retrieved from 04/16/researchers-find-out-why-some-stress-is-good-for-you/.

Sang Dol, K. (2014). Effects of yogic exercises on life stress and blood glucose levels in nursing students. *Journal of Physical Therapy Science, 26*(12), 2003–2006 4p. doi:10.1589/jpts.26.2003.

# GLOSSARY

**abstinence:** voluntary avoidance of a specific substance or behavior.

**abuse:** improper treatment; may be verbal or physical, resulting in injury to the victim; also, may be sexual, involving a child or unwilling adult.

**ADD:** acronym for *attention deficit disorder*.

**addiction:** physiological dependence on a substance; cessation results in withdrawal symptoms.

**ADHD:** acronym for *attention deficit hyperactivity disorder*.

**adjustment:** the degree to which one is dealing successfully with life situations.

**adrenalin:** the hormone produced by the adrenal glands during emotion-arousing situations; increases muscular strength and endurance; prepares the individual for "fight or flight."

**advance medical directive (AMD):** a legal document which specifies an individual's wishes in regards to end-of-life care.

**affluent:** having an abundance; wealthy.

**alcoholism:** physiological dependence on alcohol.

**allopathic:** pertaining to therapy that relies primarily on drugs; as currently used, refers to medical practice in which drug therapy and surgery are the most common forms of treatment.

**alternative therapy:** a nonallopathic therapy; term preferred by most practitioners is *complementary therapy*.

**alternatives:** two available choices.

**altruism:** concern about the well-being of others; may lead one to perform charitable acts.

**ambiguity:** vagueness or lack of clarity.

**AMD:** acronym for *advance medical directive*.

**analgesic:** substance that relieves pain without causing loss of consciousness; less potent than a narcotic.

**anticipatory grief:** grieving experienced during a terminal illness, or before the death of a loved one.

**appraisal:** an evaluation or estimate.

**aptitudes:** natural tendencies, talents, or capabilities. Those who have an aptitude for a specific area (e.g., mathematics) learn material related to that area more easily than someone who does not have that aptitude.

**aspiration:** goal, desire for achievement.

**assisted suicide:** ending one's own life with assistance from another person, who provides medication, information, or other means of ending life

**assumption:** acceptance of something as fact without evidence or proof.

**attention deficit disorder (ADD):** a chronic condition characterized by inattention, or difficulty focusing on and completing tasks.

**attention deficit hyperactivity disorder (ADHD):** a chronic condition characterized by inattention and hyperactive or impulsive behavior.

**attitude:** disposition toward something specific; includes feelings, beliefs, and behavior.

**autism spectrum disorder:** one of several related developmental disorders, which include the disorders previously referred to as classic autism, Asperger's syndrome, and pervasive development disorder—not otherwise specified (PDD-NOS).

**autonomy:** the state of functioning independently, without outside control or direction.

**ayurveda:** a traditional system of natural medicine developed in India.

**behavioral genetics:** a field of study which investigates how behavioral traits and disorders are influenced by heredity and environment.

**bereavement:** separation from or loss of someone who is very significant in one's life.

**burnout:** a state of physical and mental exhaustion due to cumulative stress.

**capabilities:** unexpressed traits that may be developed under the proper conditions.

**chiropractic:** a treatment method in which manipulation and re-alignment of the spine and other joints is used to treat pain or other symptoms.

**chromosomes:** rod-shaped bodies that carry the genes containing hereditary characteristics; each cell (except the germ cells) has 46 chromosomes in the nucleus.

**clarification:** explanation or qualification of something.

**codependency:** relationship in which the dysfunctional behavior (usually alcoholism or drug addiction) of one person meets certain needs of the other (e.g., a wife receives satisfaction from "rescuing" her alcoholic husband).

**compassion:** concern for the suffering or misfortune of another.

**compensation:** (1) a defense mechanism in which a substitution of some type provides temporary relief from the discomfort of an unmet need, but does not actually satisfy the need; (2) some form of payment or reward.

**complementary therapy:** a nonallopathic therapy.

**condolences:** expressions of sympathy.

**conformity:** tendency to be like others, to observe the conventions of a group.

**congenital:** a condition present at the time of birth.

**consequence:** the result of an action or behavior.

**conservator:** one who has been legally designated to protect the interests of a person who is unable to manage his or her affairs.

**coping skills:** the skills needed for dealing effectively with various life experiences.

**covert:** hidden, not observable; opposite of *overt*.

**cultural bias:** a misjudgment about a person or group because of his or her cultural background or social class.

**cultural competence:** knowledge and skills which enable one to work effectively with individuals from various cultural backgrounds

**cynicism:** distrustful of human nature or motives.

**debilitating:** weakening; impairing one's strength.

**dehydration:** condition in which the body lacks adequate water to maintain body functions; if severe, can lead to a life-threatening imbalance of body chemistry.

**dependency:** reliance on someone or something for support.

**derogatory:** critical or disrespectful.

**desertion reaction:** a form of withdrawal that may occur when a very young child or an elderly person is left in the care of someone other than a family member.

**developmental disorders:** physical or mental disorders which affect a child's development, often causing the individual to learn or to meet developmental milestones at a slower than typical rate.

**digital:** using the fingers or toes.

**discrimination:** different treatment of a person because of some specific characteristic, such as age, gender, race, religion, national origin, or economic status.

**disguised behavior:** behavior used by a person to cover up true feelings.

**displacement:** a defense mechanism in which strong feelings (usually anger) about one person are transferred or directed to someone else who did not initially arouse the feelings.

**DNA:** acronym for *deoxyribonucleic acid*, the substance that contains the hereditary makeup of each cell.

**DNR:** acronym for *do not resuscitate*.

**do not resuscitate (DNR) order:** a legal document that states that an individual should not be resuscitated in the event of cardiac or respiratory arrest.

**dolorology:** a medical specialty concerned with pain management.

**DPA:** acronym for *durable power of attorney*.

**durable power of attorney (DPA):** a legal document designating an agent to act on one's behalf in the event one becomes incapacitated.

**dysfunctional:** faulty or disturbed function.

**dyslexia:** a developmental disorder that affects reading.

**egocentric:** concerned primarily with self.

**empathy:** ability to identify with another person's situation and understand the feelings and reactions of that person.

**empirical:** based on observation and experience, rather than on experimental data.

**empowerment:** becoming stronger and more confident.

**enabler:** one who facilitates another's addictive behavior by helping the addict gain access to the addictive substance.

**enunciation:** the uttering of sounds; may be clear or unclear to the listener.

**ethics:** standards of conduct, a code of behavior for a specific group; medical ethics are the standards of conduct to be observed by health care providers.

**euthanasia:** administration of a lethal substance to a person who is dying and in great pain; also called *mercy killing*.

**excellence:** the quality of being extremely good.

**expectation:** something one thinks will occur.

**external locus of control:** the belief that various factors outside oneself control the events of one's life.

**family dynamics:** the interactions between and among members of a family.

**fetal alcohol syndrome (FAS):** a pattern of growth, mental, and physical problems that a child develops as a result of the mother's consumption of alcohol during pregnancy.

**fixed mindset:** the belief that one's abilities, such as intelligence or talent, are fixed and unchangeable.

**frustration:** any blocking of progress toward a desired goal.

**gene:** unit that carries a hereditary trait.

**genetic:** carried by the genes; pertaining to heredity.

**genotype:** the specific hereditary makeup of a person.

**grief work:** the process of working through the emotional reaction to loss; generally considered to last at least one year.

**growth mindset:** the belief that one's abilities can be improved and developed through practice and hard work.

**habituation:** psychological dependence, need, strong desire.

**hallucinogenic:** causing a person to hallucinate, to perceive sights and sounds that are not actually present.

**hassle:** an annoyance.

**herbalism:** the use of herbs for a variety of purposes, including medicinal uses.

**hereditary:** traits inherited from the parents.

**heredity:** the transmission of characteristics from parents to offspring.

**hierarchy:** arrangement in a specific order or rank from lowest to highest; vertical relationships.

**holism:** the belief system that encompasses holistic ideas.

**holistic health care:** perceiving the whole and all of its parts; the philosophy that healing occurs most readily when all aspects of the patient are considered.

**homeopathy:** a system of alternative medicine based on the concept that a disease can be cured by a low dose of a substance that causes similar symptoms in a healthy person.

**hospice:** a facility for the care of terminally ill patients, based on a death-with-dignity philosophy.

**hostility:** anger, either specific or general; may be the basis for aggressive tendencies.

**Human Genome Project:** a scientific research project between 1990 and 2003 that identified all the genes in human DNA.

**hypnosis:** trancelike condition usually induced by another person, in which the subject is receptive to suggestions.

**incapacitated:** incapable of functioning.

**incest:** sexual intercourse between persons whose blood relationship makes it illegal for them to marry; usually involves parent/child, brother/sister, or uncle/niece; may be an aspect of child abuse.

**incompatible:** unable to exist together harmoniously.

**inconsistency:** differing from one occurrence to another.

**individual worth:** the right to be valued and respected as a human being, regardless of personal circumstances or qualities.

**integrative medicine:** a health care approach that emphasizes wellness and treating the whole person using a combination of allopathic, complementary, and alternative therapies.

**intention:** a specific purpose (a conscious thought) for a particular action.

**internal locus of control:** the belief that one can utilize inner resources to influence events.

**I-statement:** a communication technique used to express feelings or needs by stating them in the first person.

**learning:** a change in behavior resulting from acquisition of knowledge and development of a skill.

**lethargy:** abnormal drowsiness, sluggishness.

**living will:** a document stating a person's wishes for medical care in the event that the person is incapacitated and unable to express those wishes directly.

**manipulative:** using various strategies to influence others in order to obtain something.

**martyr complex:** psychological condition in which a person derives satisfaction from being taken advantage of by another person.

**mediocre:** performance that is acceptable but not good.

**mental chatter:** the stream of thoughts and memories that runs through the mind when it is not focused on a mental task or on an experience that requires attention; may interfere with going to sleep; if uncontrolled, can be a source of stress.

**mindfulness:** a practice which involves being aware, attentive, and intentional in the present moment.

**mindset:** mental readiness to react in a specific way.

**mortality:** subject to dying.

**narcotic:** addictive type of drug used medically to relieve pain.

**naturopathy:** a form of alternative medicine that includes diet and lifestyle counseling, herbal medicine, and detoxification.

**necrosis:** death of tissues in a limited area.

**neglect:** failure to pay appropriate attention or, in the case of a child, provide essential needs.

**neurotransmitter:** chemical substances that transmit impulses in the brain and nerves.

**nocebo effect:** an inert substance or treatment which causes an adverse effect on the recipient; opposite of *placebo effect.*

**noradrenalin:** hormone produced by the adrenal medulla during emotion-arousing situations.

**osteopathy:** medical practice which focuses on prevention, wellness, and lifestyle factors. Doctors of Osteopathy are fully licensed physicians.

**overt:** obvious, observable; opposite of *covert.*

**palliative:** relieving or controlling symptoms without healing the underlying disease process.

**paraphrase:** restate; express a meaning in different words.

**paraverbal:** the tone, volume, and rate of speech, all of which can alter the meaning of a statement even when the same words are used.

**passive aggression:** indirect resistance, sometimes while giving the appearance of cooperation; may be due to covert hostility.

**Patient Self-Determination Act:** a law passed by Congress in 1990 requiring health care facilities to inform patients about advance health care directives upon admission to the facility.

**pedophilia:** sexual activity between a child under the age of 13 and someone 5 to 10 years older than the child; a type of child abuse.

**perception:** use of the senses to become aware of something.

**perfectionism:** excessive concern about order and what is right; holding *perfect* as the standard of what is acceptable.

**perpetrator:** one who commits, or has committed, some type of offense or crime.

**phenotype:** an organism's physical type; a set of characteristics that establish physical appearance.

**philosophy:** a theory or set of beliefs held by a person or group that serves as a guide for behavior.

**physiological:** dealing with the functions and vital processes of living organisms; the physical aspect of being, rather than the mental, emotional, or spiritual aspects.

**placebo:** an inactive substance administered instead of a specific therapy.

**placebo effect (placebo response):** the beneficial effect of a placebo, usually reflecting the expectations of the patient, health care provider, or both.

**potential:** hidden or undeveloped trait, quality, or talent. (*Ability* is a quality or talent that has been developed; a *characteristic* is a trait that has been developed.)

**prejudice:** a preconceived opinion held without regard for the facts; generalized negative feelings toward a person or group because of race, sex, or subculture.

**procrastinate:** to put off doing something until a later time.

**proficient:** skillful.

**prognosis:** predicted course or outcome of a disease or injury.

**projection:** a defense mechanism which involves blaming one's own shortcomings on someone else or on circumstances.

**prosthesis:** an artificial replacement for a missing body part.

**proxy:** one who has been designated to act on behalf of another person.

**PSDA:** acronym for *Patient Self-Determination Act.*

**psychoanalysis:** method of treating mental/emotional disorders by discovering and analyzing repressed memories, emotional conflicts, and past traumas.

**psychoneuroimmunology (PNI):** the study of the relationship between the the brain, nervous system, and immune system.

**psychopharmaceutical:** a class of drug that has specific effects on the mind, emotions, or mood, usually by altering brain chemistry.

**psychosocial:** related to both psychological and social factors.

**psychotherapy:** the treatment of mental and emotional illness through one or more psychological techniques.

**rapport:** a relationship in which there is mutual acceptance, understanding, and respect.

**rationalization:** a defense mechanism which involves offering a socially acceptable explanation for behavior when the true reason would be too painful to admit.

**regression:** exhibiting behaviors that are appropriate to an earlier stage of development.

**relaxation response:** in stress management, a physical response which includes lowered blood pressure and stress hormones, relaxed muscles, and a feeling of well-being.

**REM:** acronym for *rapid eye movement.*

**REM sleep:** the phase of sleep during which dreaming occurs.

**repression:** a defense mechanism which involves forcing an unpleasant memory into the subconscious mind.

**resentment:** chronic anger that is not consciously expressed, but may be an unconscious influence on behavior.

**resilience:** the ability to bounce back after a bad experience.

**role:** the duties and behaviors expected of a person in a specific situation.

**scientific method:** a systematic procedure for conducting measurements, observations, and experiments and forming and testing hypotheses.

**selective observing:** a tendency to notice certain details of a situation while ignoring or overlooking other details.

**self-confidence:** believing in oneself as a competent person.

**self-deception:** seeing oneself incorrectly; lack of self-awareness.

**self-reliant:** able to depend upon oneself; confident in one's own judgment, decisions, abilities, and coping skills.

**separation anxiety:** extreme anxiety that a child may develop when a caregiver is absent or about to leave.

**sexism:** belief or attitude that one sex is inferior to the other; often the basis for discrimination.

**sexually transmitted disease (STD):** an infectious disease which is transferred from one individual to another through sexual contact.

**socioeconomic:** relating to a combination of social and economic factors.

**stance:** a mode of standing or positioning of the body and feet.

**standard of performance:** a level of quality against which one's work can be measured.

**stress:** a physiological response (internal and adaptive) to extreme or chronic emotional states.

**stress management:** techniques which counteract the effects of stress by encouraging relaxation, lowered heart rate and blood pressure, lowered stress hormones, and a sense of well-being.

**stressors:** outside influences that arouse some type of emotional response.

**subtle:** delicate, refined, not obvious.

**suffocation:** death from lack of oxygen due to the face (nose and mouth) being covered.

**superstition:** a commonly held but unjustified belief.

**suppression:** not expressing, holding in or down.

**survivor guilt:** the tendency of a survivor of a trauma or accident to feel guilty for being alive, especially when someone else did not survive the same experience.

**sympathy:** concern for another person, especially one who is experiencing illness, trauma, or crisis.

**synergism:** increased effectiveness or potency of a substance when combined with another substance.

**thanatology:** the study of death and dying.

**trait:** a quality or characteristic.

**transference:** unconsciously directing one's feelings about one person toward another person.

**trauma-informed care:** an approach that recognizes and responds to the effects of trauma on individuals.

**value system:** the importance attached to various aspects of living, such as beliefs, ideas, objects, and relationships.

**variables:** factors that has an influence or ability to bring about change.

**verbalize:** express in words; often used to indicate oral expression, rather than written.

**vicious cycle:** recurring behaviors or events that maintain an unsatisfactory situation; will continue unless a change is made to interrupt the cycle.

**withdrawal (drug-related):** withholding a substance to which someone is addicted; the group of symptoms that occur as the body reacts to absence of the addictive substance.

# INDEX